Fractures of the distal radius

Fractures of the distal radius

Philippe Saffar, MD

Chirurgien des Hôpitaux de Paris
Institut Français de la Main
Centre Chirurgical de la Main
Paris
France

William P Cooney III, MD

Professor, Mayo Medical School
Vice Chairman of Orthopedic Surgery
Head of the Division of Hand Surgery
Mayo Clinic
Rochester
Minnesota
USA

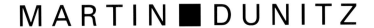

© **Martin Dunitz Ltd 1995**

First published in the United Kingdom in 1995
by Martin Dunitz Ltd, The Livery House, 7–9 Pratt Street, London NW1 0AE

All rights reserved. No part of this publication may be reproduced, stored in a retrieval system, or transmitted, in any form or by any means, without the prior permission of the publisher.

A CIP record for this book is available from the British Library.

ISBN 1 85317 178 6

The editors wish to acknowledge A. I. Kapandji for his authorization to use his drawings for the front cover.

Composition by TecSet Ltd, Wallington, Surrey, United Kingdom
Printed and bound in Spain by Grafos, S.A. Arte sobre papel

CONTENTS

Contributors vii

Fundamentals

1. Anatomy of the distal radius
   F Brunelli, A Pagliei, C Smussi 1

2. Current trends in treatment and classification of distal radial fractures
   Ph Saffar 12

3. Pathomechanisms of intra-articular distal radial fractures
   I Semaan, Ph Saffar 19

4. Biomechanical aspects of percutaneous pinning for distal radial fractures
   Thomas J Graham, Dean S Louis 28

5. A cadaveric study to determine whether ligamentotaxis restores radiopalmar tilt in intra-articular fractures of the distal radius
   RA Bartosh, MJ Saldana 37

6. Classification of distal radial fractures by mechanism of injury
   Ronald L Linscheid 41

Extra-Articular Fractures

7. Percutaneous pinning of fractures of the distal end of the radius
   MD Greatting, MB Wood 50

8. Treatment of distal radial fractures with the 'PY' isoelastic pinning procedure:
   100 consecutive cases
   M Ebelin, C Delaunay, E Lenoble, T Lebalc'h, F Mazas 56

9. Osteosynthesis of the radius by flexible double pinning: functional treatment of distal radial fractures in 130 consecutive cases
   E Desmanet 62

10. Treatment of non-articular distal radial fractures by intrafocal pinning using arum pins
    AI Kapandji 71

11. Bone cementing in distal radial fractures in the elderly
    Y Kiyoshige 84

12. Treatment of extra-articular malunions of the distal radius
    J Duparc, B Melchior, B Valtin 89

13. Multiplanar osteotomy for treatment of malunions of the distal radius
    GA Brunelli, GR Brunelli 98

Intra-Articular Fractures

14. Treatment of articular fractures of the distal radius with external fixation and pinning
    Diego L Fernandez 104

15. Open reduction of distal radial fractures: indications, classification, and functional assessment
    William P Cooney III 118

16. Classification of intra-articular fractures of the distal radius
    Ch Mathoulin, E Letrosne, Ph Saffar 126

17 Classification and treatment of intra-articular fractures of the distal radius
H Saito 131

18 Evaluation of comminuted intra-articular distal radial fractures with computerized tomography
Richard M Singer, Guy Pierret 143

19 Treatment by plates of anteriorly displaced distal radial fractures
Ph Ducloyer 148

20 The postero-medial fragment in distal radial fractures: description and treatment
JP Mortier, S Baux 153

21 Treatment of articular distal radial fractures by intrafocal pinning with arum pins
AI Kapandji 160

22 Management of comminuted distal radial fractures
Jesse B Jupiter, Craig S Williams 167

23 The role of bone grafting in comminuted distal radial fractures
KS Leung, PC Leung 184

24 Open reduction of intra-articular fractures of the distal radius
Peter C Amadio 193

25 Treatment of distal radial fractures by external fixation: techniques and indications
Frédéric Schuind, Monique Donkerwolcke, Franz Burny 203

26 Corrective osteotomy for extra-articular malunion of the distal radius
Diego L Fernandez 210

27 Fixation of distal radial fractures: intramedullary pinning versus external fixation
JL Haas, JY de la Caffinière 229

28 Indications for open treatment of intra-articular fractures of the distal radius
Ch Mathoulin, E de Thomasson, Th Judet, Ph Saffar 240

29 Treatment of complex comminuted fractures of the distal radius utilizing the internal distraction plate
Edward F Burke 246

30 Treatment of distal radial intra-articular malunions
Ph Saffar 249

31 Long-term follow-up of intra-articular fractures of the distal radius
Ph Kopylov 259

Miscellaneous

32 Galeazzi and Essex-Lopresti fractures
G Herzberg 264

33 Radiocarpal dislocations and fracture-dislocations
C Dumontier, E Lenoble, Ph Saffar 267

34 Fractures and epiphyseal fracture-separation of the distal bones of the forearm in children
S Guero 279

35 Radial styloid fractures associated with scapholunate ligament sprains
Ph Saffar 291

36 Fractures of the ulnar styloid
C Sokolow 297

37 Acute and chronic neurovascular complications of distal radial fractures
Arnold-Peter C Weiss, James B Steichen 300

38 Extensor pollicis longus tendon rupture after distal radial fractures
J Sallerin, P Bonnevialle, M Mansat 308

Index 313

CONTRIBUTORS

PC Amadio
Mayo Clinic
200 First Street SW
Rochester
Minnesota 55905
USA

S Baux
Hôpital Rothschild
33, boulevard de Picpus
75012 Paris
France

P Bonnevialle
CHU Toulouse
Place du Dr Baylac
31059 Toulouse
France

F Brunelli
Institut Français de la Main
15, rue Benjamin Franklin
75116 Paris
France

GA Brunelli
Facoltà di Medicina e Chirurgia
Università degli Studia di Brescia
Piazzale Ospedale Civile 2
25124 Brescia
Italy

GR Brunelli
Facoltà di Medicina e Chirurgia
Università degli Studia di Brescia
Piazzale Ospedale Civile 2
25124 Brescia
Italy

EF Burke
Hand Surgery Associates
Suite 1026
Harper Professional Building
4160 John R
Detroit
Michigan 48201
USA

F Burny
Hôpital Erasme ULB
Route de Lennik 808
1070 Brussels
Belgium

JY de la Caffinière
Hôpital de la Fontaine
2, rue du Dr de la Fontaine
93205 Saint-Denis
France

WP Cooney III
Mayo Clinic
200 1st Street SW
Rochester
Minnesota 55905
USA

C Delaunay
Centre Hôpital-Universitaire de Bicêtre
78, rue du Général Leclerc
94270 Le Kremlin Bicêtre
France

E Desmanet
Hôpital de Jolimont
7161 Haine Saint Paul
Belgium

M Donkerwolcke
Hôpital Erasme ULB
Route de Lennik 808
1070 Bruxelles
Belgium

Ph Ducloyer
Clinique Sud-Vendée
Rue du Dr Fleurance
BP 209
85204 Fontenay Le Comte
France

C Dumontier
Institut Français de la Main
15, rue Benjamin Franklin
75116 Paris
France

Prof J Duparc
2, place de la Porte d'Auteiul
75016 Paris
France

M Ebelin
Centre Hôpital-Universitaire de Bicêtre
78, rue du Général Leclerc
94270 Le Kremlin Bicêtre
France

DL Fernandez
Lindenhof Hospital
Bremgartenstrasse 117
3001 Berne
Switzerland

TJ Graham MD
Cleveland Clinic Foundation
9500 Euclid Avenue
Cleveland
Ohio 44195
USA

MD Greatting MD
Southern Illinois University School of Medicine
800 N. Rutledge Street
Springfield
Illinois 62794
USA

S Guero
114, boulevard St-Germain
75006 Paris
France

JL Haas
Centre Hospitalier de Longjumeau
91160 Longjumeau
France

G Herzberg
Hôpital Edouard-Herriot
5, place d'Arsonval
69437 Lyon
Cedex 3
France

Th Judet
Hôpital Tenon
4, rue de Chine
75970 Paris Cedex 20
France

JB Jupiter
Massachusetts General Hospital
15 Parkman Street
Boston
Massachusetts 02114
USA

AI Kapandji
Clinique de l'Yvette
43, route de Corbeil
91160 Longjumeau
France

Y Kiyoshige
Saisekai Yamagata Hospital
2-3-1 Kozirakawa-machi
Yamagata 990
Japan

Ph Kopylov
Hand Surgery Unit
Hospital of the University of Lund
22185 Lund
Sweden

E Lebalc'h
Centre Hôpital-Universitaire de Bicêtre
78, rue du Général Leclerc
94270 Le Kremlin Bicêtre
France

E Lenoble
Centre Hospital-Universitaire de Bicêtre
78, rue du Général Leclerc
94270 Le Kremlin Bicêtre
France

E Letrosne
Clinique Axium
Avenue Alfred Capus
13100 Aix-en-Provence
France

KS Leung
Faculty of Medicine
Chinese University of Hong Kong
Prince of Wales Hospital
Shatin
New Territories
Hong Kong

PC Leung
Faculty of Medicine
Chinese University of Hong Kong
Prince of Wales Hospital
Shatin
New Territories
Hong Kong

RL Linscheid
Mayo Clinic
200 First Street SW
Rochester
Minnesota 55905
USA

DS Louis
University of Michigan Medical Center
2912 Taubman Healthcare Center
1500 East Medical Center Drive
Ann Arbor
Michigan 48109
USA

M Mansat
CHU Purpan
Place du Dr Baylac
31059 Toulouse Cedex
France

Ch Mathoulin
Institut Français de la Main
15, rue Benjamin Franklin
75116 Paris
France

F Mazas
Centre Hôpital-Universitaire de Bicêtre
78, rue du Général Leclerc
94270 Le Kremlin Bicêtre
France

B Melchior
Poliklinik de l'Atlantique
rue Claude Bernard
44000 Nantes
France

JP Mortier
Clinique Mont-Louis
8, rue de la Folie-Régnault
75011 Paris
France

A Pagliei
Istituto di Clinica Ortopedica
Università Cattolica del Sacro Cuore
Largo A Gemelli 8
00168 Rome
Italy

G Pierret
Hand Surgery Associates
Suite 1026
Harper Professional Building G
4160 John R
Detroit
Michigan 48201
USA

Ph Saffar
Centre Chirurgical de la Main
8, square Petrarque
75116 Paris
France

H Saito
Seirei Hamamatsu General Hospital
Sumiyoshi 2-12-12
Hamamatsu
Shizuoka-ken 430
Japan

MJ Saldana
Nix Medical Center
414 Navarro, Suite 1621
San Antonio
Texas 78205
USA

J Sallerin
CHU Toulouse
Place du Dr Baylac
31059 Toulouse
France

F Schuind
Hôpital Erasme ULB
Route de Lennik 808
1070 Brussels
Belgium

I Semaan
Centre Hospitalier Général de Longjumeau
91160 Longjumeau
France

RM Singer
Hand Surgery Associates
Suite 1026
Harper Professional Building
4160 John R
Detroit
Michigan 48201
USA

C Smussi
Laboratoire d'Anatomie
Université René Descartes
45, rue des Saints Pères
75006 Paris
France

C Sokolow
Institut Français de la Main
15, rue Benjamin Franklin
75116 Paris
France

JB Steichen
The Indiana Hand Center
8501 Harcourt Road
Indianapolis
Indiana 46260
USA

E de Thomasson
Hôpital Tenon
4, rue de Chine
75970 Paris Cedex 20
France

B Valtin
72, avenue Jack-Gowevitch
94500 Champigny
France

APC Weiss
Rhode Island Hospital
593 Eddy Street
Providence
Rhode Island 02903
USA

CS Williams
Massachusetts General Hospital
15 Parkman Street
Boston
Massachusetts 02114
USA

MD Wood
Mayo Clinic
200 First Street SW
Rochester
Minnesota 55905
USA

1
Anatomy of the distal radius
F Brunelli, A Pagliei, C Smussi

In 1980, 565 Colles' fractures were reviewed at the Mayo Clinic by Cooney et al., who reported a complication rate of 31%. This has prompted a re-evaluation of the treatment of these injuries, which were previously generally regarded as benign. More than a century ago, the French surgeon and anatomist Malgaigne wrote 'I always found this fracture one of the easiest to cure, without stiffness, deformity or the least functional problem for the limb'. In fact, sequelae are not uncommon and involve soft tissue as well as bone (Dupont 1977). Injuries of the adjacent ligaments, tendons and neurovascular bundles can be a cause of post-operative complications, and secondary treatment of soft tissue problems is often difficult. A thorough knowledge of these adjacent anatomical structures is necessary to prevent the residual impairment often seen after these very common fractures.

This chapter will describe the structures most vulnerable to initial trauma or to iatrogenic injury associated with treating Colles' fracture.

The skin

Anterior aspect

This area is covered by thin, practically hairless skin which is rather adherent to the underlying fascia and has limited mobility, especially distally. The fascia about the wrist and distal radius begins in the distal forearm as antebrachial fascia and becomes thick distally as it coalesces with deeper fascia to form the flexor retinaculum and transverse carpal ligament. These tendinous longitudinal protrusions are the limits of grooves on the lateral and medial sides where the radial and ulnar arteries can be palpated. The central protrusion corresponds to the flexor tendons parallel to the median nerve, the lateral to the flexor carpi radialis (FCR) tendon and the medial to the flexor carpi ulnaris (FCU). Three transverse skin creases, proximal, middle and distal correspond respectively to the ulnar head, the radiocarpal joint, and the midcarpal joint.

Posterior aspect

The skin of the posterior aspect of the wrist is thicker and more mobile than the anterior skin and is covered by short hairs which are more numerous on the ulnar than the radial side.

When the wrist is in extension, many creases are present but their variability precludes any clinical description. The subcutaneous tissue is crossed by numerous veins coming from the dorsal aspect of the hand and going on the medial side to become the ulnar superficial vein and on the lateral side the radial superficial vein.

Three bony protuberances, which are easy to locate by palpation, elevate the dorsal skin:

1. on the ulnar side, the ulnar head, smooth and rounded, with the ulnar styloid process as a distal antero-medial bony protrusion;
2. on the radial side, the distal radius continues with another bony protrusion, the radial styloid process. A curved line of radius 1 cm and concave distally, that joins the two styloid processes with a 1 cm height of the curve can locate rather precisely the radio-ulno-carpal space;
3. on the radial part of the dorsal aspect, a third bony protrusion corresponds to Lister's tubercle. On its ulnar side, the compartment of the extensor pollicis longus (EPL) is located where it changes its course to curve radially.

If the thumb is extended and in maximum abduction, the EPL tendon protrusion is important and, together with the first compartment tendons — abductor pollicis longus (APL) and extensor pollicis brevis (EPB) — defines an oval space termed the anatomical 'snuff-box' by the ancient anatomists. The radial artery can be palpated in the depth of the snuff-box before it leaves this space to become dorsal at the level of the carpus.

The bones

The epiphysis of the distal radius usually appears at one year of age. The timing can vary, however, so that in some females it is present at birth, whereas in some males it does not appear until two or three years of age. It grows more in a lateral than a medial direction and forms the radial styloid process five facets and three articular fossae (scaphoid, lunate, and sigmoid notch) with the distal radius. It fuses to the diaphysis between 17 and 21 years of age in females and between 20 and 26 years of age in males.

The distal radius is composed of cancellous bone with trabeculae that are directed more or less perpendicular to the articular surface. This pattern is seen clearly on radiographs of the distal radius, particularly at the volar aspect. Trabeculae are densely aligned proximally on the volar cortex and diverge distally toward the articular facet, defining a triangle which corresponds to the fragment detached in volar rim fractures. The dense cortex surrounding the medullary canal covers only three-quarters of the circumference of the diaphysis. A thin layer of cortical bone extending more distally on the volar than on the dorsal aspect covers the distal one-quarter, explaining the dorsal and proximal direction of the fracture line. The strength of the epiphysis is reinforced at the dorsal aspect by the bony crests which make up the tendinous grooves.

In adults, fractures of the distal radius will occur selectively at the level where the epiphyseal crests end and the diaphyseal cortices disappear. Five facets are named after their position: distal, volar, dorsal, medial and lateral. The distal facet has two articular surfaces, the scaphoid fossa and the lunate fossa. The medial facet has one articular surface, the sigmoid fossa (notch) of the distal radius. The distal articular facet is triangular in shape, and covered completely by hyaline cartilage. It has two specific areas, the scaphoid and lunate fossae, which articulate with the proximal carpal row and the scaphoid and lunate bones. It is smooth and concave in all directions with the exception of a smooth antero-posterior interscapholunate crest which divides the two articular facets. The medial lunate fossa is quadrangular and the lateral scaphoid fossa is triangular. These two fossae transform the distal carpal facet of the radius into an antebrachial glenoid limited anteriorly and posteriorly by two rims, the posterior extending much more distally than the anterior. These rims present an anterior and posterior notch at the end of the interscapholunate crest, the anterior being deeper than the posterior. It is very important to describe accurately the orientation of the radial articular surfaces. Only a precise restoration of the orientation of both scaphoid and lunate fossae when reducing a distal radial fracture allows recovery of the normal motion of the wrist. The articular facet of the distal radius is oriented with a dorsal to volar angulation and a lateral to medial inclination. In the frontal plane, radial ulnar inclination is a mean 25°. In the sagittal plane, the dorsal to palmar inclination is 10°. The latter allows full flexion of the wrist.

Ulnar variance, which corresponds to the triangular fibro-cartilage (TFC) thickness, is approximately ±2 mm.

The anterior aspect

The anterior aspect of the distal radius is a continuation of the anterior aspect of the diaphysis. It is smooth and concave and accepts the insertion of the pronator quadratus. This muscle attachment extends distally and stops at 0.5 mm proximal to the anterior rim.

The posterior aspect

The posterior aspect of the distal radius is narrower than the anterior aspect, irregular, and crossed by longitudinal crests and grooves in which the tendons of the posterior compartments of the forearm glide. The most prominent crest (Lister's tubercle) is the pulley where the EPL turns from a medial to a lateral (ulnar to radial) direction. Injury to this tendon is one of the most frequent after fractures of the distal radius, occurring either when inserting pins to stabilize the fracture, or by tendon wear against bony prominences due to incomplete reduction and bone callus. EPL repair requires a tendon transfer in most cases (Fig. 1.1).

The medial aspect

The medial aspect of the distal radius is triangular in shape and presents at its distal part an articular facet, which is concave and extends from anterior to posterior. This is called the sigmoid notch of the radius. It articulates with the convex head of the distal ulna. The radial border or origin of the triangular fibro-cartilage (TFC) attaches at the distal border of the sigmoid fossa. On the anterior and posterior rim, two prominent crests give attachment to the distal radio-ulnar joint (DRUJ) ligaments.

The lateral aspect

The lateral aspect of the distal radius is separated from the posterior aspect by Lister's tubercle. A vertical groove forms where the APL and EPB excursion can be seen clearly. It extends distally with a pyramidal prominence, the radial styloid process, which is superficial and easily palpated just under the skin. The latter is convex posteriorly and laterally. It ends distally with a rounded end, the tip of the styloid, where the collateral radio-carpal ligament is inserted.

At the base of the radial styloid where it joins the radial diaphysis, the brachioradialis tendon is inserted. The radial styloid process extends more distally than the ulnar styloid by 1.5 cm. This difference in the level of the two styloids is helpful in the clinical diagnosis of distal radial fractures (Laugier's sign in the Pouteau–Colles' fractures).

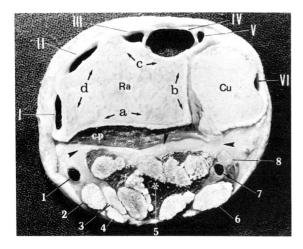

Figure 1.1

Transverse cut, at the distal radio-ulnar joint level of a left forearm injected with latex into the humeral artery and frozen in pronation. Tendons of the muscles of the posterior and lateral compartments have been removed to show the position of dorsal compartment muscles better.
I: abductor pollicis longus (APL)
extensor pollicis brevis (EPB)
II: extensor carpi radialis longus (ECRL)
extensor carpi radialis brevis (ECRB)
III: extensor pollicis longus (EPL)
IV: extensor digitorum communis (EDC)
extensor indicis proprius (EIP)
V: extensor digiti minimi (EDM)
VI: extensor carpi ulnaris (ECU)
1 arteria radialis (AR)
2 flexor carpi radialis (FCR)
3 nervus medianus (NM)
4 flexor palmaris longus (FPL)
5 flexor digitorum profundus and superficialis (FDP and FDS) and flexor pollicis longus (FPL)
6 flexor carpi ulnaris (FCU)
7 arteria cubitalis (AC)
8 nervus ulnaris (NU)
Ra: radius and its anterior (a), medial (b), posterior (c), and postero-lateral (d) aspects.
Cu: ulna
cp: pronator quadratus (PQ) and fat pads (black arrowheads)

The nerves

The area of the distal radius is crossed by numerous sensory branches of the medial cutaneous nerve of the forearm and musculocutaneous (MC) nerve which supply the anterior and posterior aspects of the wrist respectively. Three other nerves, however, are more commonly injured as a complication of distal radial fractures. On the anterior aspect, the main trunks of the ulnar and median nerves and on the posterior and lateral aspect of the wrist, the sensory branches of the radial nerve can be injured.

The median nerve

Distribution

At the level of the distal radius the median nerve has motor and sensory fibres. The sensory area is limited in the palm by a line passing through the middle of the fourth finger; the median nerve innervates the palmar aspect of the thumb, index and long fingers and the radial half of the ring finger. On the dorsum of the fingers, the median nerve extends to the two last phalanges of the index, long and lateral surface of the ring finger. The autonomous zone is the index fingertip. Muscle innervation in the thenar eminence, is supplied to the abductor pollicis brevis (APB), opponens pollicis (OP) and the deep belly of the flexor pollicis brevis (FPB). The radial two lumbricals are usually supplied by the median motor branch.

Course

This large nerve lies longitudinally in the middle of the forearm and deep to the flexor superfealis tendons. Distally it extends beneath the flexor retinaculum but gives terminal branches in the palm through the palmar cutaneous nerve which exits the main median nerve proximal to the transverse carpal ligament.

Anatomic relations

The median nerve emerges at the wrist from under the muscular belly of the flexor digitorum superficialis (FDS) and progresses to lie beneath the index finger, and lateral to the middle tendons of the FDS. The artery of the median nerve, a branch of the anterior interosseous artery, may lie directly on the median nerve and serves as a landmark of nerve orientation. The median nerve lies on the anterior aspect of the distal radius, with the pronator quadratus (PQ) between the nerve and the bone. Distally, the nerve lies near the radiocarpal joint capsule, before entering beneath the flexor retinaculum. It then enters into the carpal tunnel, keeping the same relationships with the tendons and the synovial sheaths of the flexor tendons to divide into terminal branches as it emerges from the carpal canal. Its sheath is surrounded by a net of sympathic fibres going to the hand.

Cross-innervation

The median nerve communicates with the ulnar nerve by a superficial cross-innervation between the interosseous nerves of the third and fourth spaces and by deep thenar branches to the FPB. Occasionally, the intrinsic muscles of the hand are totally innervated by the ulnar nerve (Riché–Cännau or Martin–Gruber anastomosis). The median communicates with the radial nerve on the thenar eminence by the cutaneous thenar branch of the radial nerve and by the dorsal collateral nerves at the digital level. In summary, the median nerve is most important because of its sensory supply, which covers the useful zone of prehension and because of its motor supply to the intrinsic muscles of the thumb. As a result of anatomical variance after a median nerve injury, this area can be partially reinnervated by the ulnar nerve, giving a satisfactory functional supply. The anatomical location of the median nerve exposes it directly to injuries associated with fractures of the distal radius.

The ulnar nerve

The ulnar nerve, like the median, is a mixed nerve with both motor and sensory supply to the hand. This important nerve provides a motor supply by branches to all the hypothenar muscles, the deep belly of FPB, the adductor pollicis (AP) and the two ulnar lumbricals.

The sensory area of the ulnar nerve extends from the ulnar border of the hand to a line passing through the middle of the fourth digit at the palmar aspect and at the dorsal aspect, excluding the zone innervated by the median nerve. Its autonomous sensory area is the fifth fingertip.

Course

The ulnar nerve runs along the antero-medial aspect of the forearm until the lateral aspect of the pisiform, where it divides into two terminal branches. It arises underneath the flexor carpi ulnaris (FCU) muscle and runs on the lateral side of its tendon before entering the fibro-osseous tunnel, named Guyon's canal. During its entire course, the nerve is lateral to the ulnar artery. It is separated from the median nerve by the transverse carpal ligament and hook of the hamate. The ulnar nerve lies on a narrow osseous plane composed of the ulnar head, the pisiform medially, and the hamate laterally and dorsally.

In summary, in distal radial fractures, the ulnar nerve is less exposed to injury than the median nerve. It is not directly on the fracture line and not involved in compression syndromes in the carpal tunnel, being outside it, in the relatively protected area of Guyon's canal. When distal radius fractures are associated with either ulnar fractures or dorsal or palmar dislocations, then ulnar nerve injury is more common.

The sensory branch of the radial nerve

Distribution

The dorsal cutaneous area of the hand, lateral to a line passing through the middle of the third digit (except the two distal phalanges) is innervated by the radial nerve. The radial nerve also innervates the lateral aspect of the wrist, the dorsal wrist and the entire dorsal aspect of the thumb.

Course

The sensory portion of the radial nerve perforates the superficial aponeurosis behind the tendon of the brachioradialis and penetrates the wrist area before crossing this tendon. Just proximal to the distal end of the radius, the radial sensory nerve divides into three terminal branches: lateral, middle and medial. It runs lateral to the radial artery and just superficial to the abductor pollicis longus and external pollicis brevis tendons.

Cross-innervation

At the dorsal, distal end of the forearm, there are areas of cross-innervation between the sensory portion of the radial nerve and the posterior branch of the musculocutaneous nerve (Fig. 1.2). At the thenar eminence there is an anastomosis with the palmar branch of the median nerve.

In summary, a direct injury to the radial nerve is not uncommon at the time of a distal radial fracture. In addition, it can be injured when reducing and stabilizing the fracture by pinning. Longitudinal incisions are necessary to carefully retract and preserve branches of the radial nerve. Percutaneous pinning should be avoided in these areas to prevent painful neuromas, which are difficult to cure.

The vessels

Anterior aspect

Arteries

The radial artery is situated in a groove between the brachioradialis laterally and flexor carpi radialis (FCR) medially (Fig. 1.3). It runs on the pronator quadratus and then distally on the volar aspect of the radius, where only the fascia is interposed with the skin. The radial artery can be easily palpated at this location. At the radial styloid process base, the course of the radial artery suddenly changes to reach the posterior aspect of the wrist.

There are two collateral branches of the radial artery:

1. the ramus volaris superficialis is a continuation of the radial artery and branches on the palmar aspect of the hand to anastomose with the superficial palmar arch;
2. the ramus carpeus volaris is usually a very thin branch, running along the distal limit of the pronator quadratus to anastomose with a corresponding branch of the ulnar artery.

The ulnar artery (with the ulnar nerve laterally) is situated in a gutter which is formed by the FDS laterally and the FCU medially. It is more deeply situated than the radial artery. Direct palpation, as well as the surgical approach, is more difficult than with the radial artery.

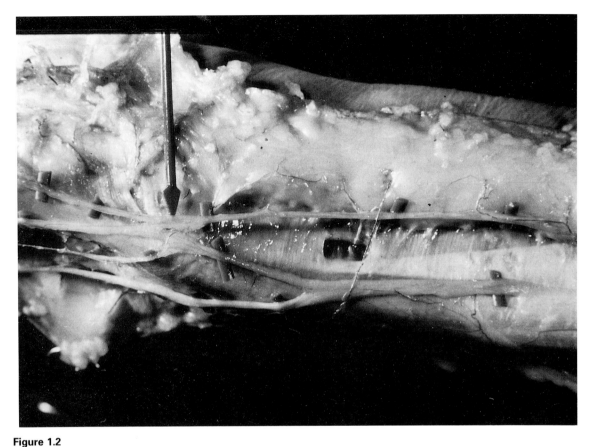

Figure 1.2

Anatomical dissection of the sensory branch of the radial nerve: the arrow shows the anastomosis with the musculocutaneous nerve.

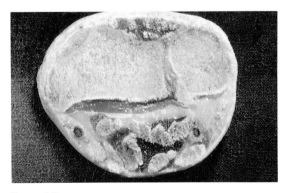

Figure 1.3

Section of the distal radius. At the bottom, adjacent to the flexor tendon, the radial artery is visible on the left and the ulnar artery on the right side.

At the pisiform bone level, the ulna artery changes to a lateral direction to supply the superficial arch.

There are two main collateral branches:

1. the ramus carpeus volaris communicates with the corresponding artery emerging from the radial artery;
2. the ulnopalmar emerges from the ulnar artery at the level of the pisiform bone and continues distally to form the deep vascular arch.

Two arteries of less magnitude cross the anterior aspect of the wrist:

1. the anterior interosseous artery runs under the pronator quadratus to perforate the interosseous membrane and end at the dorsal aspect of the wrist;

2. the median nerve artery (branch of the anterior interosseous artery) is adjacent to the median nerve and in some instances is of significant size and can replace the ulnar artery.

Veins

The superficial veins are usually of small calibre, coming from the hand and forming the median vein. Two deep veins (venae comitantes) run along the main arteries of the area.

Posterior aspect

Arteries

The radial artery is the main artery of this area. It arises at the posterior aspect of the wrist after crossing the anatomical snuff-box obliquely and passing under the APL, EPB and EPL tendons.

Three other arteries, of less importance, cross the area:

1. the anterior interosseous artery (AIA) perforates the interosseous membrane to emerge dorsally;
2. the posterior interosseous artery, which is situated along the interosseous membrane separating the ECU and extensor proprius of the fifth finger;
3. the dorsal artery of the carpus, arising from the ulnar artery, turns dorsally over the ulna and communicates with the corresponding artery branches emerging from the radial artery.

Veins

The superficial veins are variable in size and position, and are much larger than the palmar veins. They arise from the venous arcades of the dorsal aspect of the hand and form the superficial ulnar vein on the medial side and the superficial radial vein on the lateral side.

The deep veins are collateral to the arteries.

The distal radius bone vascularity

Blood supply to the distal radius is mainly from the anterior interosseous artery and the radial artery. The ulnar artery and the posterior interosseous arteries are involved only indirectly via the anastomoses between the carpal arteries (Fig. 1.4). As for all long bones, the vascularity arises from three sources:

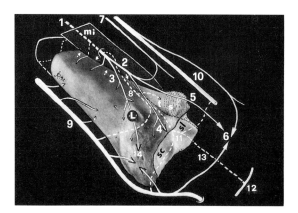

Figure 1.4

Vascularization of the distal radius seen from the posterolateral view. At the distal forearm, the AIA (1) runs under the pronator quadratus, perforates the interosseous membrane (mi) and is in the dorsal compartment: the dorsal terminal branch (2), which is in direct continuation with the AIA, produces further branches: the radial epiphyseal branch (3), the comitans branch (4) for the posterior interosseous nerve, and the anastomotic branch (5) for the dorsal carpal arch (6). The anastomotic branch produces a further branch communicating with the posterior interosseous branch (7). In the anterior compartment, a branch from the AIA continues in the same direction as the AIA. This is the terminal palmar branch (8), which communicates with the radial artery (9) and the ulnar artery (10), and produces the palmar carpal arch (11) and the deep carpal arch (12) via the palmar carpal arch (13). At the lateral aspect of the distal radius are the peristyloid vascular loop (14) and Lister's tubercle (L). The medial aspect (black broken line) is triangular, limited by the two bifurcating lines of the radius. The interosseous membrane insertion continues along the posterior line. This area is divided into two parts: proximal (t), where the deep fascicles of the PQ are attached, and distal, where the sigmoid notch (S) articulates with the ulnar head. At the distal aspect of the radius are the facets which articulate with the scaphoid (SC) and with the lunate (SL).

8   FRACTURES OF THE DISTAL RADIUS

1. nutrient arteries;
2. metaphyseal and epiphyseal perforating arteries, which can be viewed as the adult vascular pattern;
3. the periosteal plexus.

Only the latter two systems will be analysed.

The metaphyseal arteries, coming from the periosteal network, enter the cortical bone and anastomose in the medullary canal with branches coming from the nutrient artery. The epiphyseal vessels penetrate into the cortex in a circumferential way, near the epiphyseal plate, to form nets, the branches of which form a dense capillary network in the metaphyseal and subchondral areas (Crock 1980). During growth, the vessels inside the bone do not cross epiphyseal plates: the *germinal* cartilage line growth depends on the vascular supply of the epiphysis, and any vascular injury of the epiphysis can lead to an impairment of epiphyseal plate growth (Dimeglio 1983).

The periosteal plexus takes its origin from three types of vessels: direct periosteal branches, musculoperiosteal branches, and fascioperiosteal branches (Simpson 1985).

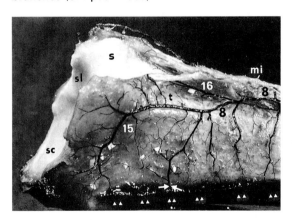

Figure 1.5

Distal radius vascularization: anterior and medial aspect. The anterior aspect and the triangular area (t) proximal to the sigmoid notch (S) are supplied by the terminal palmar branch (8) of the AIA. The lateral fibres of the PQ have been saved by the dissection (arrowheads); (mi) interosseous membrane. The arrows indicate the anastomosis between the musculoperiosteal branches of the palmar terminal branch and the radial artery branch (15) of the palmar carpal arch, which supplies the radius anterior rim branch (16) for the medial aspect of the distal radius and the DRUJ. In this specimen, coloured latex has been injected into the humeral artery.

Anterior interosseous artery (AIA)

This vessel probably plays an important role in the vascular supply to the radius. It is the main supply (Figs 1.5, 1.6) for the anterior and medial aspect of the radius (Leung 1990, Santos Rath 1990) and a principal supply to the posterior aspect through palmar to dorsal anastomoses (Fig. 1.7). Two types of dorsal endings of the AIA have been observed (Pagliei 1991).

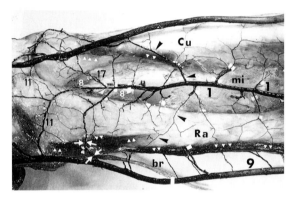

Figure 1.6

Vascularization of the distal radius: anterior aspect. The radial artery (9) produces small muscular and musculoperiosteal branches, which penetrate the flexor palmaris longus (FPL) and the pronator quadratus (PQ); the lateral fibres of these muscles inserted on the radius (Ra) and on the ulna (Cu) have been preserved (white arrowheads). These branches contribute to the palmar periosteal network of the radius, which communicates with the musculoperiosteal branches of the AIA.

The AIA (1) perforates the interosseous membrane (mi) and runs dorsally. The terminal palmar branch (8) runs under the PQ with the terminal branches of the anterior interosseous nerve, and vascularizes this nerve, the PQ and the anterior aspect of the distal radius. The ulnar epiphyseal branch (17) arises and the terminal branch runs along the radial slope to produce the palmar carpal arch (11), of which the radial branch is almost always dominant (Kuhlmann, 1986). This arch is among the three arches (dorsal and palmar) described by Gelberman (1983). The dorsal carpal arch (or dorsal intercarpal) provides the most constant direct periosteal branches for the radius and ulna (black arrowheads). These branches are present at the proximal border of the PQ and supply the two bones, at the site of the attachments of this muscle. The ulnar periosteal branch is usually more dominant. Note the anastomosis (arrows) between the musculoperiosteal branches of the palmar terminal branch and the radial artery, which branches into the attachment fibres of the PQ brachioradialis (br). In this specimen, coloured latex has been injected into the humeral artery.

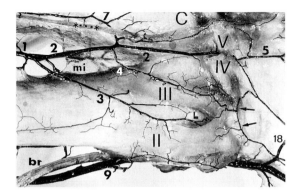

Figure 1.7

Vascularization of the distal radius: posterior aspect. The dorsal terminal branch (2) of the AIA (1) anastomoses with the posterior interosseous artery (7). The radial epiphyseal branch (3) runs towards Lister's tubercle (L). The osteoperiosteal branch (4) arborizes on the third and fourth extensor compartment gutters: its anastomosis with the carpal dorsal network is visible, producing the dorsal radiocarpal arch (arrows) described by Gelberman (1983). Small perforating vessels for the posterior rim of the radius arise from this arch. The radial artery (9) produces a transverse branch (18) for the dorsal arch of the carpus.

The dorsal terminal branch (2) runs distally (5) to contribute to the carpal dorsal arch: note its deep situation in the septum between the fourth and fifth dorsal compartments. C, ulnar head; mi, interosseous membrane; br, brachioradialis tendon; *- -*, septum between EPM and ECU. In this specimen, coloured latex has been injected into the humeral artery.

Type I

The dorsal terminal branch produces a radial epiphyseal branch, which has a proximal retrograde direction toward Lister's tubercle, in the septum separating the EPL from the EPB.

Type II

A perforating proximal branch follows the same course as the radial epiphyseal branch, but perforates the interosseous membrane proximally to the terminal dorsal branch.

The radial epiphyseal branch (type I) and the proximal perforating branch (type II) are similar in that they both anastomose with the peristyloidian vascular network (from the radial artery). They vascularize the posterior aspect of the radial epiphysis by their arborization (producing fascioperiosteal vessels) all along the septum between EPL and EPB. On the posterior aspect of the metaphysis and epiphysis of the radius covered by these muscles, vascular branches enter the third dorsal compartment and the ulnar part of the second compartment, including Lister's tubercle. These vessels supply the osteoperiosteal flap described by Martin (1989) and Baudet (1990).

Before continuing its course (in the septum separating the fourth and fifth compartments) to the dorsal arch of the carpus, and to anastomose with the posterior interosseous artery, the terminal dorsal branch produces an osteoperiosteal branch (in close contact with the posterior interosseous nerve) which arborizes on the third and fourth extensor compartment grooves. Usually of small calibre, this branch can be distal to the radiocarpal joint, where it can contribute to the anastomotic dorsal carpal network.

Radial artery (RA)

The postero-lateral aspect and the lateral part of the anterior aspect of the distal radius are supplied mainly by the radial artery (Fig. 1.8a). Small musculoperiosteal branches arise distal to the pronator teres from the radial artery to supply the FPL and PQ. These branches pass across the radial attachments of the muscles to vascularize the postero- and antero-lateral aspect of the radius and communicate with the musculoperiosteal branches of the AIA (see Fig. 1.6). These branches, coming from the radial artery, represent the vascular anatomical supply of the osteocutaneous composite radial flap of the forearm (Biemer 1987, Chacha 1987, Foucher 1984, MacCormack 1986, Marin Braun 1988).

The radial styloid process is supplied by the radial artery, significantly by the AIA, and by the dorsal carpal network, which together form the peristyloid 'vascular loop' (Fig. 1.8b).

There are two 'border lines' between the RA and AIA: one occurs at the junction between the posterior and postero-lateral areas and one at the junction between the anterior and antero-lateral areas (see Fig. 1.4). The anterior and posterior margins of the distal radius are supplied by the carpal arches (see Figs 1.5 and 1.7) and are at the junction between three arterial systems: the radial, the ulnar and the anterior

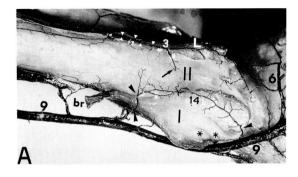

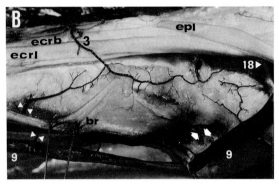

Figure 1.8

Vascularization of the distal radius: postero-lateral aspect of the radial styloid process.

a) Small osteoperiosteal branches (black arrowheads) arise from the radial artery (9) at the base and top of the radial styloid processes (recurring styloid branches). The anastomosis forms a peristyloid vascular loop (14), arborizing on the postero-lateral aspect and situated between the extensor carpi radialis longus (ECRL) and extensor carpi radialis brevis (ECRB) gutter (II) and the first compartment gutter (I), on which the distal fibres of the brachioradialis (br) end. The small longitudinal prominence (**) divides this gutter into two secondary gutters for the APL and EPB. The dorsal carpal arch (6), or dorsal intercarpal arch arises from the RA. The radial epiphyseal branch (3) of the AIA arborizes (white arrowheads) on the ECR gutters, producing the fascioperiosteal vessels. The black arrow shows a small perforating vessel penetrating the epiphyseal cortex. L, Lister's tubercle.

b) The peristyloid vascular loop is also provided by the radial epiphyseal branch (3) via its superficial anastomosis, on the ECRL and ECRB tendons. The transverse branch (18) of the radial artery (9), situated under the ECRL and ECRB tendons, provides the dorsal carpal arch. The recurring styloid branch (arrows) is in this case rather thin: the peristyloid loop is provided by the dorsal carpal network. In this specimen, coloured latex has been injected into the humeral artery.

interosseous. There are close anatomical relationships between these three arteries and the posterior interosseous system by connections at the wrist, which is actually a real 'anastomotic thoroughfare' between the four arterial systems of the forearm.

Conclusion

Fractures of the distal radius can result in permanent impairment. Every effort should be made to achieve anatomical restoration of the radiocarpal articular surface.

Radio-ulnar inclination should be around 25°, the palmar slope 10° and ulnar variance around ±2 mm.

A good knowledge of the anatomical structures around the distal radius is necessary to prevent complications due to fracture reduction manoeuvres and/or stabilization by pins, or external fixation frames.

The two main structures exposed to injury are:

1. the sensory branch of the radial nerve, which should be approached by longitudinal incisions and retracted before pinning;
2. the EPL tendon passing medial to Lister's tubercle, which can be injured by closed pinning or from wear on a prominent osseous callus.

References

Baudet J, Martin D, Hu W, Persichetti P. *Le lambeau épiphysaire radial postérieur: un nouveau site donneur en microchirurgie vasculaire.* Paris: IIème Congrès Latin de Chirurgie de la Main et du Membre Supérieur, 1990.

Biemer E, Stock W. Total thumb reconstruction: a one stage reconstruction using an osteocutaneous forearm flap. *Br J Plast Surg* 1987; **40**: 36–92.

Chacha B, Soin K, Tan C. One stage reconstruction of intercalated defect of the thumb using the osteocutaneous radial forearm flap. *J Hand Surg* 1987; **12B**: 86–92.

Colles A. On the fractures of the carpal extremity of the radius. *Edi Med Surg J* 1814; **10**: 182–86.

Cooney W, Dobyns J, Linscheid R. Complications of Colles' fractures. *J Bone Joint Surg* 1980; **62A**: 613–19.

Crock HV, Chiari PR, Crock MC. La vascularisation des os du poignet et de la main chez l'homme. In Tubiana R: *Traité de chirurgie de la main. Tome I*. Paris: Masson, 1980.

Dimeglio A, Pous JG, Bonnel F. Le cartilage de croissance. *Encycl Med Chir Paris Appareil Locomoteur* 1983; **B10**: 14009.

Duparc J, Valtin B. Complications tendino-nerveuses des fractures de l'extrémité du radius. *Ann Chir* 1977; **31(4)**: 335–39.

Foucher G, Genechten F, Merle M, Michon J. A compound radial artery forearm flap in hand surgery: an original modification of the chinese forearm flap. *Br J Plast Surg* 1984; **37**: 139–48.

MacCormack GC, Duncan J, Lamberty BGH. The blood supply of the bone component of the compound osteocutaneous radial artery forearm flap. An anatomical study. *Br J Plast Surg* 1986; **39**: 173–75.

Simpson AHRW. The blood supply of the periosteum. *J Anat* 1985; **140, 4**: 697–704.

2
Current trends in treatment and classification of distal radial fractures
Ph Saffar

Thirty years ago, distal radial fractures were considered benign and conservative treatment was the rule. The population involved supposedly consisted of osteoporotic old women who were functioning well despite poor results and exact reduction was not mandatory, since good results were not said to be correlated with good reduction. Unaesthetic malunions were noticed, but deemed unimportant.

Since then, a growing number of young male, manual workers and sport enthusiasts have suffered high-velocity injuries, often resulting in complex intra-articular fractures. Pain and disability have resulted from subsequent malunions. Recently surgical treatment has been widely recommended and performed on an emergency basis to prevent these sequelae. The aim of the treatment is to obtain a good or perfect reduction, especially for intra-articular fractures.

Redisplacement or loss of reduction after conservative treatment is another feature which was not well recognized, in the past. We are now aware that an almost inevitable shortening (2–5 mm) takes place during healing of distal radial fractures in the absence of external or internal fixation, and sometimes occurs in spite of it. The extent of this redisplacement is usually related to the initial displacement. Cast immobilization does not prevent finger movements. The contraction of the flexor tendons transmits compression forces in the axis of the forearm and the carpus abuts on the distal radius, resulting in its proximal migration and radial shortening. This factor of redisplacement was also overlooked for a long time. Furthermore, a non-displaced fracture is not always stable. One must always look for dorsal comminution and try to evaluate and anticipate a secondary displacement.

A combination of different directions of displacement have been described: dorsal tilt, loss of radial inclination, radial shortening, etc. However, it has been pointed out recently that a rotational displacement of the fractured distal radius (epiphyseal component) can also be a part of the deformity, resulting in rotational malunions and problems of incongruity at the distal radio-ulnar joint (DRUJ).

Treatment of distal radius fractures

Conservative

Different types and positions of immobilization of the wrist and hand have been described: straight, in flexion-ulnar deviation, in extension; with or without permanent cast, with a below- or over-the-elbow cast; with the forearm pronated or supinated. It seems that redisplacement during healing is not correlated with the type of immobilization but only with the dorsal comminution and the initial displacement.

Percutaneous direct pinning

An early technique, in fact one of the first used for fixation of distal radius fractures, was percutaneous pinning, usually entering at the level of the radial styloid process. Some variations in the point of penetration and the direction of the pins were presented, but the aim was always to fix the mobile fragment to the opposite cortex proximal to the fracture. This type of pinning cannot prevent redisplacement of certain fragments, and this is particularly true of intra-articular fractures. Direct pinning of the fragments, especially the postero-medial fragment (which can involve the DRUJ) through the distal ulna, adds stability to the structure.

Elastic intrafocal or extrafocal pinning

This method is popular and considered to be a reliable treatment for extra-articular fractures. The fracture is first reduced by external manoeuvres. The K-wire is then moved dorsally through the fracture site to penetrate the opposite cortex in a 45° proximal direction. The elastic force of the K-wire gives a persistent reduction and prevents redisplacement. The exact placement and direction of each K-wire is very important; two or three are inserted through separate, short approaches after protection of the nerves and tendons. One of the main complications of this technique is over-reduction if the K-wires are inserted too vertically.

In a second type of elastic pinning, pins enter through the distal epiphyseal fragment and are then directed through the medullary canal to the proximal radius, to take support from the proximal cortex without penetrating it.

External fixation

This technique was proposed for comminuted fractures, and it has improved the reduction of comminuted intra-articular fractures. Ligamentotaxis can exert influence only on fragments in which capsuloligamentous attachments are still intact. The traction is exerted mainly by the strong volar ligament plane on the anterior rim of the distal radius. The dorsal tilt is not completely reduced because dorsal ligaments are thinner and in a transverse plane. Central articular fracture fragments are not reduced.

This procedure can be complicated by problems with fixation, pin placement and also by neurosympathetic dystrophy (NSD), which occurs at an increased rate if the external fixator is maintained for more than five weeks or if distraction is too strong: the aim is to realign and not to distract. Hinged external fixators, by providing early motion of the wrist, can reduce stiffness and help to prevent the onset of NSD.

External fixation and direct pinning

The next technique which might be used to try to obtain perfect reduction in an intra-articular fracture is external fixation, associated with a short, direct and open reduction of the non-reduced fragments and direct pinning. Sometimes, reduction is possible by manipulation combined with percutaneous pinning. This relatively aggressive, open reduction procedure is reserved for comminuted intra-articular fractures in young people.

Bone grafting

In certain cases, for example when there is excessive comminution and bone loss that persists after reduction, a corticocancellous or cancellous graft is certainly the best tool to prevent proximal migration of a central fragment. This migration can occur in a die-punch fracture, or in elderly people with osteoporotic bone. It can also be present despite the use of K-wires, external fixation or both. The results of bone grafting can be almost perfect and healing is faster. In these cases, some authors have proposed the use of bone cement instead of a bone graft in elderly people to allow immediate mobilization, but this is rarely recommended.

Plate fixation

This is indicated in fractures with volar displacement, such as Barton's and Smith's fractures and in selected cases of dorsal displacement where rigid fixation can provide for early wrist motion. Plate fixation can provide either a buttress effect or hold the distal epiphysis by corticocancellous screws. Premoulded plates reproducing the distal curvature of the radius are best, as they give an automatic reduction. New distal radius fixation plates are under study.

Wrist arthroscopy

The last refinement developed to achieve perfect reduction of intra-articular fragments is wrist arthroscopy with a triangulation probe. This can detect a step-off of one or two millimetres, which is not always visible on radiographic examination; the fragments can then be directly reduced and fixed by fine K-wires.

To analyse complex fractures correctly, image intensification is recommended. After reduction and pin or plate fixation radiographic examination is mandatory: antero-posterior, lateral and oblique views should be obtained. Traction with Chinese traps can be used before treatment.

Summary of treatment options

In the literature, the results of extra- and intra-articular fractures are often mixed. It would be inappropriate to discuss these two types of fractures together here, since the treatments are different and the accuracy of reduction needed in the intra-articular fractures tends to prevent post-traumatic osteoarthritis. This disease has been documented widely, as much as for its frequency as for its correlation with pain and disability.

We have reviewed the evolution of ideas for treatment of distal radial fractures over the last 20 years, but this does not mean that every fracture should be treated by operation.

In distal radial fractures in the elderly, conservative treatment is always the rule, even if a Darrach procedure is necessary six months later to treat ulnar pain. Minimum intervention is the rule, while the redisplacement problem can be difficult to manage for both the surgeon and the patient.

This has nothing in common with a young patient's intra-articular comminuted fracture: here, the maximum treatment is mandatory. All available techniques should be used to achieve healing in the best possible anatomical position.

Distal radial fractures are often associated with carpal ligament tears. The reported frequency varies from 10% to 75%, depending mainly on the diagnostic tool used; the higher rate was reported after a series of systematic arthroscopic examinations during emergency reductions. Ligament tears do not always mean carpal instability: there is a difference between ligament tears, instability (dynamic) and dissociation (static instability) of the carpal bones. In the first two cases, ligament tears can heal in a good position with cast immobilization. In the last case, a residual carpal instability will persist. Furthermore, carpal ligament tears can pre-exist in elderly people and this has to be considered. In all distal radial fractures, the position of the carpal bones should be carefully assessed after reduction and during healing to prevent late instability and arthritis.

In conclusion, great care should be taken in every case to choose the treatment that suits the real functional needs of the patient, rather than automatically pursuing a perfect radiological result using over-aggressive treatment.

Classification of distal radius fractures

For more than 80 years, surgeons have tried to classify fractures of the distal radius. Some classifications have been forgotten or have not gained recognition, such as those of Pilcher (1917), Destot (1923), Taylor and Parsons (1938), Nissen-Lie (1939), Humphries (1948), Key (1954) and Arbeitlang and Boeckl (1963).

Others are frequently used in the literature. Frykman's classification (Table 2.1) is the most popular, but does not provide treatment options or prognosis. Other classifications have been based on:

1. radiographic appearance or fracture displacement direction: the AO classification (Table 2.2), the Sarmiento classification (Table 2.3) and the Lidström classification (Table 2.4);
2. the mechanism of injury: the Castaing classification (Table 2.5), the Fernandez classification (Table 2.6) and the Linscheid classification;

Table 2.1 Frykman's classification
Modified from: Frykman G, 1967.

Groups 1 and 2	Extra-articular with and without fracture of the distal ulna
Groups 3 and 4	Intra-articular involving the radiocarpal joint with and without fracture of the distal ulna
Groups 5 and 6	Intra-articular involving the distal radio-ulnar joint with and without fracture of the distal ulna
Groups 7 and 8	Intra-articular involving both radiocarpal and distal radio-ulnar joints with and without fracture of the distal ulna

Table 2.2 AO classification

Group 1	Extra-articular
Group 2	Partial articular
Group 3	Complete articular C1: simple articular and metaphyseal C2: simple articular and complex metaphyseal C3: complex articular and complex metaphyseal + fracture distal end

Table 2.3 Sarmiento et al. classification
Modified from: Sarmiento A, Pratt GN, Berry NC, Sinclair WF, 1975.

Group	
1	Non-displaced fractures without radiocarpal joint involvement
2	Displaced fractures without radiocarpal joint involvement
3	Non-displaced fractures with radiocarpal joint involvement
4	Displaced fractures with radiocarpal joint involvement

Table 2.4 Lidström and Anders classification
Modified from Lidström A, 1959.

Group 1	Undisplaced
Group 2a	Dorsal angulation, extra-articular
Group 2b	Dorsal angulation, intra-articular but without gross separation of fragments
Group 2c	Dorsal angulation plus dorsal displacement, extra-articular
Group 2d	Dorsal angulation plus dorsal displacement, intra-articular but without gross separation of fragments
Group 2e	Dorsal angulation plus dorsal displacement, intra-articular with separation of fragments

3. articular joint surface involvement: the Mayo classification (Table 2.7), the McMurtry and Jupiter classification (Table 2.8) and the Melone classification (Table 2.9);
4. degree of comminution: the Gartland and Werley classification (Table 2.10), the Jenkins classification (Table 2.11), and the Older classification (Table 2.12);
5. on bone calcification and resistance: the Sennwald and Segmuller classification.

More recent classifications tend to provide therapeutic options and prognosis to prevent redisplacements and malunions, for example those of Cooney (Table 2.13), Melone, and Mathoulin, Letrosne and Saffar (Table 2.14). The extent of DRUJ involvement complicates some of these classifications.

16 FRACTURES OF THE DISTAL RADIUS

Table 2.5 Castaing and le Club des Dix classification
Modified from Castaing J, le Club des Dix, 1964.

Type 1	Compression–extension (posterior displacement)
	■ Pouteau–Colles
	■ with postero-medial fragment
	■ complex
	    a) sagittal T
	    b) with medial component
	    c) with lateral component
	    d) postero-lateral rim, isolated or complex
	    e) frontal T
	    f) cross lines in two planes
	    g) comminuted
	    h) undisplaced

Type 2	Compression–flexion: ■ Goyrand–Smith ■ anterior rim, isolated or antero-lateral ■ complex anterior rim
Type 3	Associated osteo-articular injuries: ■ ulnar styloid ■ ulnar head ■ ulnar neck ■ radio-ulnar dislocation ■ radio-ulnar diastasis ■ carpal injuries ■ other injuries of the upper limb ■ open fracture ■ bilateral
Type 4	Non-classified

Table 2.6 Fernandez classification

Bending: type 1	One cortex of the metaphysis fails due to tensile stress (Colles' and Smith fractures) and the opposite undergoes a certain degree of comminution
Shearing: type 2	Fracture of the joint surface: Barton's, reversed Barton's styloid process fracture, simple articular fracture
Compression: type 3	Fracture of the surface of the joint with impaction of subchondral and metaphyseal bone (die-punch fracture), intra-articular comminuted fracture
Avulsion: type 4	Fracture of the ligament attachments to ulnar and radial styloid process, radiocarpal fracture–dislocation
Combinations: type 5	Combination of types, high-velocity injuries

Table 2.7 Mayo classification of intra-articular fractures

Type	
1	Extra-articular radiocarpal Intra-articular radio-ulnar
2	Intra-articular scaphoid fossa of distal radius
3	Intra-articular lunate fossa of distal radius + sigmoid fossa
4	Intra-articular, scaphoid fossa, lunate fossa and sigmoid fossa of the distal radius

Table 2.8 McMurtry and Jupiter classification

Modified from: McMurtry RY, Jupiter JB.
In *Skeletal Trauma*. Browner B, Jupiter JB, Levine A, and Trafton P, eds. Philadelphia: WB Saunders, 1991.

Number of parts:

Group	
1	2 parts: (the opposite portion of the radio-carpal joint remains intact) — dorsal Barton — palmar Barton — chauffeur — die-punch
2	3 parts: The lunate and scaphoid facets separate from each other and the proximal portion of the radius
3	4 parts: The same + lunate facet fractured in dorsal and volar fragment
4	5 parts or more

Table 2.9 Melone's intra-articular fractures classification

Modified from: Melone, 1986.

Type	
1	Minimal comminution — stable
2	Comminuted — stable Displacement of medial complex: posterior: die-punch, Barton anterior: Smith 2
3	Displacement of medial complex as a unit + anterior spike
4	Wide separation or rotation of the dorsal fragment and palmar fragment rotation

Types 1 and 2: reducible
Type 3:   percutaneous pinning or external fixation
Type 4:   open reduction

Table 2.10 Gartland and Werley classification
Modified from Gartland JJ, Werley CW, 1951.

Group
1 Simple Colles' fracture
2 Comminuted Colles' fracture with undisplaced intra-articular fragments
3 Comminuted Colles' fracture with displaced intra-articular fragments

Table 2.11 Jenkins classification
Modified from: Jenkins NH, 1989.

Group
1 No radiographically visible comminution
2 Comminution of the dorsal radial cortex without comminution of the fracture fragment
3 Comminution of the fracture fragment without significant involvement of the dorsal cortex
4 Comminution of both the distal fragment and the dorsal cortex. As the fracture line involves the distal fracture fragment in Groups 3 and 4, intra-articular involvement is very common within these groups. Such involvement is not, however, inevitable and nor does it affect the fracture's placement within the classification

Table 2.12 Older and Cassebaum classification
Modified from: Older TM, Cassebaum TM 1965.

Group
1 'Non-displaced' — up to 5° dorsal angulation, radial articular surface at least 2 mm distal to ulnar head
2 'Displaced with minimal comminution' — dorsal angulation or displacement, radial articular surface no lower than 3 mm proximal to ulnar head, minimal comminution of dorsal radius
3 'Displaced with comminution of dorsal radius' — comminution of dorsal radius: radial articular surface proximal to ulnar head; minimal comminution of distal fragment
4 'Displaced with severe comminution of radial head' — marked comminution of dorsal and distal radius; radial articular surface 2–8 mm proximal to ulnar head

Table 2.13 Cooney's classification
Universal classification of distal radial fractures

Type		
1	Non-articular	Undisplaced
2	Non-articular	Displaced
	■ reducible*	Stable
	■ reducible	Unstable
	■ irreducible	
3	Articular	Undisplaced
4	Articular	Displaced
	■ reducible*	Stable
	■ reducible	Unstable
	■ irreducible	

*(by ligamentotaxis only)

Table 2.14 Mathoulin, Letrosne and Saffar classification
Modified from: Mathoulin Ch, Letrosne E, Saffar Ph 1989.

Type
1 1 articular line in the coronal plane
   Barton, reverse Barton
2 1 articular line in the sagittal plane involving:
   ■ the scaphoid facet
   ■ the lunate facet
   ■ the radio-ulnar joint
3 2 lines associated:
   ■ one extra-articular horizontal
   ■ one intra-articular = type 2a, b + other fragments or dorsal comminution (T fractures, die-punch)
4 3 lines associated:
   ■ one extra-articular horizontal
   ■ two articular, one coronal, one sagittal (postero-medial fragments — T frontal and sagittal)

References

Arbeitlang E and Boeckl O. Kritische Bernerkungen zur distalen radiusfraktur. *Arch Orthop Unfall-Chir* 1963; **55**: 1.

Castaing J, le Club des Dix. Les fractures recentes de l'extrémité inférieure du radius chez l'adulte. *Rev Chir Orthop* 1964; **50**: 581–666.

Destot E. Quoted by Platt H. *Traumatisme du poignet et rayons*. Paris: Masson. 1923.

Frykman G. Fracture of the distal radius, including sequelae–shoulder–hand–finger syndrome. Disturbance in the distal radioulnar joint and impairment of nerve function. A clinical and experimental study. *Acta Orthop Scand* 1967; **suppl 108**: 1.

Gartland J, Werley C. Evaluation of healed Colles' fractures. *J Bone Joint Surg* 1951; **33A**: 895–907.

Humphries SV. Severe Colles' fractures. Report on seven cases. *Clin Proc* 1948; **7**: 339.

Jenkins NH, Jones DG, Johnson SR. External fixation of Colles fractures. *J Bone Joint Surg* 1987; **69B**: 207–11.

Key JA. Colles' fracture. *Surgery* 1954; **36**: 998.

Lidström A. Fractures of the distal end of the radius. *Acta Orthop Scand* 1959; **41 (suppl)**: 1–118.

Mathoulin Ch, Letrosne E, Saffar Ph. Fracture articulaire du radius chez le sujet jeune: revue de 112 cas avec un recul plus d'un an. Paper presented at Congress of the Goupe d'Etude de la Main, Paris, France, December 1989.

McMurtry RY, Jupiter JB. Fractures of the distal radius. In: Browner B, Jupiter J, Levine A, Trafton P, eds. *Skeletal Trauma*. Philadelphia: WB Saunders, 1991: 1063–94.

Melone CP. Articular fractures of the distal radius. *Orthop Clin North Am* 1984; **15, 2**: 217–36.

Nissen-Lie HS. Fractura radii 'typica'. *Nord Med* 1939; **1**: 293.

Older TM, Stabler GV, Casselbau WH. Colles' fracture: Evaluation and selection of therapy. *J Trauma* 1965; **5**: 469.

Pilcher LS. Fractures of the lower extremity or base of the radius. *Ann Surg* 1917; **65**: 1.

Sarmiento A, Pratt G, Berry N, Sinclair W. Colles' fracture: functional bracing in supination. *J Bone Joint Surg* 1962; **44A**: 337–51.

Taylor GW and Parsons CL. The role of discus articularis in Colles' fracture. *J Bone Joint Surg* 1938; **20**: 149.

3
Pathomechanism of intra-articular distal radial fractures

I Semaan, Ph Saffar

Introduction

Intra-articular fractures deserve to be considered as a particular sub-group of distal radial fractures because the treatment options available for them are difficult, and there is a high incidence of post-traumatic osteoarthritis (OA).

These fractures have always been studied with similar experimental designs of a bone submitted to an impact. The wrist is usually positioned in an extended or flexed position, and the displacement depends on the position at the time of the impact. This simple concept is widely accepted and cited in the literature, however, the mechanism is far from a true reproduction of the mechanism of injury. In a real situation, the bones are surrounded by active and passive stabilizers and at the time of the impact, muscle contractions and ligament restraints can modify the fracture lines.

History

Many authors have performed cadaver studies to explain the pathomechanism of distal radial fractures, most notably Dupuytren (1834), Nelaton (1844), Malgaigne (1847), Linhart (1852), Lecomte (1861), Destot and Gallois (1896), Lilienfeldt (1907), Pilcher (1917), Stevens (1920), Mayer (1940) and Lewis (1950).

The classical idea is that a fall on a hyperextended wrist is the usual cause of these fractures. Three main theories have been developed by these authors:

1. the theory of compression impaction.
2. the avulsion theory.
3. the incurvation theory.

The theory of compression impaction

Dupuytren was the first one to suggest, in 1834, that the weight of the body generates a counter-shock at the surface of the impact. This force is transmitted through the carpal bones to the distal end of the radius. The fracture is most often located at the level where the cortex is thinnest.

Nelaton in 1844 and Malgaigne in 1847 adopted this theory, as did Destot and Gallois in 1986, who showed radiographically that when the wrist is in extension the carpal bones are in contact with the surface of the impact. At the same time, the radial head is in compression against the humerus. This force is then automatically transmitted to the distal end of the radius. It is at this moment that the fracture occurs.

It is therefore a mechanism of compression–impaction and crush: the wrist is an anvil on which the radius is crushed (Fig. 3.1)

This crush theory was studied experimentally by Stevens in 1920. It is based on the very important fact that all distal radial fractures are compression fractures: the fall occurs on a wrist in extension–pronation, so that the wrist as an anatomical entity is a vault looking like the arch of a Roman bridge and, according to Stevens, the lunate bears more on the posterior than anterior part of the radius (Fig. 3.2). Tensile forces act on the anterior part and compression forces on the posterior part. The posterior constraint forces are very high.

The avulsion theory

This theory was proposed by Linhart in 1852 and analysed by Lecomte in 1861. The indirect

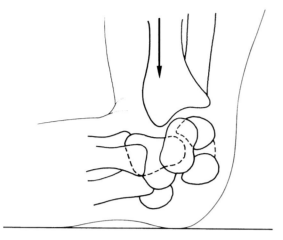

Figure 3.1

Mechanism of ulna-articular fracture according to Destot (1898). Compression and impaction.

forces presented by the body weight are transmitted through the humerus, the ulna, the interosseous membrane, the distal radius and then the volar wrist ligaments to the point of impact of the hand. The distal radial fracture is then caused by an avulsion mechanism applied by the tensile forces transmitted by the volar wrist ligaments. This theory was strongly criticized by Lobker in 1885 and Bahr in 1894. They argued that if avulsion is the principal mechanism, the fracture line should begin proximally at the palmar aspect and end distally at the dorsal aspect, which is not consistent with the facts.

To complement and adjust the two theories, Lobker came to the conclusion that the two mechanisms are associated because if the compression theory were the only explanation, more comminution of the articular surface of the radius would be seen than was actually the case.

The incurvation theory

The theory that fractures are produced by bending forces was supported by Mayer in 1940. The fracture line is affected by three factors:

1. the position of the hand;
2. the extent of the area of impact;
3. the magnitude of the applied force.

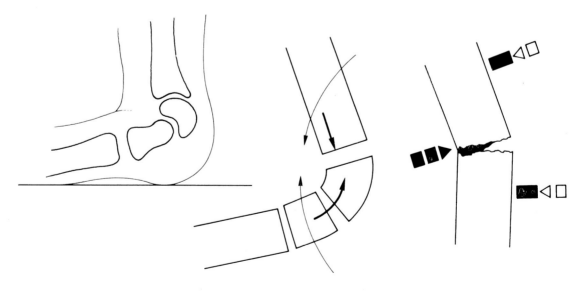

Figure 3.2

Tensile forces act on the anterior part of the radius and compression forces on the posterior part (modified from Stevens JH. In: Compression fractures at the lower end of the distal radius. 1920). For a 70 kg man falling from his height, Stevens gave the following numbers: tensile forces 900 kg/cm^2; compression forces 2000 kg/cm^2.

If tension increases at the level of the ulnar collateral ligament when the radial fracture occurs, an ulnar styloid process fracture will occur at the same time. Experimental work performed by Lewis in 1950 supported this theory and demonstrated that a fall on an open hand (with a greater area of impact than a closed hand) is sufficient to cause a distal radial fracture. The skin is usually not lacerated at the palm, implying that the hand has not slipped but was blocked on the floor. The body continues to go forward, moved by kinetic energy or inertia, and the volar wrist ligaments become tense because the wrist is placed in a hyperextended position.

If these ligaments resist, the forces are transmitted to the radiocarpal joint and the radius is in compression against the articular facets of the bones of the first carpal row. If the scaphoid and lunate are not crushed, the forces end at the level of the radius to produce a fracture at the weakest part of this bone, in the same way that a cantilever-girder breaks when charged beyond its elasticity. This explanation makes things clear for Lewis: distal radial fractures are caused by bending forces (Fig. 3.3).

Pathomechanism of anteriorly displaced fractures

These fractures are generally considered as secondary to falls on the dorsum of the hand, wrist in flexion. However, they are often the consequence of a fall on the palm of the hand, with the wrist in extension.

Two mechanisms have been proposed:

1. Axial stress on the radius with a backward fall on the palm of the hand, wrist in extension, and without displacement of the body over the hand. The radial incurved 'girder' sustains

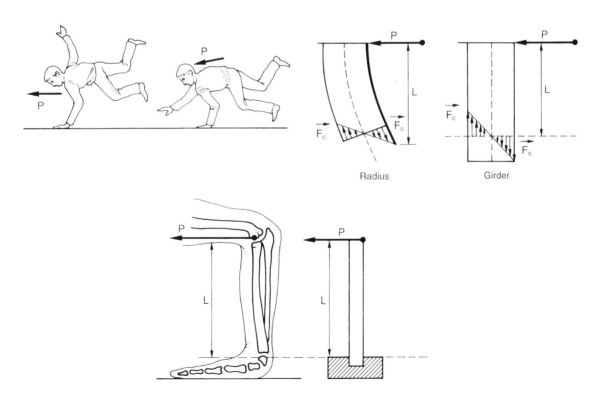

Figure 3.3

The incurvation theory. (Modified from Lewis 1950.)

compression forces on the volar cortex and tensile forces on the dorsal (Fig. 3.4a).
2. Forced flexion, where direct stress of the carpus on the volar part of the radial joint is combined with traction exerted by the dorsal ligaments. This is the reverse of the mechanism described by Lewis in the fractures with dorsal displacement, and is relatively frequent in motorbike accidents (Fig. 3.4b).

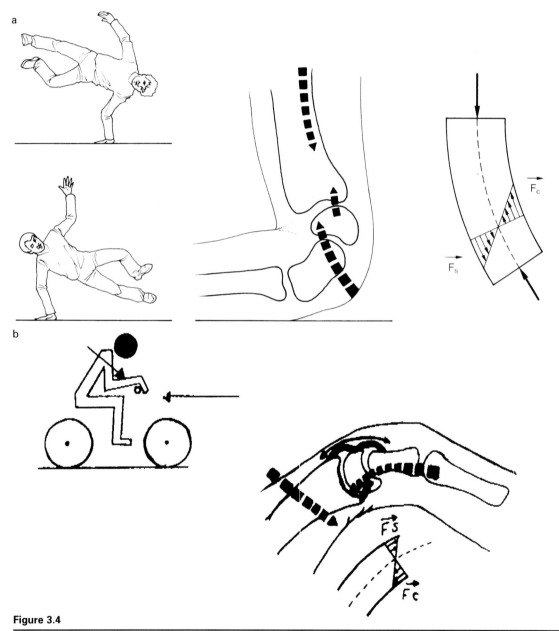

Figure 3.4
Pathomechanism of anteriorly displaced fractures. a) axial stress: compression forces act on the volar cortex and tensile forces on the dorsal cortex. b) forced flexion, with direct stress on the volar part of the radius and traction exerted by the dorsal ligaments.

Summary of the various theories

Each theory, undoubtedly, contains a part of the truth, but each is too exclusive of the others. There seem to be various pathomechanisms for distal radial fractures; that is, many factors are combined to produce each type of fracture. We will now consider each factor and its particular role in the production of each type of fracture.

Nature of the forces

Magnitude of the force

The forces resulting from a common fall from standing height are obviously different from a high-velocity impact resulting from a motorbike accident or a fall from an elevated place. In these cases the body or vehicle inertia and its different acceleration should be considered. The latter can be calculated with the following formula: the greater the force relationship to the contact area plane, the greater the decrease in compression forces. Conversely, the sheer component of the forces increase (Fig. 3.5).

Direction of the force

If a force is applied through the bone axis perpendicular to the contact area, its components are mainly compression forces. The more the force is inclined relative to the contact area plane, the greater the decrease in compression forces. Conversely, the sheer component forces increase (Fig. 3.5).

Speed of application of the force

A force applied within a period of hundredths of a second (for example in a high-velocity vehicle accident) does not allow muscle contraction to resist it; conversely, a slow and progressive injury (for example in a fall from standing height) allows muscle contraction to resist against the forces applied to the hand.

Forces relative to the situation of the impact

A force applied at the metacarpal heads has different components than one applied at the base of the palm, where the axial forces through the radius are predominant (Fig. 3.6).

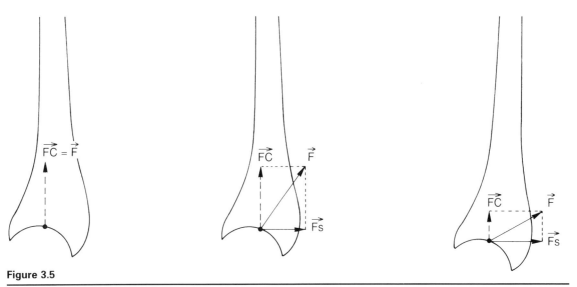

Figure 3.5

Magnitude and direction of the forces relative to the contact area.

Hand and wrist positions

Hand and wrist positions relative to the body at the time of the injury influence the pattern of the fracture lines. Wrist extension can produce posterior as well as anterior displacement, depending on the position of the body relative to the hand. For example, a fall can produce an anterior rim fracture if the wrist is in slight extension, the force axial, and the body remaining behind the hand (Fig. 3.7).

Age of the patient

The patient's age is very important and determines the bone, ligamentous and muscular structural properties: a fall from standing height often results in a comminuted fracture with bone disintegration in elderly subjects; conversely, sprains are more frequent in young people, who sustain comminuted fractures only after significant injuries.

Bone morphology

Bone morphology plays an essential role. The distal end of the radius, seen from a lateral view, is a cup with an anterior angulation of a mean of 10°, which explains why the posterior part sustains more stress than the anterior. This also explains the frequency of posteriorly displaced fractures.

From an antero-posterior view, the distal end of the radius presents a radial inclination of a mean 25°. This explains the frequency of radial displacements with a radial styloid fragment, which occasionally is present in isolation.

If the articular area is examined from the front, the medial part is seen to have a radial inclination. From a lateral view, it has a volar angulation. This area apposes the highest point of the carpal condyle of the first row formed by the lunate, which explains the frequency of the postero-medial fragment in distal radial fractures in extension.

Muscular contraction at the time of the injury

Muscle contractions change the result of the applied forces. Consider the example of a shock, with an impact on the metacarpal heads in forced extension of the wrist, without muscular contraction. This is a static state of balance which is achieved by the passive bone and ligamentous

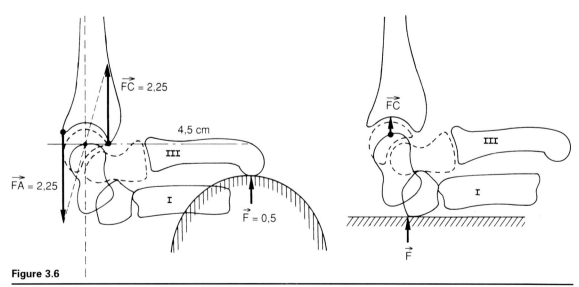

Figure 3.6

Exertion of the forces relative to the situation of the impact.

PATHOMECHANISM OF INTRA-ARTICULAR DISTAL RADIAL FRACTURES 25

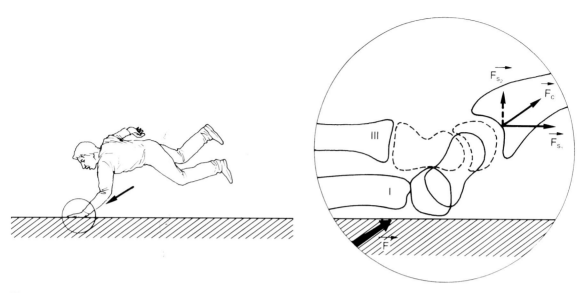

Figure 3.7

The fracture lines depend on the hand and wrist position relative to the body.

restraints. The applied force can be divided at the level of the radius into posterior compression forces and anterior tensile forces. This will result in an extra-articular posteriorly displaced force (see Fig. 3.6). If a volar muscular contraction force is added (from the flexor digitorum muscles), the wrist will be in a dynamic balance of forces. This volar force, created by the muscular contractions of the flexor muscles, will suppress the anterior tensile forces and perhaps add compression forces, which will modify the final result in an axial compression to produce an intra-articular fracture (Fig. 3.8).

Conclusion

Considering the preceding statements, it can be said that different mechanisms combining multiple factors will influence the outcome of a wrist injury. All the combinations are possible, but they can be classified by their frequency: high-velocity injuries result in intra-articular fractures because of compression forces resulting from muscular contractions and the significant impact forces. The fall of a child produces an extra-articular fracture, while the same fall, under the same conditions, will result in an intra-articular fracture in an elderly patient. Only one feature has changed, the age.

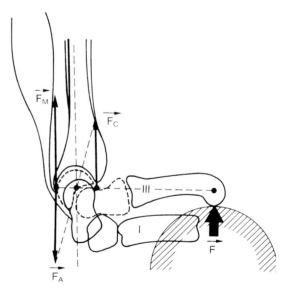

Figure 3.8

Muscle contractions modify the final result of the forces.

To conclude, several factors are involved in producing an intra-articular fracture:

- a high-velocity injury;
- predominance of compression axial forces;
- age;
- 'dynamic stabilization' by muscular contraction.

These combined factors create a significant number of mechanisms.

References

Alffram PA, Bauer GCH. Epidemiology of fractures of the forearm. A biomechanical investigation of bone strength. *J Bone Joint Surg* 1962; **44A, 1**: 105–14.

Axelrod T, Paley D, Green J, McMurtry RY. Limited open reduction of the lunate facet in comminuted intra-articular fractures of the distal radius. *J Hand Surg* 1988; **13A3**: 372–77.

Axelrod TS, McMurtry RY. Open reduction and internal fixation of comminuted, intra-articular fractures of the distal radius. *J Hand Surg* 1990; **15A**: 1–11.

Bahr F. Cited by Frykman G. Die Typische Radius Fraktur und Ihro Entstehung. *Zbl Chir* 1894; **21**: 841.

Bartosch RA, Saldana MJ. Intra-articular fractures of the distal radius: a cadaveric study to determine if ligamentotaxis restores radiopalmar tilt. *J Hand Surg* 1990; **15A**: 18–21.

Bassett RL. Displaced intra-articular fractures of the distal radius. *Clin Ortho Rel Res* 1987; **214**: 148–52.

Bradley JB, Slauterbeck J, Benjamin JB. Fracture patterns and mechanisms in pedestrian motor vehicle trauma: the ipsilateral dyad. *Orthop Trauma* 1992; **6, 3**: 279–82.

Bradway JK, Amadio PC, Cooney WP. Open reduction and internal fixation of displaced, comminuted intra-articular fractures of the distal end of the radius. *J Bone Joint Surg* 1989; **71A, 6**: 839–47.

Castaing J, le Club des Dix. Les fractures recentes de l'extrémité inférieure du radius chez l'adulte. *Rev Chir Orthop* 1964; **50**: 581–666.

Cooney WP, Linscheid RL, Dobyns JH. External pin fixation for unstable Colles' fractures. *J Bone Joint Surg* 1979; **61A, 6**: 840–5.

Cooney WP, Dobyns JH, Linscheid RL. Complications of Colles' fractures. *J Bone Joint Surg* 1980; **62, 4**: 613–19.

Cooney WP. Management of Colles' fractures (Editorial). *J Hand Surg* 1989; **14B, 2**: 137–38.

DePalma AF. Comminuted fractures of the distal end of the radius treated by ulnar pinning. *J Bone Joint Surg* 1952; **34A, 3**: 651–62.

Destot E, Gallois E. Cited by Frykman F. Recherches physiologiques et expérimentales sur les TSP fractures de l'extrémité inférieure du radius. (Radiographie). *Rev Chir* 1898; **18**: 886.

Destot E. Cited by Frykman G. *Traumatisme du poignet et rayons*. Paris: Masson, 1923: 174–8.

Dupuytren G. Cited by Castaing J. Des fractures de l'extrémité inférieure du radius simulant les luxations du poignet. *Leçons orales de clinique chirurgicale*: 1. Paris: Baillière, 1839: 323–8.

Frykman G. Fracture of the distal radius, including sequelae-shoulder-hand-finger-syndrome. Disturbance in the distal radioulnar joint and impairment of nerve function. A clinical and experimental study. *Acta Orthop Scand* 1967; **suppl 108**: 1.

Geissler WB, Fernandez DL. Percutaneous and limited open reduction of the articular surface of the distal radius. *Orthop Trauma* 1991; **5, 3**: 255–64.

Jupiter JB. Current concepts review fractures of the distal end of the radius. *J Bone Joint Surg* 1991; **73A, 3**: 461–69.

Kapandji IA. *Physiologie articulaire*, fasc I. Paris: Maloine, 1963.

Knirk JK, Jupiter JB. Intra-articular fractures of the distal end of the radius in young adults. *J Bone Joint Surg* 1986; **68A**: 647–59.

Lafontaine M, Delince Ph, Hardy D, Simons M. L'instabilité des fractures de l'extrémité inférieure du radius: à propos d'une série de 167 Cas. *Acta Orthop Belgica* 1989; **55, 2**: 203–16.

Lecomte O. Cited by Frykman G. Recherches nouvelles sur les fractures de l'extrémité inférieure du radius. *Arch Gén Méd* 1860–61; **5**: 641.

Leung KS, So WS, Chiu UDF, Leung PG. Ligamentotaxis for comminuted distal radial fractures modified by primary cancellous grafting and functional bracing: long-term results. *Orthop Trauma* 1991; **5, 3**: 265–71.

Lewis RM. Colles' fracture: causative mechanism. *Surgery* 1950; **27**: 427.

Lilienfeldt A. Cited by Frykman G. Uber den Klassischen Radius Bruch. *Arch Klin Chir* 1907; **82**: 166.

Linhart W. Cited by Frykman G. *Die Brüche der unteren Epiphyse der Radius Durch.* 2nd edition. Vienna: Gesellschaft Ärzte Wien, 1852.

Lobker K. Cited by Frykman G. Sitzung der Medicinischen Vereins zu Greifswald. *Dtsch Med Wschr* 1885; **27**: 475.

Malgaigne JF. Cited by Frykman G. *Traité des fractures et des luxations*, T1. Paris: JB Baillière, 1847: 603.

Mayer JH. Cited by Frykman G. Colles' fracture. *Br J Surg* 1940; **27**: 629.

McQueen M, Caspers J. Colles' fracture: Does the anatomical result affect the final function? *J Bone Joint Surg* 1988; **70B, 4**: 649–51.

Melone CP. Articular fractures of the distal radius. *Orthop Clin North Am* 1984; **15, 2**: 217–36.

Melone ChP. Open treatment for displaced articular fractures of the distal radius. *Clin Orthop Rel Res* 1986; **202**: 103–11.

Mortier JP, Baux S, Uhl JF, Mimoun M, Mole B. Importance du fragment postéro-interne et son brochage spécifique dans les fractures de l'extrémité inférieure du radius. *Ann Chir Main* 1983; **3**: 219–29.

Mortier JP, Kuhlmann JN, Richet C, Baux S. Brochage horizontal cubito-radial dans les fractures de l'extrémité inférieure du radius comportant un fragment postéro-interne. *R Chir Orthop* 1986; **72**: 567–71.

Nelaton A. Cited by Frykman G. *Eléments de pathologie chirurgicale*, T1. Paris: Germer Baillière, 1844: 739.

Peltier LF. Fractures of the distal end of the radius. An historical account. *Clin Orthop Rel Res* 1984; **187**: 18–22.

Pilcher LS. Cited by Frykman G. Fractures of the lower extremity or base of the radius. *Ann Surg* 1917; **65**: 1.

Scheck M. Long-term follow-up of treatment of comminuted fractures of the distal end of the radius by transfixation with Kirschner wires and cast. *J Bone Joint Surg* 1962; **44A**: 337–51.

Short WH, Palmer AK, Werner FW, Eng MG, Murphy DJ. A biomechanical study of distal radial fractures. *J Hand Surg* 1987; **12**: 529–34.

Stevens JH. Cited by Castaing J. Compression fractures of the lower end of radius. *Ann Surg* 1920; **71**: 495.

Szabo RM, Weber SC. Comminuted intra-articular fractures of the distal radius. *Clin Orthop Rel Res* 1988; **230**: 39–48.

Taleisnik J, Watson HK. Midcarpal instability caused by malunited fractures of distal radius. *J Hand Surg* 1984; **91**: 350–57.

Weber SC, Szabo RM. Severely comminuted distal radial fracture as an unsolved problem: complications associated with external fixation and pins and plaster techniques. *J Hand Surg* 1986; **11A**: 157–65.

4
Biomechanical aspects of percutaneous pinning for distal radial fractures

Thomas J Graham, Dean S Louis

Introduction

Despite the frequency of presentation of distal radial fractures, their optimal treatment continues to be debated. As the orthopaedic community recognizes the complexity of this injury and focuses attention on the anatomical restoration that is germane to optimal function, a variety of treatment options are being investigated. Regardless of patient age, vocation, or recreational interest, therapies are sought to maximize the potential for pain-free motion and acceptable cosmetic results.

Although initial reduction of the fractured distal radius is typically achieved, maintenance of anatomic alignment remains a clinical challenge (Clancy 1984, Green 1975, Rayhack et al. 1989, Stein and Katz 1975). Based on fractures treated by closed methods, Colles observed 'that the limb will again enjoy perfect freedom in all its motion, and be completely exempt from pain' (Colles 1814). However, many modern authors have described difficulties similar to those recounted by Lorenz Bohler, who wrote of the 'difficulty in maintaining the alignment of the fragments in an unpadded plaster cast' (Amadio and Botte 1987, Bacorn and Kurtze 1953, Bohler 1923, Cooney et al. 1980, Gartland and Werley 1951, Knirk and Jupiter 1986).

Closed treatment is just one of many options available to the practitioner, and is by no means alone in causing complications and contributing to suboptimal results (Bacorn and Kurtz 1953, Chapman et al. 1982, Gartland and Werley 1951, Knirk and Jupiter 1986, Weber and Szabo 1986). A variety of treatments including casting, bracing, external and internal fixation have been advocated for distal radial fractures (Axelrod and McMurtry 1990, Bennett et al. 1989, Chapman et al. 1982, Clancy 1984, Clyburn 1987, Cooney 1983, DePalma 1952, Dowling and Sawyer 1961, Green 1975, Kapandji 1982, Lortat-Jacob et al. 1982, Mortier et al 1987, Nonnenmacher and Kempf 1988, Nakata et al. 1985, Rayhack et al. 1989, Sarmiento et al. 1975, Scheck 1962, Seitz et al. 1990, Stein and Katz 1975, Willeneger and Guggenbuhl 1959), but no single technique has proved to be universally applicable or successful.

Percutaneous pinning is one therapeutic alternative that offers the advantages of safety, economy and maintenance of reduction, without the need for more invasive procedures. The evolution and biomechanical aspects of this technique will be detailed in the following sections.

Evolution of percutaneous pinning

Fracture treatment with percutaneously introduced wires had its origins at the turn of the twentieth century. Although some of the details have been obscured by history and are cloaked in controversy, the contributions of these early practitioners remain significant.

In 1903 and 1904, Alessandro Codivilla, an Italian orthopaedist, reported his method of piercing a bone with a wire and applying skeletal traction for correction of congenital deformities and fractures. These contributions are perhaps less well recognized than those of Fritz Steinman of Switzerland. In 1908, he described using a 3–5 mm pointed four-sided pin, driven percutaneously into the distal fragment of femur fractures, to apply traction.

Steinman's concept of 'nagelextension' (nail extension) was similar to that of Codivilla, with the exception that Steinman's pins did not completely traverse the distal fragment. In 1910, Codivilla set forth to clarify the issue of the origin of nagelextension and to correct the medical community, which had embraced Steinman as the originator of this concept. Their debate, 'written in language more suitable for a gossip tabloid rather than a scientific publication' is historical (Romm 1984).

Concurrently, Albin Lambotte of Belgium was performing fracture surgery in a manner that would cause him to be regarded as the 'father of modern osteosynthesis'. In 1908, Lambotte pinned a fractured clavicle with a thin, metal device and developed 'intramedullary tacks' for fracture stabilization (Brueckman 1990).

Another famous master surgeon, Berlin's Martin Kirschner, felt that Steinman's thick pin was difficult to insert, unduly traumatized local tissues, and increased the chances of infection. Thus, in 1927, Kirschner developed a 0.7 mm-thick chromium-plated steel piano wire with driving aids that permitted easier insertion. This device, used for 'drahextension' (wire extension), resembles the device that bears his name today.

In 1937, LV Rush and HC Rush reported on the use of percutaneous intramedullary fixation of the ulna and additinal cerclage wires in a Monteggia lesion. This appears to be the first report of attempted stabilization of fracture fragments by means of percutaneous fixation in the upper extremity, excluding the clavicle.

Finally, in 1952, DePalma described the technique of percutaneous pinning of distal radial fractures. His approach consisted of positioning the patient's hand in the Weinberger finger traction apparatus, reducing the fracture, and then introducing 'a threaded wire measuring three thirty-seconds of an inch ... through the ulna and radius, entering the ulna at a point one and one-half by one and three-quarter inches from the tip of the ulnar styloid process and directed obliquely upwards and outwards so it engages the radial-styloid fragment'.

The era of application of percutaneous transfixion with wires was thus begun. Some surgeons preferred this approach to stabilization of the radial fracture by first engaging the distal ulna. Authors like Dowling and Sawyer (1961), Lortat-Jacob et al. (1982), and Rayhack et al. (1989) have expanded on DePalma's original approach and reported on their experience. Trans-ulnar pinning has been reported to reduce the incidence of complications, including radial nerve injury (Castaing 1964, Docquier et al. 1982, Lortat-Jacob et al. 1982), tendon adhesion (Clancy 1984, Kerboul et al. 1986) and pin tract infection (Castaing 1964, Docquier et al. 1982, Kerboul et al. 1986, Stein and Katz 1975) it has had its share of complications too, among them loss of reduction, and pin breakage and migration (DePalma 1952, Dawling and Sawyer 1961, Ford and Key 1955).

Seven years after DePalma's description of trans-ulnar pinning, Willeneger and Guggenbuhl (1959) reported on a method of approaching the distal radial fracture by simply introducing pins obliquely into the radial styloid. Other proponents of radial pinning include Clancy (1984), and Stein and Katz (1975), who have modified Willeneger and Guggenbuhl's method by adding a pin from the ulnar side of the radius, specifically to address the frequently encountered 'die-punch' fragment.

Other important variations of trans-ulnar radial or simple radial pinning include intrafocal (transfracture) pinning, as originally described by Kapandji (1982) and later detailed by Nonnenmacher and Kempf (1988), and double elastic spring-pinning, as described by Desmanet (1989). These techniques are fully described in other chapters by their originators.

Despite the longevity and popularity of percutaneous pinning for fractures of the distal radius, there has been no systematic study of pinning methods to determine which configurations offer the most stability. The following section details the development of a biomechanical model to test the ability of various pinning configurations to stabilize a distal radial fracture, and the results of tests using this model.

Biomechanical study of percutaneous pinning for distal radial fractures

The orthopaedic community relies on biomechanical data to supplement clinical experience in its approach to fracture fixation. Knowledge of the relative abilities of various fixation methods to control fracture displacement, or the ability to identify the most biomechanically advantageous means of applying a particular method, can maximize clinical results.

In upper extremity surgery, this is especially true with respect to fractures of the small bones of the hand. The literature is replete with biomechanical studies analysing the relative merits of rigid internal fixation and percutaneous pin fixation for metacarpal and phalangeal fractures (Black et al. 1985 and 1986, Fyfe and Mason 1979, Jones 1987, Mann et al. 1985, Rayhack et al. 1984, Vanik et al. 1984). Furthermore, comparisons of particular methods of applying percutaneous pinning have appeared (Massengill et al. 1979, Viegas et al. 1988).

Fewer studies have concentrated on the biomechanics of the distal radius in normal or pathologic states. This paucity of literature probably relates to the difficulty in modeling conditions in this complex area, and the obstacles encountered in measuring change in relative fragment position. Despite these difficulties, effective biomechanical studies of external fixation methods for distal radial fractures have been conducted by some authors (Nakata et al. 1984, Short et al. 1987, Seitz et al. 1990). However, most of the information obtained from these studies has been on frame construction, pin size and position, or resultant force change at the radiocarpal joint.

Dorsal angulation, loss of radial tilt and radial shortening are well-recognized osseous sequellae to distal radial fractures (Bennett et al. 1989, Cooney et al. 1979, Friberg and Lindstrom 1976, Kapandji 1982, Sarmiento et al. 1975, Weber and Szabo 1986). These parameters have been the foundation for radiographic assessment after this injury. Yet, to date, there has been no direct assessment of the motion of the fracture fragments under the influence of stabilizing factors, nor has a biomechanical analysis identifying optimum pinning constructs been conducted.

In order to define the optimum constructs, a biomechanical study was undertaken at the Orthopaedic Research Laboratory of the University of Michigan (Graham et al. in press), investigating the relative ability of various percutaneous pinning configurations to limit dorsal displacement of an extra-articular distal radius fracture in a cadaver model.

Fresh-frozen cadaver upper extremities were denuded proximal to the wrist and a transverse extra-articular osteotomy was made in the distal radius. The distal fragment was instrumented with an eye bolt, through which a moment causing dorsal displacement could be applied by cable attachment to an Instron Machine Testing System. A clip gauge spanning the osteotomy measured the displacement of the distal fragment (Fig. 4.1).

The fractures were pinned utilizing four or fewer 1.1 mm (0.045 in.) smooth wires in a variety of constructs. The pins were introduced from one of four pin positions (Fig. 4.2):

1. **dorsal radial** — oblique pin into the radial styloid dorsal to the first extensor compartment.
2. **volar radial** — similar to 1, but with a starting point volar to the first extensor compartment;
3. **proximal trans-ulnar** — an oblique pin, engaging both the radius and ulna which crosses the osteotomy site;
4. **distal trans-ulnar** — a horizontal pin that engages both bones distal to the osteotomy.

For the constructs in which the ulna was engaged, the pins were driven from the ulnar side in the manner described by DePalma (1952), Rayhack (1989), Desmanet (1989), and others. This was found to be the easiest and most reproducible method.

A total of 28 configurations were created by combining different numbers of pins from various positions. In some, both the radius and ulna (Docquier et al. 1982) were engaged and in others, just the radius was engaged (Bohler 1923). Constructs of one, two, three, or four pins were tested repeatedly in a manner in which damage to the pinned specimen and experimental bias were minimized, while reliability of the data was maximized. Conduct of the trials on the pinned specimens consisted of controlled distraction at a constant rate (50 mm/min), which

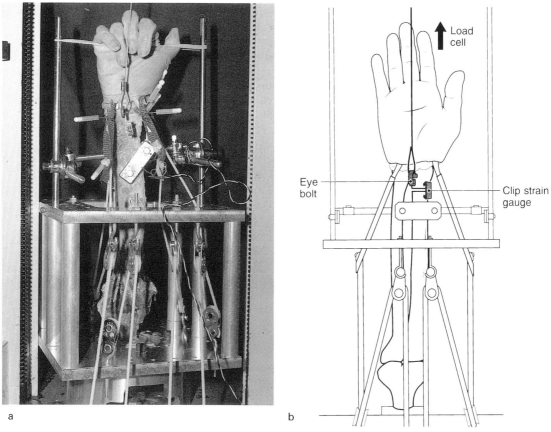

Figure 4.1

a) Photograph of prepared specimen mounted in testing apparatus. b) Schematic of experiment, showing the pull of the load cell and weights, the eye bolt, and the clip gauge.

corresponded to application of an increasing moment to the osteotomy site, causing dorsal displacement of the distal fragment. The wrist flexors and extensors were weighted with 2.27 kg (5 lbs) to simulate physiologic loads (Short et al. 1987). This testing permitted simultaneous data collection from the load cell and clip gauge (Fig. 4.3).

This experimental design and apparatus was particularly well suited for comparison of the stability imparted by each pin, and different combinations of pins. The fracture pattern was chosen both for its historical and clinical significance, as well as its reproducibility in the laboratory. The model was designed to recreate the clinical mode of failure by causing dorsal displacement. Loss of reduction due to radial shortening and rotational displacement were difficult to model, and since these modes of failure occur secondary to dorsal displacement, attempts at separate study of these parameters were abandoned.

The results indicated that when three or four pins were utilized, the moment necessary to cause a specific amount (1 mm) of displacement was significantly higher than when single or double pinning was used. The average moment needed to bring about 1 mm of displacement in the two-pin group was 22% greater than that for the single-pin group. The 'stability' of three-pin configurations exceeded that of two-pin constructs by 25% and of one-pin constructs by 53%. Four-pin patterns imparted 10% more resistance to displacement than three pins, 37% more than two, and 68% more than single-pin constructs. The difference between the stability

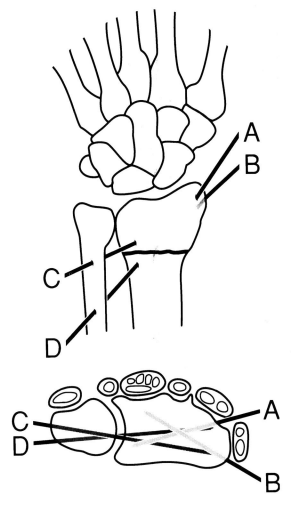

Figure 4.2

The four basic pin positions from which the 28 configurations were created. Pin A, dorsal radial; pin B, volar radial; pin C, distal trans-ulnar; pin D, proximal trans-ulnar.

imparted by four and three pins versus double and single pinning was found to be statistically significant (P < 0.001).

Constructs in which the ulna was engaged tended to limit dorsal displacement more than those with no trans-ulnar pins. In the two configurations in which the ulna was engaged, the mean moment necessary to displace the distal fragment 1 mm was 16% greater than in the seven constructs in which only the radius was pinned. A trans-ulnar pin which crossed the osteotomy (proximal trans-ulnar) appeared to lend greater stability than one driven transversely and distal to the osteotomy (distal trans-ulnar). The mean moment necessary to produce 1 mm displacement of the distal fragment in configurations with a single proximal trans-ulnar pin was 15% greater than that needed for constructs with a single distal trans-ulnar pin. No significant differences in stability were seen when comparing dorsal and volar radial pinning.

The greatest resistance to dorsal displacement was seen in configurations in which a total of four pins were entered; at least three pins crossed the radial osteotomy, and at least two trans-ulnar pins were used. Examples of pinning configurations which were shown to be among the most stable are shown in Fig. 4.4.

Conclusions

Based on the results of this study, a minimum of three pins is advocated for treatment of extra-articular distal radius fragments. Four pins provided more stability than three, but subjecting the patient to the additional risk posed by placement of the fourth pin may be unnecessary, for example in cases where the surgeon is confident with three-pin fixation and the additional security provided by the accompanying cast.

Engaging the ulna appears to provide both a biomechanical and clinical advantage. Avoidance of radial-sided structures by utilizing the trans-ulnar approach is justified by the results of this study. Engaging the ulna improved stability and, in our experience, ulnar to radial pinning is easier than the converse. The proximal trans-ulnar pin, although slightly more difficult to insert, offers some stability and avoidance of the distal radio-ulnar joint.

If stability of the fracture is gained by simply pinning the radius, using any of the described patterns, the surgeon may elect not to perform trans-ulnar pinning. This would eliminate the risks of trans-ulnar pin insertion, damage to the distal radio-ulnar joint by aberrant pin position, and possible pin breakage in the interosseous space. Clinically, we have not experienced distal radio-ulnar joint problems after trans-ulnar pinning, nor have any trans-ulnar pins broken.

At our institution, percutaneous pinning is becoming a popular treatment for displaced

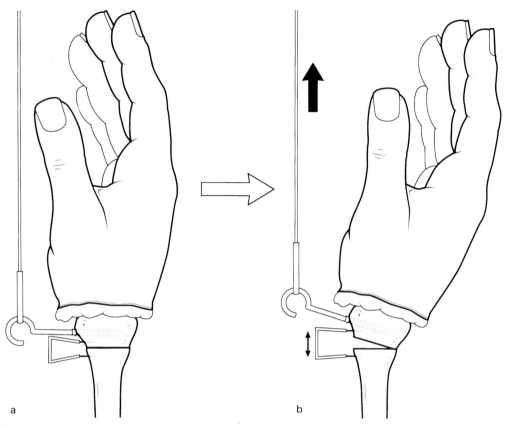

Figure 4.3

a) Lateral view of static specimen near osteotomy site prior to application of moment. b) Typical displacement created by application of moment. There is dorsal tilting and loss of congruity of the dorsal cortices, leading to shortening. (Note: for clarity, pins have been omitted from this figure.)

extra-articular distal radial fractures. In addition, 'augmented' external fixation, in which an external fixator is supplemented with percutaneous pinning, is emerging as a useful technique (Seitz et al. 1990). Thus, as the indications for percutaneous pinning expand, the need for established recommendations concerning pinning configurations are needed. Although the fracture pattern used in this study can frequently be treated by closed methods alone, it provided reliable and reproducible data concerning the ability of the various pinning constructs to resist dorsal displacement. This information can then be extrapolated when the surgeon is selecting a pinning configuration for different fracture patterns.

The results of this study permit the following recommendations to be made:

1. three- and four-pin configurations provide the greatest stability, and should be utilized;
2. constructs in which the ulna is engaged provide superior resistance to fracture displacement;
3. trans-ulnar radial pins that cross the radial fracture impart greater stability than those that do not.

Although this study does provide biomechanical evidence for the ability of percutaneous pinning to stabilize distal radial fractures and defines optimum constructs, the radiographic and clinical data presented to the surgeon, complemented by an extensive knowledge of local anatomy, should ultimately dictate the choice of pinning pattern.

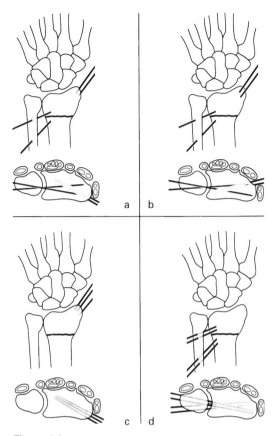

Figure 4.4

Pinning configurations which provided stability. a) Two volar radial pins with one proximal and one distal trans-ulnar pin. b) Two dorsal radial pins with one proximal and one distal trans-ulnar pin. c) Three volar radial pins, no trans-ulnar pins. d) Two proximal and two distal trans-ulnar pins.

References

Amadio P, Botte M. Treatment of malunions of the distal radius. *Hand Clin* 1987; **3**: 541–59.

Axelrod T, McMurtry R. Open reduction and internal fixation of comminuted intra-articular fractures of the distal radius. *J Hand Surg* 1990; **15A**: 1–11.

Bacorn R, Kurtze J. Colles' fracture: a study of two thousand cases from the New York State Workmen's Compensation Board. *J Bone Joint Surg* 1953; **35A**: 643–58.

Bennett G, Leeson M, Smith B. Intramedullary fixation of unstable distal radius fractures: a method of fixation allowing early motion. *Ortho Rev* 1989; **18(2)**: 210–16.

Black DM, Mann RJ, Constine RM, Daniels AU. Comparison of internal fixation technique in metacarpal fractures. *J Hand Surg* 1985; **10A**: 466–72.

Black DB, Mann RJ, Constine RM, Daniels AU. The stability of internal fixation in the proximal phalanx. *J Hand Surg* 1986; **11A**: 672–77.

Bohler LB. Die functionelle bewegungbehandlung der 'typischen radiusbrüche'. *Münch Medi Wochenschr* 1923; **20**: 387–91.

Brueckman FR. *The Art of Effective Fracture Fixation with Rush Pins*. New York: Thieme, 1990: 1.

Castaing J, le Club des Dix. Les fractures recentes de l'extrémité inférieure du radius chez l'adulte. *Rev Chir Orthop* 1964; **50**: 581–666.

Chapman D, Bennett M, Bryan W, Tullos H. Complications of distal radial fractures: pins and plaster treatment. *J Hand Surg* 1982; **7A**: 509–12.

Clancy G. Percutaneous Kirschner wire fixation of Colles' fracture. *J Bone Joint Surg* 1984; **66A**: 1008–14.

Clyburn T. Dynamic external fixation for comminuted intra-articular fractures of the distal end of the radius. *J Bone Joint Surg* 1987; **69A**: 248–54.

Colles A. On the fracture of the carpal extremity of the radius. *Edinb Med Surg J* 1814; **10**: 182–86.

Codivilla A. Sulla correzione delle deformata de fratura del femore. *Bull Sci Med Bologna* 1903; **3**: 83–87.

Codivilla A. Zur behandlung der coxa vara. *Orthop Chir* 1904; **12**: 91–95.

Cooney W. External fixation of distal radial fractures. *Clin Orthop* 1983; **180**: 44–49.

Cooney W, Dobyns J, Linscheid R. Complications of Colles' fractures. *J Bone Joint Surg* 1980; **62A**: 613–19.

Cooney W, Linscheid R, Dobyns J. External pin fixation for unstable Colles' fractures. *J Bone Joint Surg* 1979; **61A**: 840–45.

DePalma A. Comminuted fractures of the distal radius treated by ulnar pinning. *J Bone Joint Surg* 1952; **34A**: 651–62.

Desmanet E. Osteosynthesis of the radius by double elastic spring-pinning. Functional treatment of the distal end of the radius. A study of 130 cases. *Ann Chir Main* 1989; **8**: 193–206.

Docquier J, Soete P, Twahirwa J, Flament A. Kapandji's method of intrafocal pinning in Pouteau Colles' fracture (French). *J Acta Orthop Belg* 1982; **48**: 794–810.

Dowling J, Sawyer B. Comminuted Colles' fractures: evaluation of a method of treatment. *J Bone Joint Surg* 1961; **43A**: 657–68.

Ford L, Key J. Present day management of Colles' fracture. *J Iowa Med Soc* 1955; **45**: 324–27.

Friberg S, Lindstrom B. Radiographic measurements of the radiocarpal joint in normal adults. *Acta Radiol* (Stockholm) 1976; **17**: 249–53.

Fyfe IS, Mason S. The mechanical stability of internal fixation of fractured phalanges. *Hand* 1979; **11**: 50–54.

Gartland J, Werley C. Evaluation of healed Colles' fractures. *J Bone Joint Surg* 1951; **33A**: 895–907.

Graham TJ, Martins HM, Louis DS, Goldstein SA. Biomechanical evaluation of percutaneous pinning for extra-articular distal radius fractures. Paper presented at the Eighth Annual Residents' and Fellows' Conference of the American Society for Surgery of the Hand, Toronto, Canada, 1990, and *J Bone Joint Surg* (in press).

Green D. Pins and plaster treatment of comminuted fractures of the distal end of the radius. *J Bone Joint Surgery* 1975; **57A**: 304–10.

Green J, Gay F. Colles' fracture – residual disability. *Am J Surg* 1956; **91**: 636–41.

Jones WW. Biomechanics of small bone fixation. *Clin Orthop* 1987; **214**: 11–18.

Kapandji A. L'osteosynthese par double embrochage intra-focal. *Ann Chir* 1982; **11–12**: 903–8.

Kaukonen JP, Porras M, Karaharji E. Anatomical results after distal forearm fractures. *Annales Chir et Gynaecol* 1988; **77**: 21–26.

Kerboul B, LeSaout, J LeFevre C et al. Comparative study of three therapeutic methods for Pouteau Colles' fracture (French). *J Chir* 1986; **123**: 428–34.

Kirschner M. Verbesserungen der drahtextension. *Arch Klin Chir* 1927; **148**: 651–58.

Knirk J, Jupiter J. Intra-articular fractures of the distal end of the radius in young adults. *J Bone Joint Surg* 1986; **68A**: 647–59.

Lortat-Jacob A, Frank A, DeBonduwe A, Beaufils P. Pinning in Y in the treatment of fractures with posterior displacement of the inferior extremity of the radius. *Acta Orthop Belg* 1982; **48**: 936–46.

Mann RJ, Black D, Constine R, Daniels AU. A quantitative comparison of metacarpal fracture stability with five different methods of internal fixation. *J Hand Surg* 1985; **10A**: 1024–28.

Massengill JB, Alexander H, Parsons JP, Schecter MJ. Mechanical analysis of Kirschner wire fixation in a phalangeal model. *J Hand Surg* 1979; **4A**: 351–56.

Mortier J, Kuhlmann J, Richet C, Baux S. Horizontal ulnar-radial pinning in fractures of the distal radius with a postero-internal fragment. *Rev Chir Orthop* 1987; **72**: 567–71.

Nonnenmacher J, Kempf I. Place du brochage intrafocal dans la traitment des fractures du pognet. *International Orthop* 1988; **12**: 155–62.

Nakata R, Chand Y, Mitako J, Frykman G, Wood V. External fixators for wrist fractures: a biomechanical and clinical study. *J Hand Surg* 1985; **10A**: 845–51.

Rayhack JM, Belsole RJ, Skeleton WH. A strain recording model: Analysis of transverse osteotomy fixation in small bones. *J Hand Surg* 1984; **9A**: 383–87.

Rayhack J, Langworthy J, Belsole R. Transulnar percutaneous pinning of displaced distal radial fractures: a preliminary report. *J Ortho Trauma* 1989; **3**: 107–14.

Romm S. Fritz Steinman and the pin that bears his name. *Plast Reconstr Surg* 1984; **74**: 306–10.

Rush LV, Rush HC. A reconstruction operation for a comminuted fracture of the upper third of the ulna. *Am J Surg* 1937; **38**: 332–33.

Sarmiento A, Pratt G, Berry N, Sinclair W. Colles' fracture: functional bracing in supination. *J Bone Joint Surg* 1975; **57A**: 311–17.

Scheck M. Long-term follow-up of treatment of comminuted fractures of the distal end of the radius by transfixion with Kirschner wires and cast. *J Bone Joint Surg* 1962; **44A**: 337–51.

Short W, Palmer A, Werner F, Murphy D. A biomechanical study of distal radial fractures. *J Hand Surg* 1987; **12A**: 529–34.

Seitz W, Froimson A, Shapiro J. 'Augmented external fixation of unstable distal radius fractures'. Read at the annual meeting of the American Academy of Orthopaedic Surgeons, New Orleans, Louisiana. 1990.

Seitz W, Froimson A, Brooks D, Postak P, Parker R, LaPorte J, Greenwald A. Biomechanical analysis of pin placement and pin size for external fixation of distal radius fractures. *Clin Orthop* 1990; **251**: 207–12.

Stein A, Katz S. Stabilization of comminuted fractures of the distal inch of the radius: percutaneous pinning. *Clin Orthop* 1975; **108**: 174–81.

Steinman F. Eine neue Extensionsmethode in der Fracturbehandlung. *Cor-B1f schweiz Aerzte* 1908; **38**: 3–7.

Vanik RK, Weber RC, Matloub HS, Sander JR, Gingrass RP. The comparative strengths of internal fixation techniques. *J Hand Surg* 1984; **9A**: 216–21.

Viegas SF, Ferren EL, Self J, Tencer AF. Comparative mechanical properties of various Kirschner wire configurations in transverse and oblique phalangeal fractures. *J Hand Surg* 1988; **13A**: 246–53.

Weber S, Szabo R. Severely comminuted distal radial fracture as an unsolved problem: complications associated with external fixation and pins and plaster techniques. *J Hand Surg* 1986; **11A**: 157–65.

Willeneger H, Guggenbuhl A. Zur operativen Behandling bestimmer Falle von Distalen Radius Frakturen. *Helv Chir Acta* 1959; **26**: 81.

5
A cadaveric study to determine whether ligamentotaxis restores radiopalmar tilt in intra-articular fractures of the distal radius

RA Bartosh, MJ Saldana

Introduction

Intra-articular fractures of the distal radius are frequently encountered in orthopaedic practice. The classic method of treatment is closed reduction and cast support (Dobyns and Linscheid 1984). External fixation or open reduction and internal fixation techniques are recommended for comminuted or unstable distal radial fractures that fail closed reduction or have intra-articular incongruity (Cole and Obletz 1966, Cooney et al. 1979 and 1980). The preferred method of reduction is traction followed by variable amounts of palmar flexion of the wrist. This technique relies on ligamentotaxis on the fracture fragment to maintain reduction (Vidal et al. 1983).

Radial length and radio-ulnar tilt are usually easily re-established in intra-articular distal radial fractures because of the radiopalmar ligamentous attachments to the radial styloid (Gartland and Werley 1951, Melone 1984, Thomas 1957). The normal radiopalmar tilt of the distal radius is frequently lost in these fractures, and seldom restored after reduction.

The anatomic study described in this chapter was performed to determine whether the radiopalmar tilt of the distal radius following an intra-articular fracture could be returned to normal by employing ligamentotaxis.

Materials and method

Twenty wrists in ten fresh cadavers were prepared for study by sharply dissecting the skin and all soft tissues to the level of the dorsal and palmar wrist ligaments. An external fixation device was applied using two 3 mm pins in the second metacarpal and two 4 mm pins in the radius. For ease of radiographic evaluation, the external fixation device was used to lock the wrist into position after each reduction maneuver. A large threaded Steiman pin was placed through the proximal ulna and used to stabilize the forearm to a large wooden frame. Traction was achieved by pulling on a smooth 2.0 mm K-wire, placed through the base of the third metacarpal and attached to a Kirschner bow (Fig. 5.1).

Initial lateral and antero-posterior radiographs of the wrist were taken of each forearm to define the configuration of the articular surface of the distal radius.

A Frykman type VII fracture (Frykman 1967) was established, with a one-inch straight osteotome placed on the radial styloid and driven across the distal radius through the radiocarpal and radio-ulnar joints. This fracture, impacted by pushing the hand into the radius, established a dorsal intra-articular bony fragment with intact dorsal wrist ligaments.

Three positions (neutral flexion, 15° flexion, and 30° flexion), with two separate amounts of distraction (10 lb and 20 lb) were used in an attempt to reduce the fracture. A lateral radiograph was taken to determine if the radiopalmar tilt had been re-established for each position of flexion and distraction (Fig. 5.2). The entire palmar ligamentous complex was then transected at the radius and further evaluation was made in the neutral flexion position with ten pounds of distraction (Fig. 5.3).

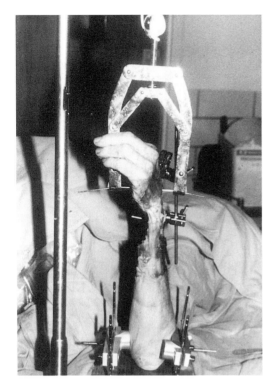

Figure 5.1

Arm secured to a board using an olecranon pin. Traction was applied on the pin inserted through the third metacarpal base.

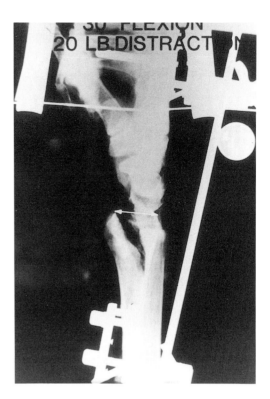

Figure 5.2

30° flexion plus 20 lb of traction failed to re-establish the radiopalmar tilt.

The length between the distal radius and the base of the third metacarpal was measured in millimetres on the antero-posterior radiograph. The increase of this length in each position measured was noted as carpal distraction.

The dorsal wrist ligaments were outlined on the radiographs by drawing three lines: one on the radio-luno-triquetral extrinsic ligament, one on the dorsal intercarpal ligament from the scaphoid, and one an interconnecting line between the first two lines. These three lines formed a 'Z' on the dorsum of the wrist (Fig. 5.4). The two acute angles formed by the 'Z' were measured in each of the positions of flexion and distraction.

Results

The appropriate fracture pattern was established in 19 out of the 20 wrists prepared. The average carpal distraction measured 3 mm on radiographs taken before the palmar wrist ligaments were cut. Normal radiopalmar tilt was re-established in neutral flexion with ten pounds of traction, only when all of the palmar wrist ligaments were transected. Flexion and distraction alone failed to re-establish radiopalmar tilt (see Fig. 5.3).

Using chi square analysis, the above findings were highly significant (chi square equalled 34.1). Allowing one degree of freedom, this was significant at the 0.001 level.

The angles created by the lines drawn on the dorsal wrist ligaments increased in size through each of the positions of flexion and distraction (Tables 5.1 and 5.2).

Discussion

Fracture fragment reduction is dependent on ligamentotaxis when external fixation or pin and

INTRA-ARTICULAR FRACTURES OF THE DISTAL RADIUS 39

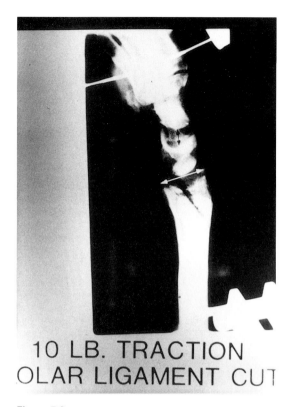

Figure 5.3
Normal radiopalmar tilt: note the increased gap between the capitate and lunate (dark arrow) and between the lunate and radius (white arrow) without the restraint of the palmar ligaments.

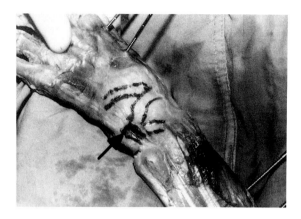

Figure 5.4
Angles drawn on the dorsum of wrist, with the arrow pointing to the triquetrum.

plaster techniques are used to reduce and maintain an intra-articular distal radial fracture (Vidal et al. 1983). The fracture produced in the experiment falls into a Frykman type VII (Frykman 1967) in that it involves the radiocarpal and radio-ulnar joints. This particular fracture pattern was chosen because it was easily reproduced and because it left the dorsal wrist ligaments intact.

The dorsal and palmar ligaments of the wrist have been fully described elsewhere (Taleisnik 1976, Mayfield 1988, Mayfield et al. 1976). The palmar wrist ligaments are arranged in two

Table 5.1 Proximal dorsal ligamentous angles between radio-luno-triquetral and dorsal intercarpal ligament

Position	10 lb	20 lb
Neutral	31–39° (31)	40–45° (41)
15° flexion	38–43° (40)	39–45° (42)
30° flexion	38–41° (40)	40–47° (43)

Table 5.2 Distal dorsal ligamentous angles between dorsal intercarpal ligament and line drawn on intrinsic distal row ligaments

Position	10 lb	20 lb
Neutral	25–39° (34)	35–37° (36)
15° flexion	38–40° (39)	39–44° (41)
30° flexion	39–42° (41)	40–48° (43)

Figures given in parentheses are averages.

'V'-shaped configurations. The apex of the 'V' formed by the radiolunate ligament and the ulnolunate ligament is located at the lunate. The apex of the radioscaphocapitate ligament and the arcuate ligament is located at the capitate. These ligaments are stout, strong and short (Mayfield et al. 1976). The average carpal distraction of 3 mm seen in 19 wrists was directly related to these short palmar ligaments coming to full stretch and arresting any further distraction.

On the other hand, the 'Z' shape configuration describes the location of the dorsal wrist ligaments, which are thinner and fewer in number than the palmar wrists ligaments (Mayfield 1988, Mayfield et al. 1976). When traction on the hand was applied through the K-wire and pulled on the dorsal wrist ligaments, the limbs of the 'Z' opened only to the length permitted by the arresting short palmar wrist ligaments. When transection of the palmar wrist ligaments eliminated their arresting effect, ligamentotaxis effectively pulled the dorsal bony fragment to the appropriate radiopalmar tilt (see Fig. 5.3).

The ligaments of the wrists, like other ligaments, are static structures. When pulled out to length they can limit the motion of the joint that they bridge. During ligamentotaxis for distal radial fractures, the palmar wrist ligaments are pulled out to length and pull on the distal radial fragment before the dorsal wrist ligaments have any traction effect on the dorsal distal radial fragment. Flexion of the wrist, while applying traction, only increases the accordion-like action of the dorsal wrist ligaments, and prevents effective ligamentotasis dorsally.

Regardless of the amount of traction or flexion, the average distraction of the 19 wrists studied was 3 mm. The palmar ligaments of these wrists were not involved in the fracture pattern and, when pulled to maximum length, arrested any further distraction. Only when the arresting effect of the palmar wrist ligaments was eliminated by transection of these ligaments, and then traction was applied to the dorsal wrist ligaments alone, was radiopalmar tilt resolved.

Conclusion

The short, stout nature of the palmar wrist ligaments and the tendency of the dorsal ligaments to stretch during traction with flexion of the wrist, limits ligamentotaxis as the sole method for re-establishing radiopalmar tilt of the distal radius, and suggests that other methods of closed or open reduction are required in the treatment of intra-articular fractures of the distal radius.

References

Cole JM, Obletz BE. Comminuted fractures of the distal end of the radius treated by skeletal transfixion in plaster cast: an end result study of thirty-three cases. *J Bone Joint Surg* 1966; **48A**: 931.

Cooney WP III, Dobyns JH, Linscheid RL. External pin fixation for unstable Colles' fractures. *J Bone Joint Surg* 1980; **62A**: 613.

Cooney WP III, Dobyns JH, Linscheid RL. External pin fixation for unstable Colles' fracture. *J Bone Joint Surg* 1979; **61A**: 840–45.

Dobyns JH, Linscheid RL. Fractures and dislocations of the carpus. In: Rockwood CA, Green DP. *Fractures in adults*. Philadelphia: Lippincott, 1984: 423–50.

Frykman G. Fracture of the distal radius including sequelae — shoulder-hand-finger syndrome, disturbance of the distal radioulnar joint and impairment of nerve function: a clinical and experimental study. *Act Ortho Scand* 1967; **108 (Suppl)**: 1–153.

Gartland JJ Jr, Werley CW. Evaluation of healed Colles' fracture. *J Bone Joint Surg* 1951; **33A**: 895.

Mayfield JK. *The wrist and its disorders*. Philadelphia: WB Saunders, 1988: Chapter 5.

Mayfield JK, Johnson RP, Kilcoyne RF. The ligaments of the wrist and their functional significance. *Anat Rec* 1976; **186**: 417.

Melone CP Jr. Articular fractures of the distal radius. *Orthop Clin N Am* 1984; **15**: 217.

Taleisnik J. The ligaments of the wrist. *J Hand Surg* 1976; **1**: 110.

Thomas FB. Reduction of Smith's fracture. *J Bone Joint Surg* 1957; **39B**: 463.

Vidal J, Buscayret C, Paran M et al. Ligamentotaxis. In Mears DC, ed. *External skeletal fixation*. Baltimore, London: Williams & Wilkins, 1983.

6
Classification of distal radial fractures by mechanism of injury
Ronald L Linscheid

Introduction

Fractures of the distal radius were seldom recognized as distinct from dislocations until the descriptions of Pouteau (1783) and later Colles (1814, Desault 1805, Malgaigne 1859). The latter suggested that little disability was to be anticipated after the fracture had healed, but we now recognize that these fractures often result in a number of complications, even when recognized early and treated appropriately by modern standards. Indeed, the treatment for this fracture, once relegated to a low priority and often consigned to a junior trauma officer, is increasingly seen as a challenge even to the experienced surgeon. Part of the problem is the use of eponymic descriptions rather than a precise detailing of the severity of fracture, the degree of displacement, the amount of comminution, the status of the adjacent carpals and associated injuries (Anderson and O'Neill 1944, Bacorn and Kurtzke 1953, Calert and Issacson 1978, Cooney et al. 1980, Dawling and Sawyer 1961, Green 1975, Idler and Lourie 1991, McQueen and Caspers 1988). The purpose of this chapter is to emphasize these aspects of distal radial fractures to aid a rational approach to treatment, based on the mechanism of injury.

Anatomy

The distal radius is expanded at its distal end to provide adjacent shallow concavoconcave articular facets for the scaphoid and lunate. These facets are angled in an ulnar and palmar direction. The metaphyseal flare has its primary sagittal arc of curvature on the palmar aspect. This flattened area which is covered by the pronator quadratus muscle is susceptible to fracture. The cortices narrow progressively over the metaphyses where they are supported by trabecular bone. Osteopenia, which weakens this structure, increases with age, systemic disease, inactivity and hormonal depletion (Burstein et al. 1972).

The carpal bones transmit on average approximately 80% of the force across the wrist onto the radial articular surfaces (Palmer and Werner 1984). Their area of contact represents approximately 30% of the articular surfaces of the fossae. The contact area changes with altering positions of the wrist (Pogue et al. 1990). With increasing extension, as likely occurs with a fall on the outstretched hand, the contact area is displaced palmarly. The palmar capsule is strengthened by two arcades of fibers that, although set obliquely to the longitudinal axis of the forearm, are capable of transmitting considerable tensile stress to the palmar cortex of the radius when the carpus is extended or forcibly translated in a dorsal direction.

Standard classifications

It is reasonable to include those fractures of the proximal aspect of the distal third of the radius that are often associated with dorsal angulation, supination of the radial fragment, and dislocation of the radius and carpus from the distal ulna (usually referred to as Galeazzi fractures), with the more common distal fractures, as they are part of the same spectrum of injury (Alexander and Lichtman 1981, Hughston 1957, Mikic 1975). The latter, often referred to as Pouteau-Colles' fractures, are fractures through the radial metaphyses associated with dorsal and radial angulation and displacement. A number of approaches to classify this injury have been made. One of the most commonly cited is that of Frykman (1967). Types I, III, V, and VII are progressive degrees of involvement of the distal radius. Type I is a simple transverse fracture, III is a fracture into the distal surface, V a fracture into the sigmoid notch, and VII a fracture into both articular surfaces. Types II, IV, VI, and VIII are identical fractures of the radius with additional fractures of the ulnar head or styloid. Although this scheme obviously indicates increasing articular surface involvement, it does not adequately indicate the degree of severity or provide guidelines for directing treatment. It also fails to account for fractures that are angulated palmarly, commonly termed Smith's or volar Barton's fractures (Smith 1854, Aufranc et al. 1966).

The AO group has addressed this problem with a comprehensive classification that focuses on the severity of the injury, but it is somewhat unwieldy (Müller et al. 1979).

Melone's classification (1986) addresses the severity by proposing a four-part injury to the distal radius. Type I fractures exhibit minimal comminution and are stable. Type II injuries are comminuted and unstable, and there is displacement of the medial fragments, which can be dorsally or palmarly or both. Type III fractures have displacement of the medial fragment as a unit, but there is also a displaced spike fragment from the shaft. Type IV fractures represent wide displacement of the four parts and are associated with extensive soft tissue injury. Both the AO and Melone classifications help in deciding when internal fixation is appropriate and provide a rationale for certain methods of treatment.

Sennwald and Segmüller (1987) base their classification on the strength of bone relative to the degree of mineralization. They can classify most fractures as 'monoblock' or 'split block' depending on the integrity of the epiphyseal fragment.

A modification of the Gartland and Werley classification has also been proposed by Cooney et al. (1980), as shown in Table 6.1. This classification is treatment-based with recommended alternatives for stable, unstable, and reducible or irreducible intra-articular fractures (see Chapter 15). An ideal classification may be based on the mechanism of injury, the resultant displacement, and the functional outcome based on different types of treatment.

Table 6.1 Classification of distal radial fractures by Cooney et al. (1980)

I.	non-articular, non-displaced
II.	non-articular, displaced
	A. reducible
	B. reducible but unstable
	C. irreducible
III.	intra-articular, non-displaced
IV.	intra-articular, displaced
	A. reducible, stable
	B. reducible, unstable
	C. irreducible

Mechanisms of injury

Most radial fractures occur from decelerating injuries with the arm positioned in front or to the side of the body. The wrist is generally in extension as a protective posture. In older individuals muscular weakness, arthritis, lack of coordination, and diminished sensory acuity are often responsible for falls. In younger individuals, in whom there is greater cortical thickness and more condensed trabecular bone, more forceful injuries are the rule. Sports, vehicular accidents, construction injuries, and industrial misadventures are more likely causes.

Frykman's work (1967) suggested that a fracture of the distal radius was more likely to occur in modest wrist extension, whereas scaphoid fractures were more likely to occur in hyperextension and radial deviation. The amount of force capable of creating such an injury varies considerably. Many additional factors such as peak force, rapidity of application, point of application and direction are also involved. The rotational position of the radius relative to the ulna may play some role. Although Koebke (1983) has shown experimentally that the interosseous membrane dissipates only a small amount of force from radius to ulna during longitudinal loading, even at its greatest length, it may nevertheless have some influence on the ultimate prefracture internal stresses. There is nearly always a component of torque around the longitudinal axis of the forearm in addition to the bending stresses (Alexander and Lichtman 1981, Cetti 1977) (Fig. 6.1).

CLASSIFICATION BY MECHANISM OF INJURY 43

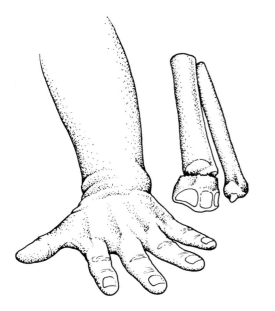

Figure 6.1

Decelerating injuries to the distal forearm result in an accumulation of tensile forces in the metaphyseal area which exceed the strength of the bone. Various degrees of torque also occur around the longitudinal axis of the radius. The severity of the fracture is dependent on the amount of force and the strength of the bone.

The probable mechanisms of injury to produce the modified Gartland-Werley classification of injuries are as follows. In the simplest two-dimensional model of a fracture of the radius, the extensile bending stresses are applied to the palmar aspect of the distal radius. This creates large tensile stresses along the palmar cortex, which diminish in strength until a null point is reached below the dorsal cortex (Fig. 6.2a and b). At this point, the forces become increasingly compressive. When failure occurs, a transverse sharp fracture extends dorsally to the null point and then extends dorsally and obliquely, in both a distal and proximal direction, in the shear mode (Fig. 6.2b).

Type I: Non-articular non-displaced fracture

A type I fracture is apparent but virtually undisplaced and stable. A simple protection splint or cast will usually suffice until healing is complete.

Type II: Non-articular displaced fracture

When the force is greater, it produces the commonly noted comminution of the dorsal cortex. It is also responsible for crushing of cancellous bone as the distal fragment is displaced proximally and dorsally (Frykman 1967, Dobyns and Linscheid 1975). This is a type II A fracture (Fig. 6.2c).

If comminution is greater, the fracture may be reducible but the forces across the fracture site acting on an unstable bony structure leads to recurrent deformity. This is a type II B fracture (Fig. 6.2d, e and f).

Occasionally, it is not possible to obtain a satisfactory reduction, despite adequate traction and manipulation. Interposition of periosteum, the pronator quadratus, or a bony fragment may be responsible. Open reduction may be necessary. This is classified as a type II C fracture.

Type III: Intra-articular, non-displaced fractures

This simple model of bending failure is inadequate to explain other components of the fractures that involve the articular surface of the radius. In this group of fractures, a compressive load is directed axially through the carpus and impacts against the distal articular surface. If the impact displaces, supinates, and ulnarly deviates the carpus, the strong radiocarpal ligaments are placed under marked tension at their origin from the radiovolar facet of the radial styloid. At the same time, the lunate fossa is placed under a marked compressive load as the radiolunate joint becomes the fulcrum of motion. This uneven distribution of internal stresses initiates a tensile fracture at the lateral aspect of the radial styloid, which propagates toward the radiolunate interfossal crest (Fig. 6.3a).

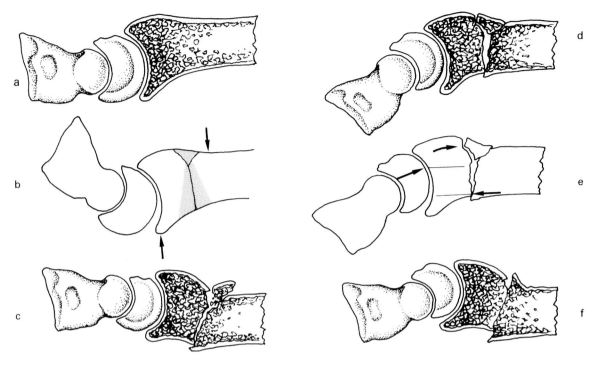

Figure 6.2

a) Sagittal cross-section of distal radius, emphasizing the narrowing cortex of the metaphyseal area, supported by varying densities of cancellous bone. b) The bone will initiate a fracture in tension until the null point is reached, at which time the fracture will progress along the oblique shear stress lines. An undisplaced fracture corresponds to type I. c) Type II A, reducible displaced extra-articular fracture. The distal fragment is dorsally rotated and supinated. d) The fracture is reduced, but failure to lock or overcorrect the palmar cortices may render this reduction unstable. e) Immobilization in the conventional position of palmar flexion and ulnar deviation may increase the force acting around the proximal palmar cortex and thus increase the likelihood that the distal fragment will redisplace. f) Redisplacement has occurred, indicating that this is a type II B, extra-articular unstable fracture. If complete reduction was not possible due to impaction of the fragments or interposition of soft tissues it would be a type II C extra-articular irreducible fracture.

Type IV: Intra-articular displaced fractures

The fracture line, if continued, progresses through the interosseous membrane, between the scaphoid and lunate, and may result in a scapholunate dissociation (Fig. 6.3b). The association of the latter with a radial styloid fracture (Fig. 6.3c) has only recently been commonly recognized (Bassett 1987, Bickerstaff 1989, Destot 1926). The lunate fossa then assumes all of the compressive load and is easily depressed as the support of the scaphoid fossa and radial styloid are lost (Fig. 6.3d and e). This mechanism of injury may also account for the occurrence of chauffeur's fracture, a nostalgic description derived from the predilection of hand-cranked automobile engines to backfire, in which the hand is displaced dorso-ulnarly (deQuervain 1913).

Palmar displaced fractures

The compressive forces acting through the carpus onto the articular surfaces may be directed more palmarly than dorsally (Fig. 6.4a). This may result in a spectrum of injuries in which the carpus is displaced palmarly. At one extreme is a fracture of the palmar rim of the radius with dislocation of the carpus volarly, sometimes referred to as a palmar Barton's fracture (Aufranc et al. 1966, De Oliveira 1973, Pattee and Thompson 1988, Thomas 1957). At the other extreme an extra-articular fracture with palmar displacement may

CLASSIFICATION BY MECHANISM OF INJURY   45

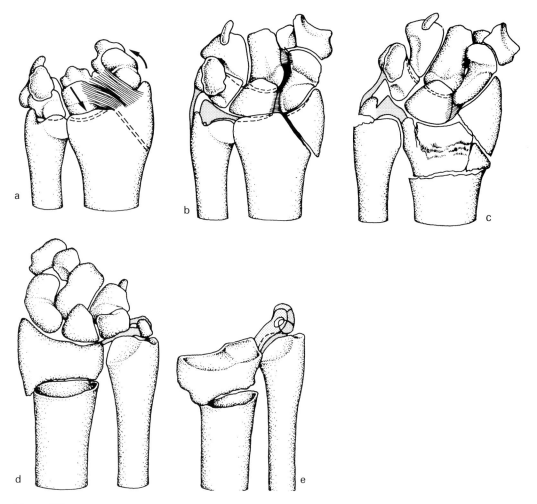

Figure 6.3

a) Type III, non-displaced intra-articular fractures. The forces acting on the distal radius may be distributed quite variably, depending on the attitude of the carpus relative to the forearm. If the hand is ulnarly deviated and extended, the lunate fossa may be under considerable compressive load while the scaphoid fossa is unloaded and the palmar radiocarpal ligaments are placing tensile stresses on the metaphysis proximal to the radial styloid. This may provoke a shear fracture obliquely into the interfossal crest region. b) Type IV, displaced intra-articular fractures. An oblique styloid fracture will displace in a proximal direction. It is usually reducible, but stability is difficult to assess at first. The force that caused such a fracture will often continue through the scapholunate interosseous ligament, producing a secondary dissociation. Such a fracture is often unstable and will redisplace without internal fixation (type IV B). c) A comminuted intra-articular fracture is invariably an unstable type IV B or irreducible type IV C. A depressed lunate fossa, or so-called 'die-punch' fracture, is usually unresponsive to external manipulation. Further comminution usually involves the radial styloid and may cause an additional transverse fracture through the lunate fossa (see Figure 6.4c). d) Disruption of the insertions of the triangular fibrocartilage renders the complex more unstable. e) Failure to fully correct the radial displacement allows the proximal radial cortex to progressively impale the cancellous bone in the distal fragment, resulting in further subsidence.

result. Any palmar (rather than dorsal) angulation or displacement is considered a type of the so-called Smith's fracture (Fig. 6.4b).

A very energetic injury may also result in a combination of fractures in which vertical fractures occur in both the scaphoid and lunate fossa of the distal radius (see Fig. 6.3d). These vertical fractures may occur alone, or combined with a horizontal split fracture of the lunate fossa (Fig. 6.4c). The latter fractures (type IV C) are referred to in the four-part fracture classification of Melone (1986). Under large compressive loads, the lunate fossa may split into dorsal and volar halves with occasional rotational displacement.

Comminution of the palmar cortex (Fig. 6.4d) adds a substantial complication to the maintenance of stability (Auffray and Comtet 1968). In most instances of distal radial fractures, the palmar cortex is used as the fulcrum about which the fragments may be manipulated. When this stability is compromised, the radius is liable not only to shorten but also to angulate unpredictably.

Anatomic status post-fracture

Shortening, malalignment and malangulation are frequent sequelae of distal radial fractures. This occasionally persists, despite our best efforts at reduction and immobilization (Bacorn and Kurtzke 1953, Dowling and Sawyer 1961, Green 1975, McQueen and Caspers 1988, Altissimi et al. 1986, Fourier et al. 1981, Lidström 1959, Parisien 1973). The distal fragment has an inherent tendency to displace proximally. The greater the cortical comminution and trabecular compression, the more certain this becomes. In most instances, the fragment tends to displace and angulate dorsally as its rotates around the structurally more secure palmar cortices. The dorsal cortices, even with a good closed reduction, are liable to collapse.

In the classic reduction of this type of fracture (see Fig. 6.2d), it has been considered desirable to palmarly flex and ulnarly deviate the wrist and to hold the reduction in this position (de Quervain 1913, Böhler 1956). The rationale for this, besides the obvious greater ease in manipulating the fragment, is that a dorsal ligamentotaxis and dorsal tendon tension should aid in holding the reduction (Bartosh and Saldana 1990). Unfortunately, quite the opposite consequence may result. This position encourages dorsoradial displacement of the radiocarpal contact areas, while at the same time increasing the tensile forces across the dorsum (see Fig. 6.2e). Assuming the moments of the fragment are acting about the fulcrum of the palmar cortices, any dorsal displacement of contact will increase the dorsal rotating moment arms (Sarmiento et al. 1975). Any collapse will only serve to increase

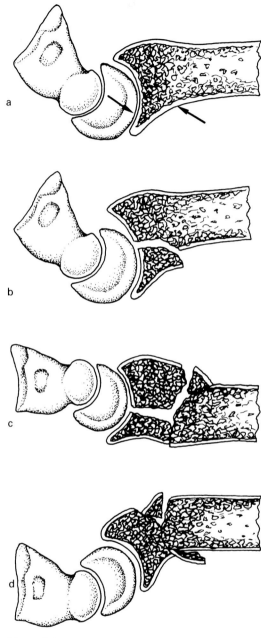

Figure 6.4

Palmar displaced fractures. a) The forces operating on the distal radius may be centered distally, such that the fracture is induced into the articular surface. b) The palmar fragment displacing proximally carries the lunate with it. c) A more comminuted fracture will 'hinge open' as the lunate displaces and rotates the fragments, making a closed reduction virtually impossible. d) Palmar comminution often results in instability, as the palmar cortex cannot be used as the stabilizing fulcrum on which to hold a reduction.

this tendency, as the radial articular surface slopes further and encourages greater carpal displacement. This accounts for the frequent redisplacement that is often observed during the first few weeks of cast immobilization (see Fig. 6.2f).

By the same token, when the carpus and hand are ulnarly deviated, the carpal contact area is displaced radially and with it, the moment arm of the joint compressive forces increases. The radial or lateral cortex of the shaft fragment is usually ulnar to the cortex of the radial styloid fragment, allowing it to impale and erode into the trabecular bone of the styloid (see Fig. 6.3e). An ideal classification may be based on the mechanism of injury as well as the resultant displacement.

A dorsally displaced distal fragment may be converted to a palmarly displaced and angulated posture with an overzealous reduction, in which the palmar cortex of the distal fragment is lying well volar to the proximal cortex. The proximal shaft can erode directly into the metaphyseal trabeculae, increasing the deformity with time (see Fig. 6.3c). If there is comminution of the palmar cortex, this problem is even more likely (see Fig. 6.4d).

Intra-articular fracture components are also apt to remain or continue displacement (Bassett and Ray 1984). Standard plain films are notorious for hiding or underemphasizing such disparities. This is often due to the fact that while a portion of the cortical rim appears to be well aligned, the step-off at a different level is two or more millimeters. A more accurate appraisal may be obtained while the radius is under distraction (traction) during the reduction maneuvers or with tomography (Dobyns and Linscheid 1975, Linscheid et al. 1984). The former is also more likely to disclose intracarpal pathology such as scaphoid fracture, scapholunate dissociation and more subtle injuries.

It is easy to forget the stability provided the distal radius by the ulna (Hughston 1957, Dymond 1984, Ekenstam 1984). Displacement of the distal radius by necessity imposes stress to the triangular fibrocartilage, the margins of which are the strong dorsal and palmar radio-ulnar ligaments. These may avulse a portion or all of the ulnar styloid. At times, the fracture includes the fovea (or base) of the ulnar styloid, ensuring that the proximal insertion of the triangular fibrocartilage is detached (see Fig. 6.3d). Alternatively, the attachments of the triangular fibrocartilage to the rim of the sigmoid notch may be avulsed. A very energetic injury will fracture and comminute the ulnar neck, greatly decreasing the stability of the construct. The ulnar head may be dislocated either dorsally or palmarly. This is especially notable in Galaezzi injuries, where the greater length of the distal radial fragment produces a more effective moment of force on the distal radio-ulnar joint (Alexander and Lichtman 1981, Cetti 1977).

The effect of malangulation on carpal kinematics has received only sporadic attention. With dorsal angulation, the carpus slides up the resulting inclined plane (Pogue et al. 1990, Bassett 1987, Bickerstaff and Bell 1989, Taleisnik and Watson 1984). Usually, the lunate balances itself in alignment with the radial articular surface and thus appears extended (see Fig. 6.2f). The capitate aligns with the forearm, thus being flexed on the lunate. The lunate becomes fixed in this position, and is unable to rotate into flexion during either wrist flexion or ulnar deviation, as the capitate is in contact with dorsal cup of the lunate concavity. The aforementioned motions are therefore greatly reduced.

With a palmar flexed posture of the epiphyseal fragment, the carpus displaces palmarly. When the palmar half of the articular surface is displaced proximally, the proximal row displaces with it, locking itself under the dorsal fracture facet. Conjunct rotation of the carpus is severely restricted (see Fig. 6.4c).

An understanding of the mechanisms of injury in distal radial fractures and the consequences to the stability of the structures may be of value in assessment and planning for treatment. I have attempted to show the probable underlying biomechanical mechanisms for the modified Gartland–Werley classification of distal radial fractures, as well as the continuing influence of these factors in maintaining reduction and stabilization.

References

Alexander AH, Lichtman DM. Irreducible distal radio-ulnar joint occurring in a Galeazzi fracture. Case report. *J Hand Surg* 1981; **6**: 258–61.

Altissimi M, Antenucci R, Fiacca C, Mancini G. Long term results of conservative treatment of fractures of the distal radius. *Clin Orthop* 1986; **206**: 202–10.

Anderson R, O'Neill G. Comminuted fractures of the distal end of the radius. *Surg Gynecol Obstet* 1944; **78**: 434–40.

Auffray Y, Comtet JJ. The role of osteosynthesis of the anterior surface in fractures of the distal end of the radius. *Lyon Med* 1968; **219**: 193–98.

Aufranc OE, Jones WN, Turner RH. Anterior marginal articular fracture of distal radius. *JAMA* 1966; **196**: 788–91.

Bacorn RW, Kurtzke JF. Colles' fractures: A study of two thousand cases from the New York State Workmen's Compensation Board. *J Bone Joint Surg* 1953; **35A**: 643–58.

Bartosh RA, Saldana MJ. Intraarticular fractures of the distal radius: a cadaveric study to determine if ligamentotaxis restores radiopalmar tilt. *J Hand Surg* 1990; **15A**: 18–21.

Bassett, RL. Displaced intraarticular fractures of the distal radius. *Clin Orthop* 1987; **214**: 148–52.

Bassett RL, Ray MJ. Carpal instability associated with radial styloid fracture. *Orthopedics* 1984; **7**: 1356–61.

Bickerstaff DR, Bell MJ. Carpal malalignment in Colles' fractures. *J. Hand Surg* 1989; **14B**: 155–60.

Böhler L. *The treatment of fractures.* (Translated by Tretter H, Luchini HB, Kreuz K, Russe OA and Björnson RGB. 13th German ed.) New York, London: Grune and Stratton, 1956.

Burstein AH, et al. Bone strength: the effect of screw holes. *J Bone Joint Surg* 1972; **54A**: 1143–56.

Cetti NE. An unusual cause of blocked reduction of the Galeazzi injury. *Injury* 1977; **9**: 59–61.

Collert S, Isacson J. Management of redisolocated Colles' fractures. *Clin Orthop* 1978; **135**: 183–86.

Colles A. On the fracture of the carpal extremity of the radius. *Edinb Med Surg J* 1814; **10**: 182–86.

Cooney WP, Dobyns JH, Linscheid RL. Complications of Colles' fractures. *J Bone Joint Surg* 1980; **62A**: 613–19.

De Oliveira JC. Barton's fractures. *J Bone Joint Surg* 1973; **55A**: 586–94.

de Quervain F. *Clinical surgical diagnosis for students and practitioners.* (Translated from 4th edn by J Snowman.) New York: William Wood & Co, 1913.

Desault PJ. In Bichet X, ed. *A treatise on fractures, luxations and other affections of the bones.* (Translated by C Caldwell.) Philadelphia: Fry & Kammerer, 1805: 160–1.

Destot EAJ. *Injuries of the wrist. A radiological study.* New York: Paul B Hoeber, 1926: 160–1.

Dobyns JH, Linscheid RL. Fractures and dislocations of the wrist. In Rockwood CA Jr, Green DP, eds. *Fractures.* Philadelphia: JB Lippincott, 1975: 345–440.

Dowling JJ, Sawyer B. Comminuted Colles' fractures: evaluation of a method of treatment. *J Bone Joint Surg* 1961; **43A**: 657.

Dymond IWD. The treatment of isolated fractures of the distal ulna. *J Bone Joint Surg* 1984; **66B**: 408–10.

Ekenstam FW. The distal radio-ulnar joint: an anatomical, experimental and clinical study with special reference to malunited fractures of the distal radius. Thesis. Uppsala Universitet, 1984: 1–55.

Fourrier P, Bardy A, Roche G, Cisterne JP, Chambon A. Approach to a definition of malunion callus after Pouteau–Colles' fractures (author's transl). *Int Orthop* 1981; **4**: 299–305.

Frykman G. Fracture of the distal radius including sequelae — shoulder hand-finger syndrome, disturbance in the distal radio-ulnar joint, and impairment of nerve function: a clinical and experimental study. *Acta Orthop Scand* 1967; **108(Suppl)**: 1–153.

Green DP. Pins and plaster treatment of comminuted fractures of the distal end of the radius. *J Bone Joint Surg* 1975; **57A**: 304.

Hughston JC. Fracture of the distal radial shaft: mistakes in management. *J Bone Joint Surg* 1957; **39A**: 249–64.

Idler RS, Lourie GM. Management concepts for fractures of the distal radius. *Adv Orthop Surg* 1991; **15**: 1–12.

Koebke J. Biomechanical & morphological analysis of human hand joints. *Advances in anatomy, embryology & cell biology* (80). Berlin, Heidelberg, New York, Tokyo: Springer-Verlag, 1983: 1–85.

Lidström A. Fractures of the distal end of the radius. A clinical and statistical study of end results. *Acta Orthop Scand* 1959; **41(Suppl)**: 1–118.

Linscheid RL, Dobyns JH, Younge DK. Trispiral tomography in the evaluation of wrist injury. *Bull Hosp Joint Dis* 1984; **44**: 297–308.

McQueen M, Caspers J. Colles' fracture: Does the anatomical result affect the final function? *J Bone Joint Surg* 1988; **70B**: 649–51.

Malgaigne JF. *A treatise on fractures*. (Translated by JH Packard.) Philadelphia: JB Lippincott Company, 1859.

Melone CP. Open treatment for displaced articular fractures of the distal radius. *Clin Orthop* 1986; **202**: 103–11.

Mikic ZD. Galeazzi fracture-dislocations. *J Bone Joint Surg* 1975; **57A**: 1071.

Müller ME, Algöwer M, Schneider R, Willengger H. *Manual of internal fixation* 2nd edn. Berlin, Heidelberg, New York: Springer-Verlag, 1979.

Palmer AK, Werner FW. Biomechanics of the distal radioulnar joint. *Clin Orthop* 1984; **187**: 26–35.

Parisien S. Settling in Colles' fracture: a review of the literature. *Bull Hosp Joint Dis* 1973; **34**: 117–25.

Pattee GA, Thompson GH. Anterior and posterior marginal fracture dislocations of the distal radius: an analysis of the results of treatment. *Clin Orthop* 1988; **231**: 183–95.

Pogue DJ. Viegas SF, Patterson RM, Peterson PD, Jenkins DK. Sweo TD, Hokanson JA. Effects of distal radius fracture malunion on wrist joint mechanics. *J Hand Surg* 1990; **15A**: 721–27.

Pouteau C. Cited by Eskelund. *Oeuvres posthumes de M Pouteau*. Vol. 2. Paris: PD Pierres, 1783; 251.

Sarmiento A, Pratt GW, Berry NC, Sinclair WF. Colles' fractures: functional bracing in supination. *J Bone Joint Surg* 1975; **57A**: 311–17.

Sennwald G. *The wrist, anatomical and pathophysiological approach to diagnosis and treatment*. Berlin, Heidelberg, New York, London, Paris, Tokyo: Springer-Verlag, 1987.

Smith RW. *A treatise on fractures in the vicinity of joints, and on certain forms of accidental and congenital dislocations*. Dublin: Hodges & Smith, 1854.

Taleisnik J, Watson HK. Midcarpal instability caused by malunited fractures of the distal radius. *J Hand Surg* 1984; **9A**: 350–57.

Thomas FB. Reduction of Smith's fracture. *J Bone Joint Surg* 1957; **39B**: 463–70.

7
Percutaneous pinning of fractures of the distal end of the radius

MD Greatting, MB Wood

Fracture of the distal radius is one of the most common fractures of the upper extremity. Several treatment options exist. These include closed reduction and plaster immobilization, percutaneous pinning, intrafocal pinning, pins and plaster, external fixation, open reduction and internal fixation and various combinations of these options. Percutaneous pinning is a useful technique for the treatment of selected fractures of the distal radius. The purpose of this chapter will be to review the various techniques of percutaneous pinning, the biomechanical data relevant to these techniques and the indications for their use.

Fracture classification

Several fracture classifications exist to assist in defining distal radius fractures (Cooney 1990, Cooney et al. 1991, Frykman 1967, Gartland and Werley 1951, Melone 1984). The more recent systems have been more helpful in the decision process concerning treatment of specific types of distal radius fractures (Cooney 1990, Cooney et al. 1991). The classification system presented in Fig. 7.1 is helpful in determining which distal radius fractures can be treated by percutaneous pinning. Fractures are classified as non-articular or articular, non-displaced or displaced, and reducible or irreducible. Percutaneous pinning is useful in fractures which can be classified as non-articular displaced, articular non-displaced and articular displaced, all of which are reducible and stable after reduction.

Rationale for treatment

In previous years, it was felt that maintenance of an anatomic reduction was not necessary to achieve a good functional result when treating fractures of the distal radius. Several modern series have reported a high incidence of complications related to plaster treatment of displaced unstable distal radius fractures (Ahstrom 1981, Aro and Koiuuner 1991, Bickerstaff and Bell 1989, Cooney et al. 1980, Frykman 1967, Lucas and Sachtjen 1977, Older et al. 1965, Taleisnik and Watson 1984, Waugh 1962). Malunion is one of these complications that is not well tolerated and often requires treatment (Fernandez 1982, Posner and Ambrose 1991, Taleisnik and Watson 1984). Biomechanical studies have supported the fact that malunion will affect the function of the wrist (Kazuki et al. 1991, Short et al. 1987). It is now generally agreed that the goal of treatment of distal radius fractures should be to obtain and maintain an anatomic reduction (Cooney 1989). Percutaneous pinning should be utilized for fractures of the distal radius where this is an obtainable goal. A useful classification system will help define which fractures can best be treated by percutaneous pinning (Cooney 1990, Cooney et al. 1991).

Literature review

One of the earliest reports of percutaneous pinning was by DePalma in 1952. He described a tech-nique using a single-threaded 2.4 mm (3/32 inch) Steinman pin inserted obliquely across the distal ulna and directed towards the radial styloid (Fig. 7.2). A short arm cast was used

PERCUTANEOUS PINNING OF FRACTURES OF THE DISTAL END OF THE RADIUS 51

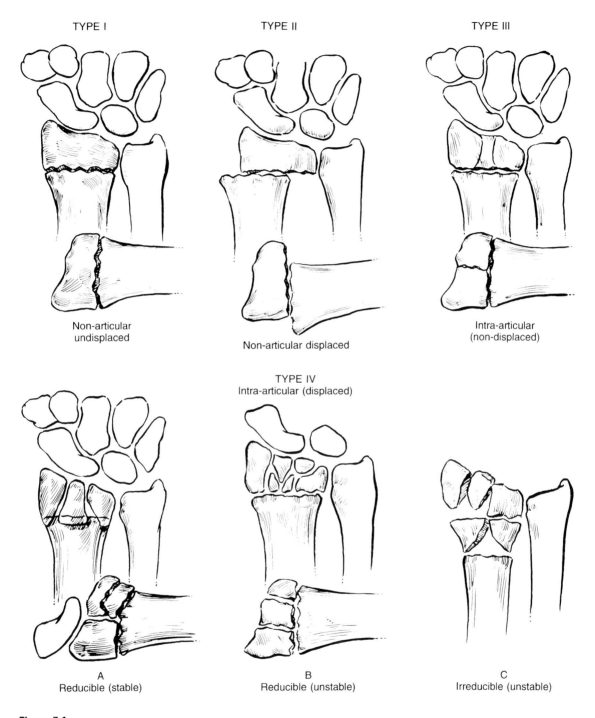

Figure 7.1

Universal classification of distal radius fractures.

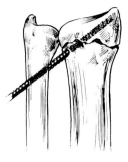

DePalma, 1952
Dowling, 1961

Figure 7.2

Transulnar techniques of percutaneous pinning of distal radius fractures.

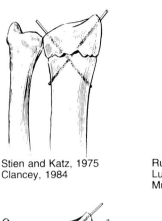

Stien and Katz, 1975
Clancey, 1984

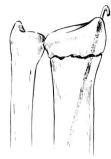

Rush, 1954
Lucas and Sachtjan, 1981
Munson and Gainor, 1981

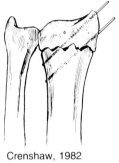

Crenshaw, 1982

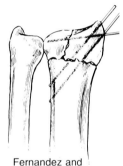

Fernandez and Geissler, 1991

Figure 7.3

Radial techniques of percutaneous pinning of distal radius fractures.

postoperatively, and the pin and cast were left in place for eight weeks. The fractures were classified using the Gartland and Werley system and all fractures were comminuted with varying degrees of involvement of the articular surface. DePalma reported 82% good and excellent results and also stated that these results were superior to a similar group of fractures treated by plaster immobilization. Complications were limited to pin-tract infections and late fracture displacement where the pin was removed before eight weeks.

Dowling reported a second series of fractures treated by the same technique in 1961 (Fig. 7.2). All fractures were again comminuted and most involved the articular surface. Excellent or good clinical results were obtained in 84% of patients but the radiographic results were markedly worse if the articular surface was involved. Postoperative immobilization was again for eight weeks but a long cast was used in this series. Complications in this series included loss of reduction in seven cases due to early removal of the pin and breakage of the pin in two cases. A more recent review of this technique was reported by Garner and Grimes in 1977.

A different technique of percutaneous pinning using a single large pin inserted through the radial styloid and down the medullary canal of the radius was reported by Rush in 1954. This technique is performed by placing a 3.2 mm or 2.4 mm (1/8 or 3/32 inch) Rush rod percutaneously through the radial styloid after performing a closed reduction (Fig. 7.3). The pin is then passed down the medullary canal of the radius and does not engage the cortical bone. Postoperative splinting is maintained for just several days. The pin was removed only if it caused symptoms after fracture healing. The majority of the fractures were stated to be comminuted but no mention was made of articular involvement. Range of motion was reported to be satisfactory in a large percentage of patients, but little other clinical information is available. Complications included one case of extensor tendon adhesions, two cases of pin-site irritation and several cases of overcorrection of the distal fracture fragment.

Two more recent series have been reported using this technique. In 1982 Munson and Gainor reported the radiographic results of 22 fractures treated by this technique (Fig. 7.3). The fractures were stated to be due to high-energy trauma but no mention was made of the extent of articular involvement. Short arm immobilization was used postoperatively and the pin was removed at eight weeks. Radiographic results were excellent and good in 21 of 22 patients; no clinical results were reported. Complications included one superficial pin-tract infection, one pin migration and one case of pain localized to the site of pin insertion.

Lucas and Sachtjen (1981) reported the results of 33 fractures treated with the same technique (Fig. 7.3). The fractures were all comminuted and displaced. Postoperative immobilization consisted of a removable wrist splint worn for two to three weeks. Using a modification of Sarmiento's evaluation system, 32 excellent and good results were reported out of 33 cases.

Another method of percutaneous pinning of distal radius fractures was reported by Stein and Katz in 1975 (Fig. 7.3). This method utilizes two 1 mm or 1.2 mm (0.035 or 0.045 inch) Kirschner wires. A closed reduction is performed and then one pin is inserted through the radial styloid and a second pin is inserted dorso-ulnarly. Both pins engage cortical bone of the radius proximally. A long cast was used postoperatively and immobilization was continued for approximately 7.5 weeks. Radiographic and clinical results appeared to be improved over a similar group treated by plaster immobilization alone. Complications related to the pins were minimal.

A second report using the same technique was reported by Clancey in 1984 (Fig. 7.3). Half of the fractures involved the articular surface of the radius. Two 1.6 mm (0.062 inch) Kirschner wires were introduced in the same manner as described in the previous study. Plaster immobilization was used for six weeks postoperatively and the pins were removed at eight weeks. Satisfactory anatomic results were achieved in 28 out of 30 patients and 27 out of 28 were found to have good or excellent functional results. Complications in this series included two cases of pin migration, loss of reduction in one patient and one case of flexor pollicus longus tendon adhesions, secondary to overpenetration of a pin proximally.

A similar technique utilizing two pins inserted obliquely through the radial styloid, has been reported (Crenshaw, 1992) but no information is available concerning the results using this method of treatment (Fig. 7.3).

Another variation of percutaneous pinning has recently been reported by Rayhack et al. (1991). This technique consists of the use of four to eight 1.2 mm (0.045 inch) Kirschner wires, inserted obliquely from the distal ulnar shaft to the radius (see Fig. 7.2). Plaster immobilization is used for three weeks postoperatively and then motion is allowed in a lightweight splint. Good and excellent results were reported in 25 out of 27 cases, using the clinical evaluation criteria of Scheck. Pins were left in place for eight to ten weeks. Complications included loss of reduction in one patient after pin removal and four broken pins in three patients.

Most recently, percutaneous pinning has been used to treat selected distal radius fractures with displaced articular fragments. Fernandez and Geissler (1991) have reported the treatment of 21 fractures with articular displacement treated by two Kirschner wires inserted obliquely through the radial styloid and a third pin inserted transversely, stabilizing the ulnar articular fragment after reduction has been obtained (Fig. 7.3). Postoperative immobilization consists of either casting or external fixation. A high percentage of satisfactory anatomic and clinical results were obtained. Complications in this series included five pin-tract infections and one superficial radial nerve lesion.

A similar technique has also recently been reported by Seitz et al. (1991) Initial reduction and stabilization was performed by use of an external fixator. Stabilization of the radial styloid is performed using percutaneously placed 1.6 mm (0.062 inch) Kitschner wires. The ulnar articular fragment is then reduced by manipulation with a dorsally placed ulnar wire and stabilized by a transversely placed pin supporting the subchrondral bone (Fig. 7.4). Bone grafting is performed if a large dorsal defect is present post-reduction. Satisfactory results were obtained in 92% of patients. Complications related to this technique included one loss of reduction and five cases of superficial pin-tract infection.

Biomechanical data

Little biomechanical data is available concerning the various techniques of percutaneous pinning of distal radius fractures. A recent report by Graham et al. (1990) makes several recommendations concerning percutaneous pinning. Their data suggests that percutaneous pinning is effective in preventing dorsal displacement of extra-articular distal radius fractures, that multiple pins (three or four) should be used and that

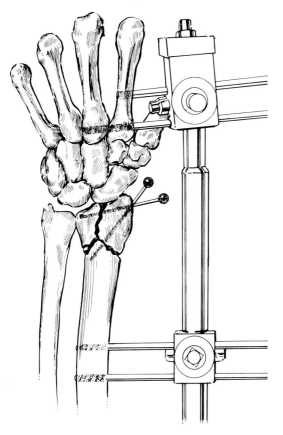

Figure 7.4

External fixation and percutaneous pinning of distal radius fractures. (From Seitz et al. 1991.)

techniques which involve transulnar pinning are more stable than techniques involving radial pins alone.

Indications and contraindications for percutaneous pinning

It is generally agreed that the goal of treatment of distal radius fractures is obtaining and maintaining an anatomic reduction and restoring normal function to the involved upper extremity (Cooney 1989). Many options exist to obtain this goal. Recent publications suggest that percutaneous pinning is most useful for an unstable extra-articular fracture or in an unstable fracture with intra-articular involvement which is not significantly displaced or can be reduced by traction alone (Cooney 1990, Cooney et al. 1991). Relative contraindications to percutaneous pinning include osteoporosis and severe comminution (Cooney et al. 1991, Palmer 1988, Szabo and Weber 1988, Weber 1987). Percutaneous pins have also recently been shown to be useful in obtaining and maintaining reduction of displaced intra-articular fragments and have been used in combination with external fixation (Fernandez and Geissler 1991, Seitz et al. 1991).

Conclusions

Percutaneous pinning is a useful and effective technique in the treatment of selected unstable fractures of the distal radius. Various types of percutaneous pinning exist and acceptable results can be obtained with all of the variations described. As with all other methods of treatment of unstable fractures of the distal radius, the goals of treatment should be anatomic reduction of the fracture fragments and restoration of normal function of the involved upper extremity.

References

Ahstrom JP. Results of treatment of Colles' fractures by posterior plaster splint immobilization. *Orthop Trans* 1981; **5**: 434.

Aro HT, Koiuuner T. Minor axial shortening of the radius affects outcome of Colles' fracture treatment. *J Hand Surg* 1991; **16A**: 392–98.

Bickerstaff DR, Bell MJ. Carpal malalignment in Colles' fractures. *J Hand Surg* 1989; **14B**: 155–60.

Clancey GJ. Percutaneous Kirschner-wire fixation of Colles' fractures. *J Bone Joint Surg* 1984; **66A**: 1088–14.

Cooney WP. Management of Colles' fractures, editorial. *J Hand Surg* 1989; **14B**: 137–38.

Cooney WP, moderator. Symposium. Management of intra-articular fractures of the distal radius. *Contemp Orthop* 1990; **21**: 71–104.

Cooney WP, Dobyns JH, Linscheid RL. Complications of Colles fractures. *Bone Joint Surg* 1980; **62A**: 613–19.

Cooney WP, Linscheid RL, Dobyns JH. Fractures and dislocations of the wrist. In Rockwood CA, Green DP, Buchulz RW, eds. *Fractures in Adults*. New York: Lippincott, 1991: 563–678.

Crenshaw AH Jr. Fractures of the shoulder, girdle, arm and forearm. In Crenshaw AH, ed. *Campbell's Operative Orthopaedics*. St. Louis: Mosby, 1992: 989–1052.

DePalma AF. Comminuted fractures of the distal end of the radius treated by ulnar pinning. *J Bone Joint Surg* 1952; **34A**: 651–662.

Dowling JJ. Comminuted Colles' fractures. *Bone Joint Surg* 1961; **43A**: 657–68.

Fernandez DL. Correction of post-traumatic wrist deformity in adults by osteotomy, bone grafting, and internal fixation. *J Bone Joint Surg* 1982; **64A**: 1164–78.

Fernandez DL, Geissler WB. Treatment of displaced articular fractures of the radius. *J Hand Surg* 1991; **16A**: 375–84.

Frykman G. Fractures of the distal radius including sequelae – shoulder-hand-finger syndrome, disturbance in the distal radio-ulnar joint and impairment of nerve function. *Acta Orthop Scan (Suppl)* 1967; **108**: 1–153.

Garner RW, Grimes DW. Percutaneous pinning of displaced fractures of the distal radius. *Orthop Rev*. 1977; **5**: 87–88.

Gartland JJ, Werley CW. Evaluation of healed Colles' fractures. *J Bone Joint Surg* 1951; **33A**: 895–951.

Graham TJ, et al. Biomechanical evaluation of percutaneous pinning for extra-articular distal radius fractures. Presentation, American Society for Surgery of the Hand 45th Annual Meeting. Toronto, 1990.

Kazuki K, Kusunaki M, Shimazu A. Pressure distribution in the radiocarpal joint measured with a densitometer designed for pressure sensitive film. *J Hand Surg* 1991; **16A**: 401–8.

Lucas GL, Sachtjen KM. Thomas Jefferson therapeutic nihilism, and Colles' fracture. *Orthop Rev* 1977; **6**: 83.

Lucas GL, Sachtjen KM. An analysis of hand function in patients with Colles' fracture treated by Rush rod fixation. *Clin Orthop Rel Res* 1981; **155**: 172–79.

Melone CP. Articular fracture of the distal radius. *Orthop Clin North Am* 1984; **15**: 217–36.

Munson GO, Gainor BJ. Percutaneous pinning of distal radius fractures. *J Trauma* 1981; **21**: 1032–35.

Older TM, Stabler GV, Casselbaum WH. Colles' fracture: Evaluation and selection of therapy. *J Trauma* 1965; **5**: 469.

Palmer AK. Fractures of the distal radius. In Green DP ed. *Operative Hand Surgery*. New York: Churchill Livingstone, 1988: 991–1026.

Posner MA, Ambrose L. Malunited Colles' fractures: correction with a biplanar closing wedge osteotomy. *J Hand Surg* 1991; **16A**: 1017–26.

Rayhack JM, Langworthy JN, Belsole RJ. Transulnar percutaneous pinning of displaced radial articular fractures — A prospective study of 32 patients. Presentation, American Society for Surgery of the Hand 46th Annual Meeting. Orlando, 1991.

Rush LV. Closed medullary pinning of Colles' fracture. *Clin Orthop Rel Res* 1954; **3**: 152–62.

Seitz WH, Frohmson AI, Leb R, Shapiro JD. Augmented external fixation of unstable distal radius fractures. *J Hand Surg* 1991; **16A**: 1010–16.

Short WH, Palmer AK, Werner FW, Murphy DJ. A biomechanical study of distal radius fractures. *J Hand Surg* 1987; **12A**: 529–34.

Stein AH, Katz SF. Stabilization of comminuted fractures of the distal inch of the radius: percutaneous pinning. *Clin Orthop Rel Res* 1975; **108**: 174–81.

Szabo RM, Weber SC. Comminuted intra-articular fractures of the distal radius. *Clin Orthop Rel Res* 1988; **230**: 39–48.

Taleisnik J, Watson HK. Midcarpal instability caused by malunited fractures of the distal radius. *J Hand Surg* 1984; **9A**: 350–57.

Waugh TR. Unreduced Colles' fractures. *J Trauma* 1962; **3**: 254.

Weber ER. A rational approach for the recognition and treatment of Colles' fractures. *Hand Clinics* 1987; **3**: 13–21.

8
Treatment of distal radial fractures with the 'Py' isoelastic pinning procedure: 100 consecutive cases

M Ebelin, C Delaunay, E Lenoble, T Lebalc'h, F Mazas

Introduction

This chapter describes the authors' experience with isoelastic pinning of fractures of the distal radial epiphysis. This technique was first described by Claude Py in 1969 and updated by Desmanet in 1989. The study described below was initiated in 1986. The technique, as described in the literature, is easy to perform and provides good and stable results, however, some modifications were necessary.

Operative technique

In most cases, reduction is achieved under local and regional anaesthesia with manipulation under fluoroscopic control. Two 10 mm incisions are made with a sharp surgical scalpel (15# blade), one at the level of the radial styloid and the second at the dorsal margin, medial to the extensor pollicis longus and Lister's tubercle. The pins are equal in length and size (1.8 or 2 mm) and have speared or smooth ends that are shaped like a spatula distally.

The distal radial nerve branches, the abductor pollicis longus and extensor pollicis brevis tendons are retracted. Using a manual handle, the first pin is inserted so that it penetrates the tip of the radial styloid process and is pushed all along the medullary canal until it reaches the radial head subchondral plate. Thanks to its spatula-shaped end, the pin can 'slide' along the cortex wall without penetrating it.

To prevent injury to the extensor tendons, a short incision is made in the dorsal retinaculum. Thus, the second pin is inserted in the medial third of the dorsal margin of the radius and is pushed to the level of the radial head (Fig. 8.1). Once the two pins are placed, reduction stability is checked under fluoroscopy in both frontal and sagittal views. The pins are bent close to their bony penetration points and cut a few millimetres proximally, and the incisions are closed. The pins are subcutaneous but are long enough to avoid injuring the extensor tendons and can be easily located to facilitate their removal.

In some cases, for example with significant comminution, poor bone stock or non-compliant patients, additional stabilization can be provided with an anterior splint or a circular cast. In most cases, however, immediate stability is achieved and the treatment avoids extra immobilization and allows early wrist and finger rehabilitation.

Radiographic evaluation is carried out on the second day after surgery to examine for loss of reduction (Figs 8.2 and 8.3). Pin removal is performed around the 40th day, usually on a one-day (outpatient) surgery programme. Local or regional anaesthesia is needed to remove the pins through their long intramedullary tracks: to do so without anaesthesia would be too painful.

Material and methods

The subjects of the study included 26 men and 74 women with an average age of 55.4 years (age range 17 to 94 years old). The dominant wrist (right wrist) was involved in 57 patients. There were only a few work-related injuries (11 cases). The study started at the end of 1986, and the

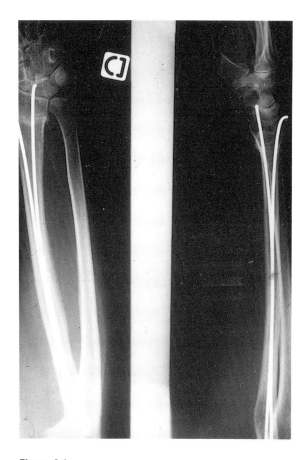

Figure 8.1

Standard double pinning of a distal radius fracture.

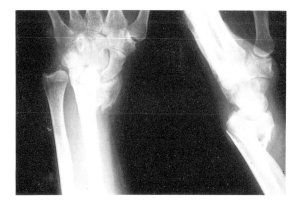

Figure 8.2

Pre-operative radiograph of a distal radius fracture.

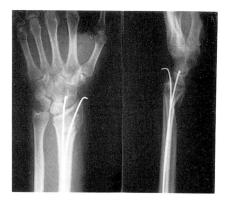

Figure 8.3

Post-operative radiographic evaluation of the fracture shown in Fig. 8.2.

average follow-up period was five months. Of those studied, 90 patients were clinically and radiologically assessed, one patient died and nine patients were lost to follow-up.

Using the Castaing classification (Castaing 1964), the balance between articular and extra-articular fractures was found to be identical: 50 extra-articular fractures (27 Pouteau–Colles, 21 Gerard–Marchand and two Goyrand–Smith types), and 50 articular fractures (19 Pouteau–Colles with an articular medial-posterior fragment, 12 frontal T, seven sagittal T, six cross-fractures, five with extensive comminution and one isolated radial styloid fracture). In 29 cases a fracture of the ulnar styloid was associated with the radial fracture.

In 90% of the patients, surgery was performed within 48 hours of the injury. Three fractures were treated by operation between the 8th and 21st day because of secondary fracture displacement after initial conservative treatment.

In 88 of the cases, the elastic pinning procedure, as described above, was used. Some modifications were necessary in other cases: a third, short pin was inserted in the frontal plane to stabilize the distal radio-ulnar joint in four cases (Fig. 8.4); a third, long intramedullary dorsal pin (the triple elastic procedure) was used in four other cases, and a lateral bicortical 'classic' pin was used instead of the radial styloid elastic one in the remaining four cases.

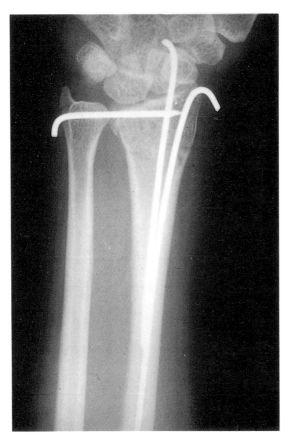

Figure 8.4

A radio-ulnar pin complementing the two standard pins.

Postoperative complications

Postoperatively, immediate mobilization was allowed in 45 cases, whereas it was postponed to the 8th or 10th day in 25 cases. A circular cast was maintained until pin removal in 30 patients.

Postoperative complications are frequent, and may be unavoidable with this technique. In this study, secondary displacements occurred in 27 cases including:

- lateral opening in three cases;
- anterior shift in three cases and posterior shift in four cases;
- 'en bloc' epiphyseal medial translation in four cases;
- postero-medial marginal fragment displacement in four cases; and
- epiphyseal impaction in nine cases.

Some of these secondary displacements (lateral opening, anterior shift, epiphyseal medial translation) have no perjorative influence on the final result. Others (postero-medial marginal fragment displacement, posterior shift, epiphyseal impaction) develop more prejudicial consequences. No early reoperation was necessary, but three procedures (two Sauvé–Kapandji and one ulnar head resection) were performed later due to distal radio-ulnar joint problems which caused a loss of the prono-supination range of motion.

Other complications were less specific, including three cases of neurosympathetic syndrome, three cutaneous infections leading to early pin removal, five radial nerve paresthesias (diagnosed after pin removal) and two extensor tendon ruptures (one index and one long finger extensor digitorum) due to pins.

The overall review of the cases in this study revealed a significant complication rate: 20 benign and 16 with harmful consequences (secondary displacement impairing wrist range of motion or functional result, extensor tendon rupture, and severe neurosympathetic syndrome).

Results

According to the clinical examination (pain, strength, range of motion) and radiological criteria defined by Castaing, the results of the 90 cases available for review were as follows: very good in 43 cases (47.7%), good in 21 cases (23.4%), fair in 12 cases (13.4%) and poor in 14 cases (15.5%). Thus, overall, 71.1% of the cases showed excellent or good results.

Factors suggesting a poor prognosis are described below.

Age. Eighty per cent of very good and good results were in patients under 40 years of age and 36% of poor results occurred in patients over 80 years of age.

Type of fracture. The results fell into two groups:

1. Fractures with a good prognosis, leading to less than one third of fair or bad results. These included Pouteau–Colles fractures, even with a marginal postero-medial fragment and T-frontal fractures.
2. Fractures with a poor prognosis, leading to more than one third of fair or bad results. These included, by increasing range of severity, T sagittal fractures, lateral styloid fractures, cross-type fractures and comminuted fractures.

Quality of immediate postoperative reduction. Immediate reduction was achieved in 80 cases: the results were deemed very good and good in 75.3% of the cases with anatomic reduction but in only 55% of the cases without.

Association with a distal radio-ulnar joint incongruity. This was observed in 18 cases. It occurred immediately in six cases (because of lack of adequate reduction) and after secondary displacement in 12 cases. When distal radio-ulnar joint incongruity was present, very good and good results decreased to 33.3% and poor results increased to 38.8%.

Postoperative immobilization. When applied until the pins were removed, very good and good results occurred in only 55.5% of cases. However, this must be balanced by the fact that immobilization has always been applied in the worst cases, such as fractures of a difficult type, insufficient pre-operative stability, or non-compliant patients. Conversely, 88% of cases without immobilization and with early rehabilitation obtained very good and good results.

Overall, analysis of the poor results (23 cases) shows different reasons for failure, listed here in order of decreasing frequency: distal radio-ulnar joint incongruity (47%), malunion (21%), painful stiff wrist (13%), neurosympathetic syndrome (13%), and injury to the sensory branch of the radial nerve (4%).

Discussion

The elastic pinning method allows some residual flexibility at the fracture site (Firica et al., 1981). The pins' dynamic effect is seated on the larger distal radial epiphysis, thus preventing posterior shift with the postero-medial marginal pin and lateral translation and/or epiphyseal impaction with the styloid pin. The elastic effect produced on the epiphysis by the distal pin is well illustrated by the curved shape of the pins extending down along the medullary canal. This effect is possible so long as there are some intact parts of the radial posterior margin and a preserved styloid tip. This situation is frequently encountered.

We have found that this technique has not yet solved several problems. The study of the results and the difficulties met during team training have revealed that certain modifications should be added to the standard 'Py' technique in some cases:

1. use of a third sagittal or centro-medullar pin to fix the reduction of a postero-medial marginal fragment (Figs 8.5 & 8.6) as shown by Mortier et al., 1983;
2. use of a frontal radio-ulnar pin, taking care to avoid the ulnar nerve posterior branch. This pin is driven under power, the wrist being placed in a position of half-pronation. This is used in cases in which there is a high risk of postero-medial fragment migration along the conventional 'Py' longitudinal dorsal pin. Such

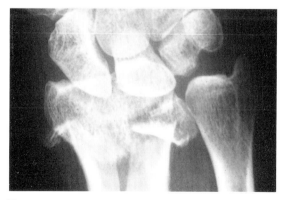

Figure 8.5

Fracture with a postero-medial fragment and dislocation, shown radiographically in the inferior radio-ulnar view.

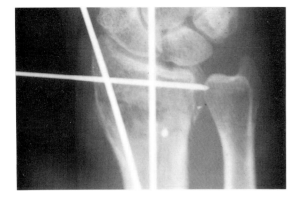

Figure 8.6

Triple pinning of the fracture shown in Fig. 8.5, with a transverse pin maintaining the postero-medial fragment.

cases include those with significant posterior comminution (Figs 8.7 and 8.8), or with an associated fracture of the ulnar styloid, where the postero-medial fragment is no longer connected with the triangular ligament;

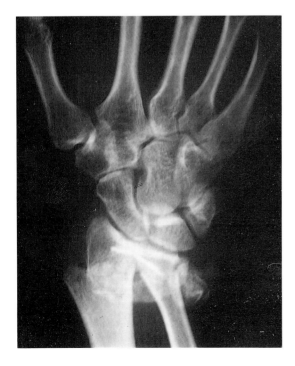

Figure 8.7

Comminuted fracture of the distal radius and of the ulna.

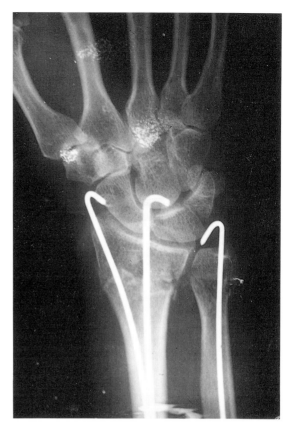

Figure 8.8

Triple pinning of the fracture shown in Fig. 8.7.

3. use of a 'classic' bicortical styloid pin in cases of unstable lateral fracture in which the dynamic effect of the 'Py' lateral pin could yield to secondary lateral opening with displacement due to excessive elastic force;
4. finally, avoid elastic 'Py' pinning in the rare associated displaced fracture of the distal ulnar shaft.

Conclusions

This review provided a good indication of the efficiency of the 'Py' elastic pinning procedure in the treatment of distal radial epiphysis fractures. The main drawback of the procedure is that it necessitates a second operation to remove the pins. The advantages, however, are numerous:

good quality and stability of reduction, short operative time and immediate post-operative rehabilitation in most cases. Consequently, the 'Py' elastic pinning procedure, along with several technical adjustments as reported above, is recommended for the treatment of extra-articular distal radial fractures. The exception is severe comminuted fractures, for which distraction with an external fixator is still indicated.

References

Castaing J, le Club des Dix. Les fractures récentes de l'extrémité inférieure du radius chez l'adulte. *Rev Chir Orthop* 1964; **50**: 581–666.

Desmanet E. L'ostéosynthèse par double embrochage souple du radius. Traitement fonctionnel des fractures de l'extrémité inférieure du radius: à propos d'un suivi de 130 cas. *Ann Chir Main* 1989; **8**: 193–206.

Firica A, Popescu R, Scarlet M. L'ostéosynthèse stable élastique; nouveau concept biomécanique. *Rev Chir Orthop* 1981; **67, suppl. II**: 82–91.

Mortier JP, Baux S, Uhl JF, Mimoun M, Mole B. Importance du fragment postéro-interne et son brochage spécifique dans les fractures de l'extrémité inférieure du radius. *Ann Chir Main* 1983; **2**: 219–29.

Py C, Churet JP. Tentative de mobilisation immédiate des fractures de l'extrémité inférieure du radius. Personal communication, Tours and Western Center Surgical Society Meeting, 18 June, 1969.

9
Osteosynthesis of the radius by flexible double pinning: functional treatment of distal radial fractures in 130 consecutive cases

E Desmanet

Introduction

Displacement in both the frontal and sagittal planes characterizes fractures of the distal radius. Traction and compression are necessary to obtain reduction and restore radial length (Fig. 9.1). To stabilize this reduction, continuous traction and compression should be maintained during the period of healing.

The principle of flexible double pinning (FDP) consists of replacing the surgeon's hand, which reduces the fracture, and the application of a cast, which maintains this reduction, by two flexible K-wires with a spring effect. The distal radial epiphysis enlarges like a funnel. When K-wires are inserted at the distal-most points of the epiphysis, they are distorted and a spring effect is obtained. This leverage effect (F) can be divided into a compression component (F′) and a traction component (F″). When added together, these two components act on the wrist like a continuous extension force (Fig. 9.2). Whilst other techniques rely on pin rigidity, this method utilizes the flexibility of the pin, transforming it into a spring.

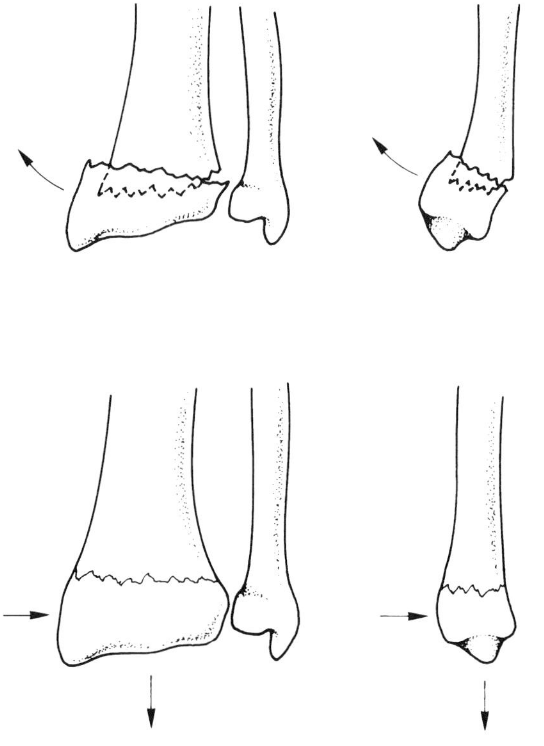

Figure 9.1

Reduction manoeuvres.

Operative treatment

K-wires of 18/10 mm are inserted either using a limited open surgical approach, or percutaneously into the medullary canal of the radius through the radial styloid process and the postero-medial end of the distal epiphysis. It is at times useful to curve the pins to make them slip on the medial cortex. During their progression along the medullary canal, the K-wires gradually obtain the fracture reduction (Fig. 9.3). They stabilize once they have contacted the radial head or the proximal radial

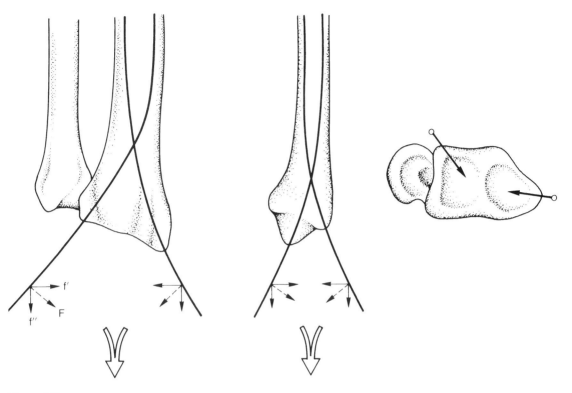

Figure 9.2

Pin effect.

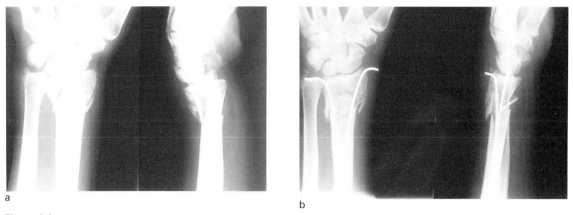

Figure 9.3

a) Unstable fracture of the distal radius with a postero-medial fragment. b) The fracture is successfully reduced and stabilized by the insertion of two K-wires.

epiphysis, and after the proximal end of the pin has been curved like a hook (Fig. 9.4).

Wrist mobility is checked to make sure the tendons have been avoided. Good reduction and stability are checked by fluoroscopy. On the lateral view, the epiphysis should not be translated forward relative to the metaphysis. If this is the case, gentle manoeuvres may often allow realignment of the fragments. If the anterior rim is unstable, a third K-wire will be inserted in the

64 FRACTURES OF THE DISTAL RADIUS

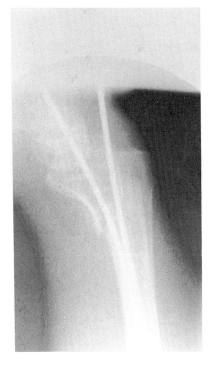

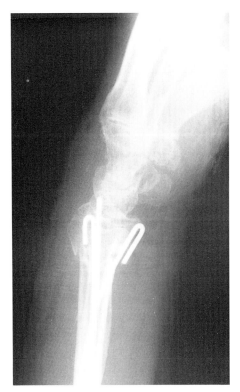

Figure 9.4

Extra-articular fracture in flexion-compression. a) Anterior instability and anterior radio-ulnar dislocation are present in spite of the flexible double-pinning. b) Anterior intrafocal pinning reduces the radio-ulnar dislocation. c) Frontal view showing the extension effect on the fragment.

fracture line using an anterior approach to stabilize the antero-medial fragment. This pin is inserted without power in a position lateral to the ulnar neurovascular bundle. If the volar fragment is stable, the pin is inserted percutaneously and fixed in the dorsal cortex, as described by Kapandji (1976), to provide an anterior buttress. If comminuted, the pin is inserted by an antero-medial approach into the medullary canal to reinforce the volar buttress effect (Fig. 9.4). There is no cast immobilization and antibiotics are not utilized. The patients are encouraged to use their hands without wrist immobilization. Radiographs are taken sequentially at two weeks. The pins are removed after the sixth week, when the bone has healed.

Material

Over a period of two consecutive years, all displaced distal radial fractures were treated by flexible double pinning (Desmanet, 1989). The pins were always inserted percutaneously, penetrating through the intramedullary canal proximally until the radial head engaged. They were then bent to be perpendicular to the skin and cut just under the skin. A total of 16 surgeons treated 130 fractures, which is the most complete study of the technique in this field. Of the 130 fractures studied, 97 (75%) were tested as emergencies by the resident. The proportion of female patients was 73%, and the left hand was injured in 61% of the cases. The mean age of the patients was 63 years old (age range 17–86 years).

Classification

The fractures were classified according to Castaing's method (1964):

- 50% extra-articular fractures: Pouteau–Colles' fractures;
- 17% intra-articular fractures with posteromedial fragment;
- 18% intra-articular fractures with sagittal T;
- 9% comminuted fractures;
- 6% compression-flexion fractures with a volar displacement (Goyrand–Smith).

Associated injuries

The ulnar styloid was fractured in 53% of the cases (Gerard–Marchand fractures). In 6% (eight) of the cases, an associated fracture of the ulna distal was found. One case was an open fracture. Two patients had a shoulder dislocation on the same side as the distal radial fracture. The radial head was fractured in one patient. Two cases had a proximal femur fracture: both returned to walking fairly early, using crutches and the osteosynthesized wrist.

Complications

The following complications were found:

- nine cases of neurosympathetic dystrophy (NSD), which were cured by physiotherapy;
- one carpal tunnel syndrome, which required operation;
- one rotator cuff syndrome, which resulted from manipulation during the plexus block;
- three cases of pin tract infection. The pins were removed early (between the third and sixth week);
- five cases of tendon rupture, which required operation on: two extensor pollicis longus (EPL), and three extensor digitorum communis (EDC) tendons.

Two slight extensor lags were also observed without functional impairment. Some paresthesiae of the sensory branches of the radial nerve have also been noted, but without the need for neurolysis.

Results

The Castaing classification was used to study the anatomical results: the four criteria, each having 4 points were as follows:

1. radial inclination (RI);
2. palmar slope (PS) or dorsal angulation;
3. radial shift (RS);
4. radial length (ulnar variance).

When all the indices are normal, the result is 'excellent', when one or several indices are slightly modified, the result is 'good'. It is considered as 'fair' if any one index shows a significant anatomical deformity. The result is 'poor' if one index shows a large variation, or if several indices show significant variations from normal (Table 9.1).

Good and excellent results were obtained in 71% of cases (Table 9.1). However, the simplest fractures obtained the best results: 81.5% for extra-articular and 60% for intra-articular fractures. Extra-articular fractures treated by FDP had six poor results: four patients had a complete

Table 9.1 Overall anatomical results

	Excellent	Good	Fair	Poor
Number of patients	22	70	22	16
%	17%	54%	17%	12%
	71%		29%	
Definition	Restored to normal	Slight deformation	Noticeable deformation	Significant deformation
Radiological score	AM indices normal, scoring 4	Indices subnormal, scoring 3	One index at 2, the others at 3	One index at 1 or several at 2

distal radio-ulnar joint (DRUJ) dislocation since the radial length had shortened; the fifth poor result was a fracture through an old malunion and the posterior pin was rapidly removed (in the third week) because it was badly tolerated. The remaining poor result was an unexplained unusual dorsal angulation (Table 9.2).

The functional results were also evaluated with Castaing's criteria (1964) noting the range of motion, grip strength and pain (Table 9.3). Each criterion was evaluated from 1 to 6, giving a possible total of 18 points. The results were categorized as follows:

- 'excellent' results score 15–18 points;
- 'good' results score 12–14 points;
- 'fair' results score 9–11 points;
- 'poor' results score ⩽ 8 points.

After six weeks, functional results were good or excellent for 74% of the patients. At the end of the third month, this figure had risen to 92% (Table 9.4). After one year, no poor functional result was present.

Table 9.2 Fair and poor anatomical results

	Fair					Poor			
	RI	PS	RS	UV		RI	PS	RS	UV
Dub.	4	3	4	2					
Jad.	3	4	4	2					
Can.	4	3	4	2					
Car.	4	3	4	2					
Evr.	4	4	4	2					
Ham.	4	4	4	2					
Ver.	4	3	3	2	Bou.	4	4	4	1
Par.	4	4	4	2	Dec.	4	3	4	1
Gla.	4	3	4	2	Car.	4	4	4	1
Hav.	4	4	4	2	Van.	4	3	4	1
DeK.	4	4	4	2	Lau.	4	4	4	1
Del.	4	4	4	2	Par.	4	4	3	1
And.	4	4	4	2	Pod.	3	4	3	1
Ver.	3	4	4	2	Pau.	3	4	3	1
Leb.	3	4	4	2	Col.	4	4	4	1
Mau.	4	3	4	2	Ber.	4	2	3	2
Dem.	4	4	4	2	Vau.	4	3	2	2
Rim.	3	4	4	2	Piu.	4	2	4	2
Ras.	4	3	2	3	Bin.	3	1	3	3
Gon.	2	3	4	3	San.	2	1	3	3
Mas.	2	4	4	3	Lel.	1	4	4	2
Abs.	3	2	4	3	Pia.	1	4	1	1

RI = Radial inclination; PS = Palmer slope or dorsal angulation; RS = Radial shift; UV = Ulnar variance or radial length.

Table 9.3 Functional results

Pain	6:	no pain
	5:	mild pain, not interfering with function
	4:	normal function possible, but painful
	3:	normal movements, work not possible
	2:	interferes with daily activity
	1:	hand unusable
Grip strength	6:	normal grip
	5:	grip slightly diminished
	4:	grip significantly diminished
	3:	grip impossible
	2:	normal movements, no grip
	1:	hand unusable
Range of motion	6:	normal
	5:	flexion extension 90° PS 160°
	4:	flexion extension 60° PS 110°
	3:	flexion extension 45° PS 60°
	2:	flexion extension 30° PS 60°
	1:	none

PS = Pronation–Supination.

Analysis of the results

Detailed analysis of fair and poor anatomical results showed several with alterations of the articular surface orientation. Out of 130 fractures, five malalignments were noted: two in the frontal and three in the sagittal plane. The anatomical deformity was significant in four cases: two in the frontal plane and two in the sagittal. Most of these secondary displacements were the consequences of a technical mistake: the pins which were poorly fixed in the radial head had loosened in the medullary canal, losing their spring effect and allowing the fracture to redisplace. In one case, the secondary displacement occurred after pin removal, after the sixth week. The anterior buttress of the radius was not initially reduced. The other fair and poor results were due to an isolated modification of the radial length by radial shortening at the fracture site. The radiographs showed that secondary impaction was present mainly when there was a lack of support at the anterior part of the distal radius: that is, when the distal epiphysis was translated backwards relative to the metaphysis by insufficient reduction or, more often, when it was translated forwards by excessive reduction (see Figs 9.4a and 9.6b).

Stabilization of this anterior distal buttress fragment of the radius is important to prevent impaction and the consequences of loss of radial length and decreased pronosupination. A third K-wire should be inserted in the fracture line to fix the antero-medial fragment, passing between the neurovascular ulnar bundle and the median nerve. The concavity of the distal radius anterior aspect requires an intrafocal K-wire to prevent rotation of the articular fragment (Fig. 9.5).

When the fracture line of the antero-medial fragment is simple, the pin is inserted percutaneously. A lever movement allows realignment of the fragment and the pin then penetrates the opposite cortex (Kapandji, 1976) to achieve a volar buttress effect. When the fragment is comminuted, the pin is introduced intrafocally into the medullary canal to have a spring effect on the antero-medial fragment (Fig. 9.6). An antero-medial approach is used to insert the K-wire. The anatomical results have improved since the introduction of this third pin. It has not caused complications and seems less dangerous than transfixing external fixators. In the opinion of the author, the importance of this antero-medial fragment has been underestimated.

Table 9.4 Global functional results

		at 6 weeks		at 12 weeks	
Functional result	Score (out of 18)	Number of patients	%	Number of patients	%
Excellent	15–18	35	27%	85	65%
Good	12–14	61	47% (74%)	35	27% (92%)
Fair	9–11	21	16% (28%)	5	4% (8%)
Poor	3–8	13	10%	5	4%

68 FRACTURES OF THE DISTAL RADIUS

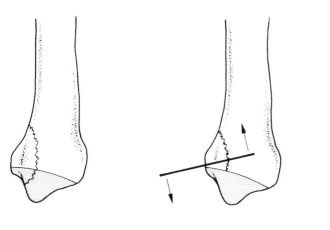

Figure 9.5
Beware of displacement of the anterior articular fragment.

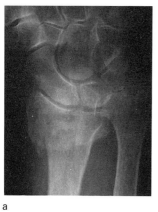
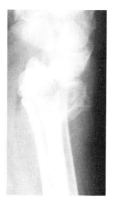
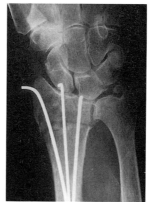
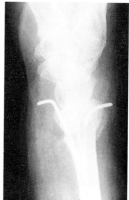
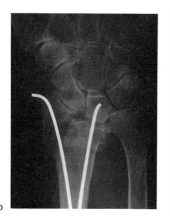
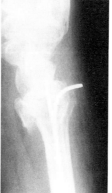

Figure 9.6

Pinning a comminuted fracture. a) T-type fracture with an ulnar component. b) Anterior instability of the antero-medial fragment. c) Reduction and stabilization by an intrafocal anterior pin.

Following FDP, there is a fast functional improvement. Early mobilization without a cast probably explains these results. However, an early return to usual activities can result in bone resorption and a decrease in radial length. This may be the price to pay for a good functional result.

Residual pain usually causes no impairment unless NSD is present (nine cases). The ulnar compartment of the wrist is often the site of this pain. It is not possible to say whether its real cause is the modification of the ulnar variance, or the ulnar styloid fracture (53%). However, after surgical treatment of ulnar styloid pseudoarthrosis, pain has disappeared immediately in some cases. Conversely, a painless wrist is often observed with positive ulnar variance.

It seems likely that the pain is caused by the ulnar styloid or its ligamentous attachments, as it decreases with time. There were no additional procedures in this series requested by the patients; however, if osteotomy had been performed late to correct radial shortening, the excellent results should have shifted from 71% to 91%.

Indications

The ideal indication for the intramedullary flexible double pin (FDP) technique is an extra-articular fracture, irrespective of the magnitude of the dorsal comminution, with a dorso-medial fragment which can be reduced by the insertion of the dorsal pin.

For the other types of fractures, it is often necessary to add a third antero-medial pin if an anterior instability is present. It seems best to correctly stabilize the three main fragments — styloid, postero-medial and antero-medial — at the time of initial treatment. These fragments are in permanent compression due to the spring effect of the pins, and the other fragments will be reduced by the capsuloligamentous attachments.

When many fragments exist and articular fragments are not reduced by the two flexible pins, a third pin can be inserted transversely from the radial styloid process. This pin is used as a lever to reduce the impacted central fragments and/or to give the right alignment to a styloid fragment displaced by the spring effect of the lateral pin. This transverse pin is then fixed in one of the medial fragments, but without restricting pronosupination (Fig. 9.7). These complex cases require a short arm-cast for one to three weeks.

Compression-flexion fractures (Smith type) with a volar displacement, can be divided into two types, depending on whether or not the volar articular fragment is still coherent with the radial styloid process (Fig. 9.8). In the first type, with a volar styloid fragment, the styloid fixation by the external pin is usually sufficient to stabilize the fracture. In the second type, an antero-medial pin will be necessary. This allows the functional treatment of almost all distal radial fractures. In addition, early mobilization of the radiocarpal joint allows realignment of the radial joint surface by the proximal carpus. The non-weight-bearing radiocarpal joint has a low rate of post-traumatic osteoarthritis. Furthermore, the usual patient is a low-demand elderly subject. In such elderly patients, it seems more rewarding to try the functional method by early mobilization than to look for a perfect anatomical reduction with an extensive osteosynthesis requiring long periods of immobilization.

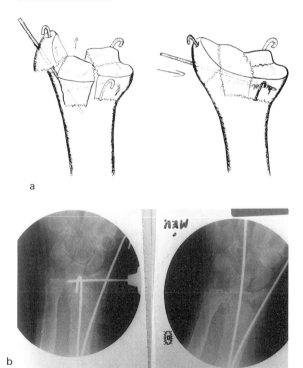

Figure 9.7

a) Effect of the transverse leverage pin. b) Styloid fragment reduced by the transverse pin.

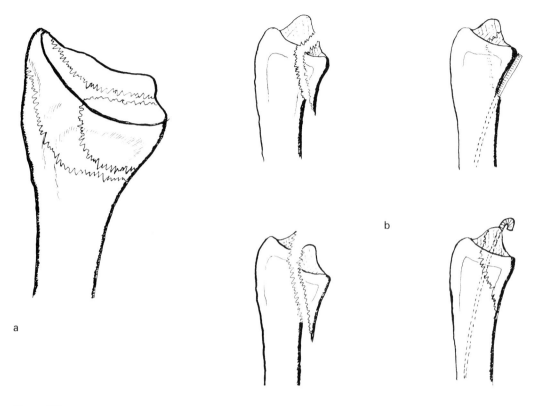

Figure 9.8

Intra-articular fracture in flexion-compression. a) Anterior rim fragment and a styloid anterior fragment. b) Stabilization by a pin.

Conclusions

Treatment of distal radial fractures by the flexible double pin method with 18/10 mm K-wires is an easy and relatively fast procedure which, even when used by a large number of different surgeons, has given a significant number of good anatomical and overall functional results, whatever the fracture type.

It is worthwhile to stabilize the antero-medial fragment and to buttress the radius using a third intrafocal antero-medial K-wire. When a multifragment intra-articular fracture is present, a transverse pin can be useful to realign and fix some of the fragments.

The stabilization obtained by this technique is such that cast immobilization is not necessary, thus allowing an early return to normal activity. This is an important factor affecting the functional result.

References

Castaing J, Le club des dix. Les fractures récentes de l'extrémité inférieure du radius chez l'adulte. *Rev Chir Orthop* 1964; **50**: 581–696.

Desmanet E. L'ostéosynthèse par double embrochage souple du radius. Traitement fonctionnel des fractures de l'extrémité inférieure du radius. A propos d'une série de 130 cas. *Ann Chir Main* 1989; **8, 3**: 193–206.

Kapandji A. L'ostéosynthèse par double embrochage intrafocal. Traitement fonctionnel des fractures non articulaires de l'extrémité inférieure du radius. *Ann Chir* 1976; **30**: 903–8.

10
Treatment of non-articular distal radial fractures by intrafocal pinning with arum pins
AI Kapandji

Distal radius fractures are the most frequently encountered type of fracture. A simple reduction and cast is not always a satisfactory treatment, so many surgeons use osteosynthesis with K-wire pinning set into the distal fragment. However this technique does not always avoid secondary displacement (Castaing 1964; Bleton in press, Di Benedetto et al. 1991, Dunaud 1983–1984, Dunaud 1989, Epinette 1982, Grumillier 1976, Hoël 1991, Kapandji 1976, Kapandji 1987, Kapandji 1991, McQueen 1980, Petit 1976). For this a new kind of osteosynthesis was proposed — intrafocal pinning (Kapandji 1976, Kapandji 1987). A subsequent improvement to this method is the use of special pins termed 'arum' pins (Fig. 10.1) because of their resemblance of its nuts to an arum flower (Kapandji, 1991).

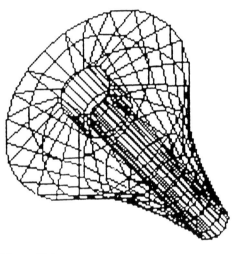

Figure 10.1

The arum nut. Computer-drawn nut, showing the concave conical extremity and smoothly convex base, which prevents tendon damage. On the base is carved a cruciform groove for the special screwdriver. A small 'room', in the nut allows the blunt cut edge of the pin to be hidden, so that it cannot injure the tendons.

Principles of intrafocal pinning

Traditionally, fractures of the distal end of the radius were fixed, after manual reduction, with pins drilled through the distal fragment and pinned into the proximal one (Fig. 10.2). Very quickly, because of the pins' flexibility, the distal fragment moves back (Fig. 10.3) until the pins bump into the inferior edge of the proximal fragment.

In the original method of intrafocal pinning a smooth K-wire is inserted after a manual reduction, through a short skin incision, directly into the fracture line (Fig. 10.4). In this way, any subsequent tilt of the distal fragment is prevented. Secondary displacement is made impossible by the immediate contact of the distal fragment with the pins, which are working as an abutment, not as a resistance component. Additional cast immobilization is not necessary with this technique, allowing immediate rehabilitation, and therefore better functional results. A good fixation needs three pins, inserted at precise points (Fig. 10.5). The first pin is pushed laterally between the tendons of the extensor carpi radialis and that of the extensor pollicis brevis; the second pin is inserted postero-laterally, close to Lister's tubercle, and taking great care to avoid the extensor pollicis longus; the third is postero-medially set,

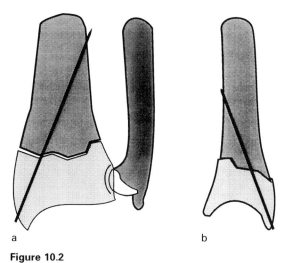

Figure 10.2

Classical pinning of a distal radius fracture. Note that the pin, inserted in the distal part, is located far away from the edge of the proximal part. a) Front view; b) Side view.

passing between the extensor digitorum tendons and the extensor carpi ulnaris tendon. Clearly, this approach needs to avoid the tendons.

Unfortunately, with this first method, it was possible that one of the pins could move either too deeply or too far towards the surface, where it threatened the skin. For this reason, smooth pins were exchanged for threaded ones, using first full-length, and then just end-threaded pins, which ensured their tightening in the opposite wall of the radius. This prevented any secondary displacement of the pins.

An important problem remained unsolved: the damage to the tendons caused by the blunt severed edge of the pin. A tentative solution was the application of small metal or plastic caps, 'hooding' the undesirable spike of the pin pointing under the skin. The positioning of these caps was difficult, however, and often they were dislodged, migrating from their pins.

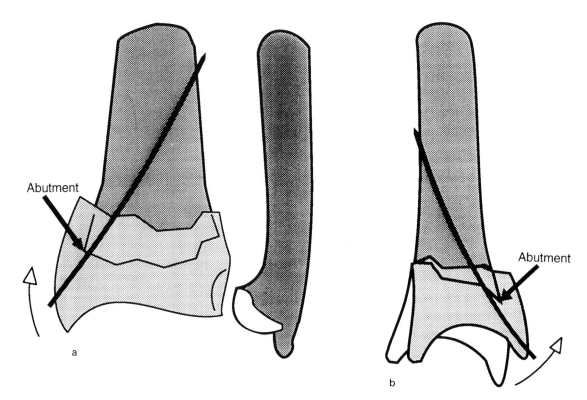

Figure 10.3

Secondary displacement after classical pinning. The pin bends until it is stopped by the edge of the proximal part, which constitutes an impassable barrier. a) Front view; b) Side view.

TREATMENT BY INTRAFOCAL PINNING WITH ARUM PINS

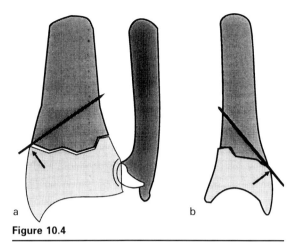

Figure 10.4

Principle of intrafocal pinning. The pin, directly set in the fracture line, makes an immediate abutment, preventing secondary displacement of the distal part. a) Front view; b) side view.

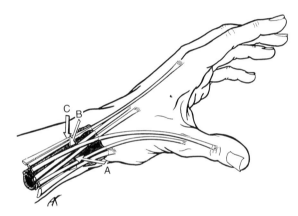

Figure 10.5

The 3 insertion points of the dorsal pins. On this 'transparent' wrist, the 3 points are defined with regard to the tendons: a) the lateral pin is set between the extensor carpi radialis brevis and the extensor pollicis brevis; b) the postero-lateral pin is inserted between the extensor pollicis longus and the extensor indicis; c) the postero-medial pin is set close to the medial side of the tendons of the extensor digitorum, sometimes between those of the fourth and fifth fingers.

Use of arum pins

The solution to all of these problems was found in a new type of intrafocal pin (Kapandji, 1991) — the arum pin (Fig. 10.6). These are full-length-threaded pins with an arum nut (again, so called

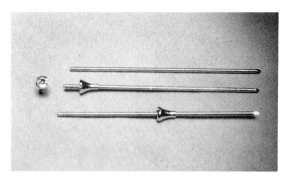

Figure 10.6

Three arum pins. These are 20/10 mm full-length-threaded pins, held with an arum nut. The isolated nut on the left shows the groove and the small 'room' in its base.

because of its resemblance to an arum flower). As it is threaded, the pin cannot be expelled. The nut provides two advantages:

1. As it penetrates, like a wedge, within the fracture line, it has a 'hyper-reduction effect' on the fracture (Fig. 10.7), which compensates in advance for the posterior compression;

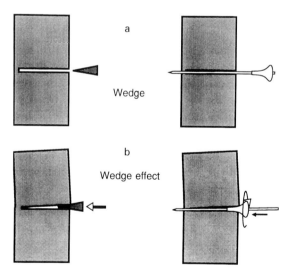

Figure 10.7

The 'wedge effect' of the arum pin. a) A wedge inserted between two pieces widens the space between them. b) When the conical nut of the arum is screwed into the fracture line, it widens this space and has a 'hyper-reduction' effect.

2. The sharp end of the pin is potentially very damaging to the tendons, but both the rounded shape of the nut and the housing of the pin's sharp edge within the base of the nut protect the tendons from any threat (Fig. 10.8).

<u>It is essential to use three pins, and not two, even in the case of a non-articular fracture, because the posterior blocking of the distal fragment is more easily achieved with two posterior pins rather than just one.</u>

Operation method

Setting the arum pins

The operation is performed under tourniquet and general or regional anaesthesia. X-ray amplification is useful but not indispensable. In every case, radiographs must be taken when the pinning is complete.

Fractures with posterior tilt

Fractures with posterior tilt are pinned as follows.

The manual reduction is the same as usual. The placement of each pin is made through three short transverse incisions located on the fracture line, localized by palpation. They should be long enough (7–8 mm) to render the tendons visible. This point is very important. Pins should never be inserted through a simple skin puncture.

The skin is divided, but only the skin, and the subcutaneous tissues are spread with the tip of a small forceps to prevent injury to the subcutaneous nerves. Tendons are separated from each other in the same way or with a haemostat clamp, introduced into an intertendinous interval. As the tips of the first forceps or haemostat are widened, a second one is inserted between them. This second closed forceps is used to scratch the bone in an up-to-down direction (Fig. 10.9a) to find the fracture line as the reduction is slightly improved. When the fracture line is detected, this second forceps or haemostat is gently introduced into the fracture focus (Fig. 10.9b), and its tips are widened so that the pin may be introduced between them and into the fracture.

The pin is held and inserted with a pin-holder, never with a power inserter or K-wire driver. Prior to being firmly positioned in the pin-holder, each threaded pin is prepared with the arum nut in good position. The nut should be at least 1 cm away from the thickness of the bone and in line with the proposed oblique direction of the pin as, visualized on the radiographs. Remember that the pin segment caught in the pin-holder becomes unusable, the threading being squeezed by the chuck.

The pins are inserted in six different stages (Fig. 10.10). From the initial position (Fig. 10.10a):

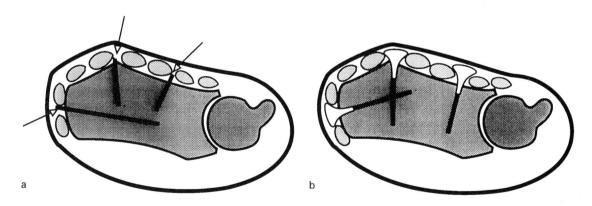

Figure 10.8

Damage to the tendons. a) In the initial technique of intrafocal pinning, the rough cut end of the pins could damage the tendons. b) The smooth shape of the arum nut is designed so that it cannot injure tendons.

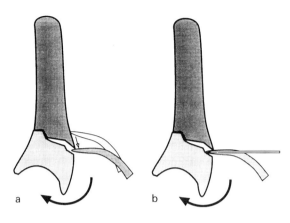

Figure 10.9

Introducing the pin into the fracture line. a) Scratching the dorsal aspect of the radius with a small forceps (or haemostat) allows location of the fracture line. b) The pin is slipped between the two edges of the forceps (or haemostat) and introduced in the fracture site.

Stage 1: the fracture is reduced manually and the pin inserted, first perpendicularly into the bone (Fig. 10.10b).

Stage 2: The pin is then moved obliquely upwards through 45°, until it touches the opposite wall (Fig. 10.10c).

Stage 3: The pin is pointed and screwed into the bone with alternative rotation motions (Fig. 10.10d). Thereafter, any dorsal displacement is impossible and the edges of the two bone's fragments are blocked onto the pin (Fig. 10.10e).

Stage 4: The arum nut is now screwed down while the fracture reduction is slightly improved (Fig. 10.10f). The cone of the arum safely penetrates the interval between the tendons, then moves between the two edges of the fracture, creating the 'reduction effect', until the narrow part of the cone is completely inside. If a greater widening of the fracture edges is desired, it is possible to insert the beginning of the larger part of the cone. Note that the nut must be screwed in a little bit over 2 mm — three or four turns more — so that it can be unscrewed later. A special pin-holder chuck with a screwdriver fitting has been specially made for this procedure (Fig. 10.11) When the pin is correctly mounted, it is possible to do the pinning without changing position. The advantage of this is that the pin is firmly held as the arum nut is screwed or unscrewed.

Stage 5: Special shears, fitted with asymetrical jaws, have also been developed to cut the pin (Fig. 10.10g) very close to the nut (less than 2 mm). With these shears, it is also possible to adjust the depth of the cut: incompletely cut, the pin can be held during the unscrewing of the nut and after unscrewing it can be bent and broken in the nut.

Stage 6: The arum nut is gently unscrewed (Fig. 10.10h) — three or four turns should be enough. This allows the freshly cut pin end to house itself into the small room prepared in the base of the arum, so that it will not harm the tendons. If the adjustment has been properly done, the base of the arum is now located at the level of the subcutaneous tissues.

The skin is closed with an intradermal suture which is not only an aesthetic mode of closure, but also the most innocuous because the stitches do not take a large amount of skin on each side. Thus, the cutaneous circumference is not diminished and the risk of oedema is reduced. It is for this reason that transverse incisions are now recommended.

Figure 10.12 shows the optimim positioning of the three pins. Compare this with the radiographs taken before reduction (Fig. 10.13a and b) and after pinning (Fig. 10.13c and d).

Never put on a cast with this technique; it is a sin against the spirit of the method! Doing so would negate the principal advantage of this technique, the immediate mobilization and rehabilitation. If there is discomfort or pain, it must be controlled with drugs. Even a temporary cast is likely to cause neurosympathetic dystrophy.

It is interesting to note that, when the pins are removed after five weeks, the unscrewing of the arum simultaneously takes off the pin, because the squeezing of the threading by the shears is blocked by the nut. General or regional anaesthesia and tourniquet are necessary for this removal, because of the risk of nerve damage with local anaesthesia.

Fractures with anterior tilt (Smith fracture)

Following the work of Hoël (1991) and Hoël and Kapandji (in press), we now know that it is

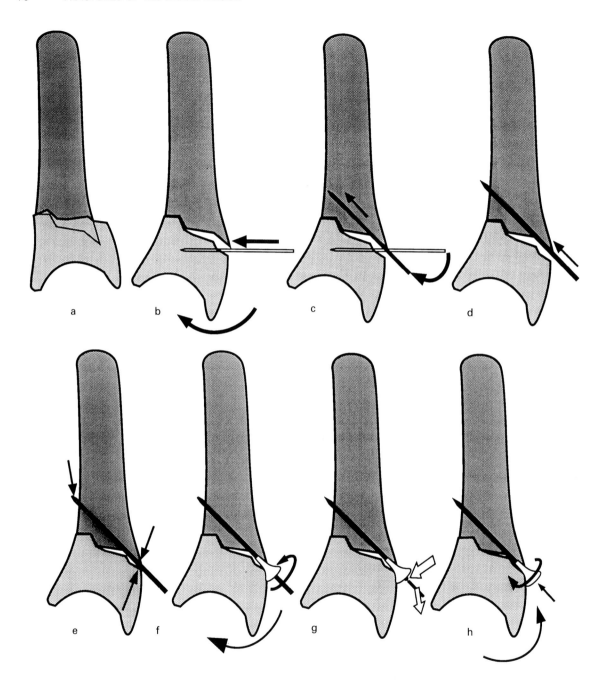

Figure 10.10

The stages of intrafocal pinning (side views). a) The displacement of the fracture is reduced first. b) The pin is introduced, first perpendicularly into the fracture gap. c) The pin is then moved obliquely upwards, until it touches the opposite wall. d) With some alternative rotation motions, it is screwed into the bone. e) Further dorsal displacement is impossible and the two edges of the fragments are blocked onto the pin. f) The arum nut is screwed into the fracture line, as the reduction is improved. g) The pin is cut as close as possible to the nut with the special shears. h) The arum nut is unscrewed until its cut end is housed in the bottom of the nut.

TREATMENT BY INTRAFOCAL PINNING WITH ARUM PINS 77

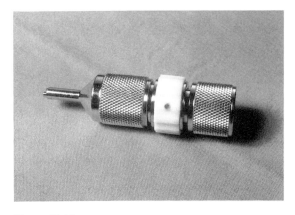

Figure 10.11

The special pin-holder is composed of three parts: on the right, the handle; in the middle, the white piece is the knob for tightening the pin into the chuck; on the left, the screwdriver, which turns freely around the handle. The entire device may be firmly held in the palm of the hand to allow precise direction of the arum pin.

of the wrist, at the lateral side of the flexor carpi radialis (FCR). Here, the subcutaneous tissues are spread with a small forceps or haemostat until they touch the palmar surface of the radius between the FCR tendon and the radial artery, which is clearly seen and protected. The fracture line is found using the forceps or haemostat. The pin is introduced perpendicularly, then obliquely and inserted into the opposite wall. The arum screwed between the two borders is perfectly tolerated by the tendon and the artery.

2. An alternative approach uses an antero-medial pin (Fig. 10.14b), placed by the method described by Kapandji at the lateral

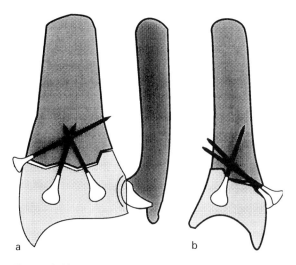

Figure 10.12

The ideal location of the 3 dorsal arum pins. a) Front view. b) Side view.

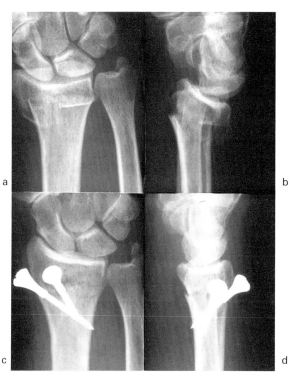

Figure 10.13

Radiographs of a Colles' fracture before and after arum pins. a) Front (AP) view of the fracture: note the shortening with lateral (radial) tilt, the positive ulnar variance, the integrity of the articular surface and the small dorsal fragment. b) Lateral view of the fracture: the dorsal tilt is clearly seen, as is the posterior (dorsal) comminution. c) Front (AP) view after reduction with only 2 arum pins: the shape of the radial epiphysis is restored; the ulnar variance is slightly negative. d) Lateral view after reduction: the dorsal tilt is completely reduced and the articular surface orientation is restored.

possible to insert anterior pins, only the approach is different. Two pins may be inserted as follows (Fig. 10.14):

1. One antero-lateral pin (Fig. 10.14a), is inserted by the method described by Hoël using a short vertical or, even better, a horizontal (radial) incision made at the anterior (palmar) aspect

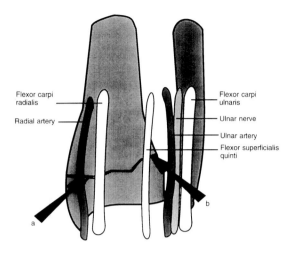

Figure 10.14

The two anterior (palmar) approaches for arum pins. a) The antero-lateral approach: between the tendon of the flexor carpi radialis and the radial artery. b) The antero-medial approach: between the tendons of the flexors digitorum, communis, ulnarly and the ulnar nerve and artery flanked by the tendon of the flexor carpi ulnaris.

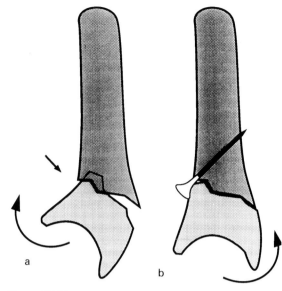

Figure 10.15

Inserting an arum pin in a fracture with anterior tilt. a) The fracture with an anterior tilt; lateral view. b) The inserted arum pin; lateral view. Note that the nut makes an abutment to the distal fragment.

(radial) side of the flexor carpi ulnaris, and moved through the interval between ulnar artery and nerve and the tendons of the flexor quinti superficialis and profundus. Once more, there is no concern regarding injury to the tendon, nerve and artery because of the smooth shape of the arum nut.

These methods can be used to reduce and fix fractures with anterior tilt (Fig. 10.15).

Evaluation of operation results

For a good evaluation of the immediate results provided by the radiographs, it is indispensable to use objective criteria with angles and millimetres.

On radiographic examination (antero-posterior view), the normal (or anatomically reduced) radius shows the following (Fig. 10.16a):

- the bistyloid line (BSL) is tilted at +10–15° on the horizontal line;
- the front articular (or glenoid) line (FGL), also called the radial inclination angle (Di Benedetto 1991) is tilted at +21–24° on the horizontal line;
- the ulnar variance (UV) is normally equal to −2 mm (the negative value is taken when the level of the ulnar head is located above the level of the inferior edge of the sigmoid notch).

An imperfect reduction is characterized radiographically by the following (Fig. 10.16b):

- the bistyloid line (BSL) becomes horizontal or inverted to negative values (−10°);
- the front articular (glenoid) line (FGL), or radial inclination angle, also tends to be horizontal or even inverted, to a measurement of −10°;
- the ulnar variance (UV) becomes positive (+4), indicating a compression of the distal part of the radius onto the proximal radius;
- a radio-ulnar diastasis (d) may be noted eventually, indicating a rupture or a tearing of the triangular fibrocartilage.

On lateral radiographs (Fig. 10.17a) the normal criterion is:

- the side glenoid line (SGL) or lateral articular surface is +15°. The articular surface of the radius is oriented downwards and slightly forwards.

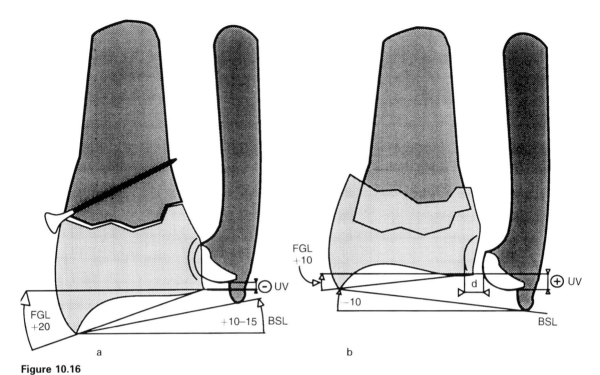

Figure 10.16

Criteria of reduction from radiographic examination: front (AP) view. a) Normal (or anatomically reduced) radius. BSL, bistyloid line is +10–15°; FGL, radial inclination angle is +20° UV, ulnar variance is −2 mm; b) Poor reduction, or non-reduction of radius. The tilt of the BSL is inverted, and may become negative. The FGL value diminishes or becomes negative. The UV value becomes positive.

An imperfect reduction (Fig. 10.17b) is characterized by:

- tilting of the lateral articular surface (side glenoid line) to neutral or with dorsal angulation. The measurement of the SGL is −10°, which indicates the dorsal or posterior tilt. Note that even a zero value for the GL indicates a posterior tilt;
- when the UV becomes positive, it allows measurement of the degree of compression of the distal fragment.

These values may be noted on a Patient Evaluation Form: a table with the values of the angles defined above, measured before and after reduction and pinning, and also after removal of the pins. The direction and angles of the secondary displacements may be easily appreciated by comparing normal, pre- and post-reduction measurements.

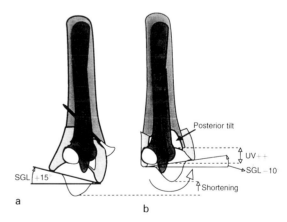

Figure 10.17

Criteria for reduction on a lateral radiograph. a) Normal. SGL, side glenoid line (lateral articular surface) is +15° palmar, so that the articular surface faces downwards and slightly forwards. b) Poor reduction, or non-reduction. SGL side glenoid line (lateral articular surface) becomes negative (i.e. dorsal angulation). UV becomes positive, as an impaction is visible and associated with a posterior (dorsal) tilt.

Complications

Intraoperative complications

Injury to a cutaneous nervous branch may be avoided by making a large enough incision: the skin incision must not be smaller than 7–8 mm and the subcutaneous tissues must be spread, not sharply divided. Injury of extensor or flexor tendons is not possible if they are seen and gently retracted so that one can pass in a safe interval. Some surgeons have pointed out that an over-reduction, with an undesired anterior tilt, has sometimes occurred. This complication may happen when the pin is set too vertically: its tilt must not be greater than 45°. When anterior tilt does occur, it is always possible to insert an anterior pin to correct the over-reduction.

Postoperative complications

With the new arum pins, there are no longer problems with loosening pins or tendon damage, but it is always important to be very careful to avoid the subcutaneous nerves, as subcutaneous neuromas are serious complications.

Malunions may occur with dorsal or lateral tilt loss of reduction. Less than ideal reductions may not compromise good function: on the whole, the functional results are less poor than with closed reduction procedures, except when the distal radio-ulnar joint (DRUJ) is displaced with a compression of the distal medial fracture fragment dorsally or laterally. Dislocation of the DRUJ may compromise pronation-supination motion, a complication observed in all types of treatment for Colles' fracture. Paradoxically, the main trouble with malunions are not the flexion-extension restrictions, but the pronation-supination problems which require specific treatment at the DRUJ and not particularly at the radius malunion itself.

Neurosympathetic dystrophy, which is the most severe complication following all kinds of treatment, is rare with this technique (Dunaud 1983–1984, Dunaud et al. 1989, Epinette et al. 1982, Grumillier 1976), probably partly because of the continuous motion of the wrist that prevents disuse and a poor mental picture of the fracture and hand function.

Results

The results of this technique were first evaluated by Epinette et al. (1982) based on a study of 72 cases treated using the first technique (that is, with smooth K-wires). An important aspect of the results was that the mobility was good or excellent in 88% and the rate of neurosympathetic dystrophy was less than one-third of our previous experience. After three to six months, the pain had totally disappeared in 95% of patients, the grip strength was normal in 67%, and finger mobility was normal in 80%. The previous activity level was recovered in 80% (by four weeks for 21%, by six weeks for 53% and by eight weeks for 93%).

Secondary displacements were less frequent than in closed reduction and casting procedures (25%), but even when they did occur the functional results were better (Petit 1976) because of the immediate rehabilitation.

Malunions occurred in 29% but the functional results were still good, except when there was disruption of the DRUJ. Radiological results were excellent to good in 70%. The patients were satisfied with excellent results in 75% and good results in 13%. There were only 1.5% of patients with poor results and 10.5% with fair results.

The superiority of the intrafocal procedure is confirmed by recent publications (Bleton et al. in press, Di Benedetto et al. 1991, Dunaud 1983–1984). Most of the authors draw attention to the decreased rate of the neurosympathetic dystrophy, the frequency of which falls to 1.3%. It appeared occasionally when a 'security cast' had been applied at the start of treatment. The most recent work by Dunaud and colleagues (1989) based on 233 cases, points out the excellence of the results (Table 10.1).

Indications

In this chapter, we have considered only non-articular (extra-articular) fractures of the distal radius. We believe that intrafocal pinning with arum pins is indicated in every case, whatever the type or the degree of the displacement. The procedure gives excellent and secure results thanks to the immediate rehabilitation. In any

Table 10.1 Results of a study of 233 cases of distal radius fracture treated with intrafocal pinning (Dunaud et al. 1989)

Functional results (in %)
Excellent	37%	total 93% excellent and good
Good	56%	
Poor	6%	
Bad	1%	

Objective results
Excellent	63%	total 92% excellent and good
Good	29%	
Poor	6.5%	
Bad	1.5%	

The small difference between these and the functional results is due to pain and loss of grip strength

Radiological results
Excellent	67%	total 89% excellent and good
Good	22%	
Poor	6%	
Bad	5%	

Complications
2 sepsis cases resolved with pins removal.
1% suffered neurosympathetic dystrophy.

Most of complications were due to technical mistakes at the beginning of the practice.

---

other technique, the treatment requires four or five weeks of immobilization; the patient then begins the rehabilitation programme, which needs weeks to compensate for and eliminate the stiffness of the initial functional block of motion (that is, the cast or splint). On the other hand, with intrafocal pinning, a fracture of the distal radius recovering a function that was never really lost. At times as soon as three weeks after operation, at the first clinical follow-up review, the function is already almost normal and some patients have returned to their previous activities. For this simple reason, the final functional result is much better: the cases treated with intrafocal pinning are cured, whereas those treated with other methods are just beginning to recover.

Is it necessary to use this procedure in case of fractures without any displacement? Previously, I would have said no, but now, I would say yes, for two reasons: first, the non-displaced fractures often displace later in spite of a good cast; and secondly, because immobilization in a cast is used for undisplaced fractures, even for a short time period, may cause functional troubles, often which are hard to overcome. In fractures with posterior (dorsal) comminution, it is also possible to use this procedure, especially with arum pins, because the cone penetration compensates, in advance, for the posterior tilt reduction. The larger diameter of the cone, compared to a simple pin, gives better support to the border of the distal fragment.

In fractures with an anterior tilt, it is quite possible to set one or two anterior pins that control the displacement perfectly, without any injury or loss of function of the tendons or other important structures like nerves and arteries. The palmar approach is more limited than the one needed for the setting of an anterior plate, and the fixation is as firm with pins as with a plate.

In children, Salter II fractures must be cared for with orthopaedic reduction and a cast, but if a secondary displacement does occur, the use of two arum pins, kept in place for only two weeks, is a good procedure to help maintain the reduction. The technique can also be used with two-bone distal fractures (Fig. 10.18).

Conclusions

The results of the treatment of distal radius fractures have been greatly improved by intrafocal pinning, especially with the arum pin

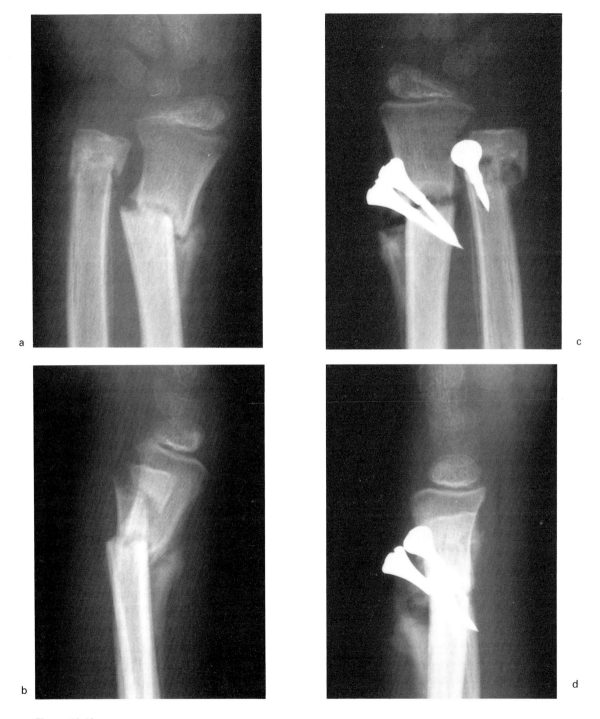

Figure 10.18

Radiographs of a secondary displacement in a distal 2-bone fracture in a child. a) Malunion of a distal 2-bone fracture in a child after 2 weeks: front (AP) view. b) Lateral view of the same case. c) Front (AP) view of this fracture after breaking the malunion and arum pinning. d) Lateral view of the same case with arum pins.

procedure. The functional results are not always parallel to the anatomical ones. Non-interruption of the function of the hand and wrist is the explanation of this paradox; motion and function are made possible thanks to this precise and firm fixation which does not need a wide exposure and is easy to do. This procedure needs only care and precision.

References

Castaing J. Les fractures récentes de l'extrémité inférieure du radius chez l'adulte. *Rev Chir Orthop* 1964; **50**: 581–666.

Bleton R, Boulate M, Alnot JY. Etude comparative de trois traitements de fractures de l'extrémité inférieure du radius. *Ann Chir Main* (in press).

Di Benedetto MR, Lubbers LM, Ruff ME, Nappi JF, Coleman CR. Quantification of error in measurement of radial inclination angle and radial-carpal distance. *J Hand Surg* 1991; **16A**: 399–400.

Dunaud JL. L'embrochage intra-focale 'en berceau' des fractures de l'extrémité inférieure du radius. Incidence de ce traitement en matière de réparation des dommages corporels. Memoire pour le CES de réparation juridique du dommage corporel (N° 02100 Saint Quentin), Université R. Descartes Paris V. 1983–1984.

Dunaud JL, Moughabghab M, Caron M, Ben Slama H. Bilan d'une série de 233 fractures de l'extrémité inférieure du radius traitées selon la technique de Kapandji. In *11ème cours de chirurgie de la main.* Paris: Hôpital Bichat. 1989.

Epinette JA, Lehut JM, Cavenaille M, Bouretz JC, Decoulx J. Fractures de Pouteau–Colles: double embrochage intra-focal 'en berceau' selon Kapandji. A propos d'une série homogène de 72 cas. *Ann Chir Main* 1982; **1**: 71–83.

Grumillier P. Fractures de l'extrémité inférieure du radius. Thèse de Médecine. Nancy, 1976.

Hoël G. La voie antero-externe pour le brochage intra-focal des fracture de l'extrémité inférieure du radius à déplacement antérieur. Communication at The International Symposium on the Wrist. Nagoya. 1991.

Hoël G, Kapandji A. Ostéosynthèse par broches intra-focales des fractures à déplacement antérieur de l'épiphyse radiale inférieure. *Ann Chir Main* (in press).

Kapandji A. Ostéosynthèse par double embrochage intra-focal. Traitement fonctionnel des fractures non articulaires de l'extrémité inférieure du radius. *Ann Chir* 1976; **30**: 903–8.

Kapandji A. L'embrochage intra-focal des fractures de l'extrémité inférieure du radius ans après. *Ann Chir Main* 1987; **6**: 57–63.

Kapandji A. Les broches intra-focales à 'effet de réduction' de type 'Arum' dans l'ostéosynthèse des fractures de l'extrémité inférieure du Radius. *Ann Chir Main* 1991; **10**: 138–45.

McQueen M, Caspers J. Colles' fractures: does the anatomic result affect the final function? *J Bone Joint Surg* 1980; **70B**: 649–51.

Petit J, et le GECO. Fractures de l'extrémité inférieure du radius. Rapport de la première réunion du Groupe d'Etude de Chirurgie Osseuse. 1976.

11
Bone cementing of distal radial fractures in the elderly

Y Kiyoshige

Distal radial fractures in elderly individuals are frequently encountered in orthopaedic practice, but unfortunately these fractures tend to be treated without any particular awareness of the nature of geriatric physiology.

Osteoporosis is an underlying condition in many older patients, and it is not unusual for this kind of fracture to become unstable and redislocate, with loss of fracture reduction. If the orthopaedic surgeon's concern is confined to anatomical reduction and preservation of that reduction, severe reflex sympathetic dystrophy can occur, even when bone union is obtained. Obviously, these complications can impair the function of the hand.

Treatment options, both conservative and surgical, for distal radial fractures in younger patients have been developed with recent advances in knowledge of the biomechanics of the wrist joint. However, these treatment options are not applicable to elderly patients because of the physiological differences between elderly and younger patients.

Orthopaedic surgeons face an apparent dilemma in the treatment of elderly patients: the problem of achieving stability whilst counteracting joint stiffness. As a result of this dilemma, elderly patients often experience deformity, pain and restricted range of motion after treatment.

For that reason, the author has developed a technique in which intramedullary fixation with bone cement is used for elderly patients with distal radial fractures in an effort to keep the alignment of fracture and produce a rigid fixation. This method has yielded excellent results, allowing patients to use the affected hand immediately after operation and without external fixation.

Materials and methods

During the period 1990 to 1991 ten patients, all women over 75 years old, were treated for distal radial fracture. Their ages ranged from 75 to 91 years (mean age: 81.6 years). The right wrist was affected in five cases and the left in the other five cases.

All patients were right-handed. An associated fracture of the distal ulnar shaft was present in two cases. Within two days of the injury, intramedullary fixation with bone cement was performed. In each case, manual reduction was performed under an axillary block, and the reduced position was transcutaneously maintained with a K-wire. To insert the K-wires, a dorsal longitudinal incision was made, separating the extensor carpi radialis (ECR) and extensor pollicis longus (EPL) tendons. When necessary, the proximal portion of the extensor retinaculum was partially divided to expose the fractured area. The dorsal cortex of the fractured area was incised over an area of about 15 mm by 10 mm, while the periosteum was preserved as much as possible.

The fracture often had the appearance of a bone window already. As the bone in these elderly patients is osteoporotic, the cancellous bone in the fractured area had already collapsed. The medullary cavity was enlarged with a bone curette, so that a sufficient amount of cement could be introduced. After careful irrigation of the fracture site and removal of blood by suction, the bone cavity was filled with bone cement. The dorsal cortical bone removed to create the bone window was placed back on top of the bone cement (Fig. 11.1).

In earlier cases, the K-wire (used to maintain the reduced position) was cut at a point very close to the cortex, and left within the bone to serve as a 'prop'. In recent cases, however, the K-wire is removed completely before the cement has hardened. After replacing the bone window, as much of the periosteum as possible was sutured to cover this area. Finally, the subcutaneous tissue and skin were closed.

After the operation, some patients were given a splint, which was used for four weeks, following the procedure described by Nilsson (1979) and by Schmalholz (1989). For the remaining cases, only an elastic bandage was used after the operation. All patients were instructed to put their wrist through the full range of motions, so long as this activity could be performed without pain. They were also told not to lift themselves using the operated wrist. Active range of motion (ROM) exercise was started within the framework of physical therapy such that the patients could return to normal life without the need for passive exercises to increase the range of motion.

Results

In this study, the range of motion of wrist joint (dorsiflexion, volar flexion, radial deviation, ulnar deviation, supination and pronation), the pulp–palm distance and the grip strength were evaluated. Radiographically, the author tried to determine when bone fusion was complete and how bone atrophy had advanced. Out of the 10 cases, three (one in which a splint was applied for four weeks, one which was complicated by dementia, and one which dropped out of the study) were excluded from evaluation.

Normal mobility of the wrist was obtained within three weeks. Grip strength tended to improve after resolution of pain, and maximum strength was achieved within six weeks. The pulp–palm distance reached 0 mm for all fingers within one week in all but one case, which was affected by fractures of both bones in one forearm. Cortical bone healing, measured radiographically, was completed in six to seven weeks; callus formation also occurred around the cortex of the bone window. The postoperative alignment of fractures was preserved throughout the follow-up period. When the extent of bone atrophy was assessed with the microdensitometry method (GSmin, which reflects cancerous bone density), the cemented cases were comparable to cast-wearing middle-aged patients (Fig. 11.2).

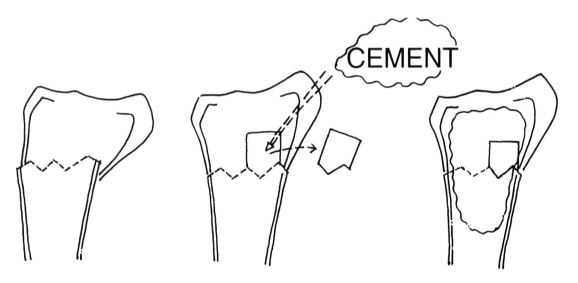

Figure 11.1

Surgical procedure. The fracture is exposed between the ECR and EPL tendons. The dorsal cortex of the fracture area is opened with a bone window. The medullary bone deficiency is filled with bone cement, and the dorsal cortex replaced on top of the cement.

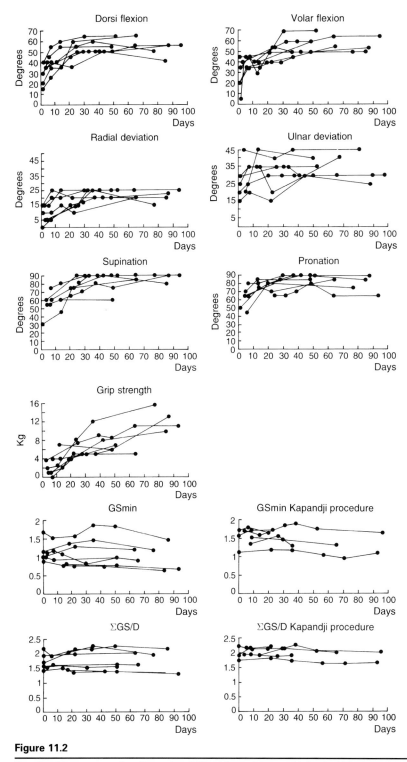

Figure 11.2

Results of bone cementing. Normal mobility of the wrist was obtained within three weeks, and grip strength within six weeks. The degree of bone atrophy was assessed with the microdensitometry method (Inoue et al. 1983) (GSmin and ΣGS/D, which reflect mineral content) and compared with that of middle-aged cases treated with the Kapandji procedure. The extent of bone atrophy in the cemented cases was comparable with that of the Kapandji cases.

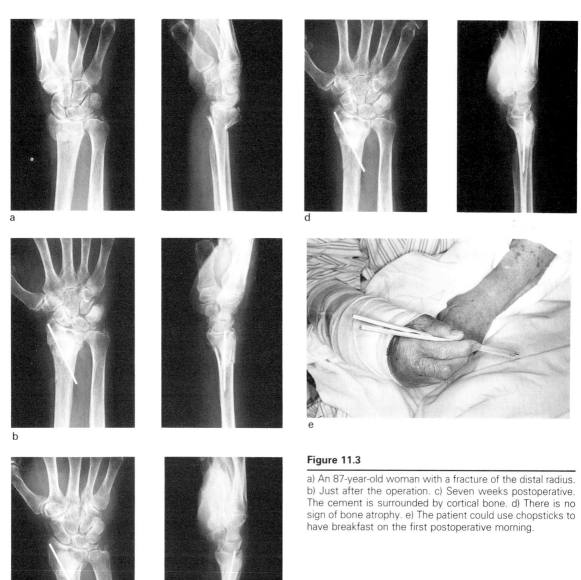

Figure 11.3

a) An 87-year-old woman with a fracture of the distal radius. b) Just after the operation. c) Seven weeks postoperative. The cement is surrounded by cortical bone. d) There is no sign of bone atrophy. e) The patient could use chopsticks to have breakfast on the first postoperative morning.

Conclusions

The use of bone cement in cases of distal radial fracture was first reported in 1970 by Charnley. Thereafter, only a few cases in Scandinavian countries were treated with this method (Nilsson 1979, Schmalholz 1989, Kofoed 1983). According to Charnley, bone formation did not occur in the region where the cement had not been covered with cortex bone. In the Scandinavian cases, the cement was used as an intramedullary core for primary fixation, after which the bone window was closed again and the periosteum was repaired as well as possible. In these cases, periosteal bone formation occurred, and bone union was complete in six to seven weeks.

As bone cement is used for core support within the distal radius, it can loosen as a result of progression of osteoporosis. It is therefore recommended that bone cement be used only for patients over 75 years of age. However, if a bioactive cement, which is now under development (Kitsugi, 1983), becomes clinically available, the indication for this therapy may be expanded. This could apply to comminuted fractures in younger patients, which are difficult to reduce and hold with current techniques. Rigid fixation allows use of the hand very soon after injury, and early mobilization leads to better functional recovery. In elderly patients, the only means of preventing reflex sympathetic dystrophy is to permit early use of the affected hand. At present, only bone cementing can produce the rigid fixation of the porotic bone needed for early use.

This therapy allows for rapid and excellent functional recovery (in terms of range of motion and grip strength) without necessitating postoperative external fixation. Bear in mind, however, that bone atrophy may occur. Overall, bone cementing can be considered to be especially suitable for elderly patients with a good quality of life.

References

Charnley J. *Acrylic cement in orthopedic surgery.* Edinburgh: Churchill Livingstone. 1970: 67–71.

Inoue T, Miyamoto S, Kusida K, Sumi Y, Orimo H, Yamashita G. Quantitative assessment of bone density on x-ray picture. *J Jap Orth Assoc 1983*; **57**: 1923–36.

Kitsugi T. Bone behaviour between two bioactive ceramics in vivo. *J Biomed Mater Res* 1983; **21**: 1109–23.

Kofoed H. Communited displaced Colles' fracture. Treatment with intramedullary methyl metacrylate stabilization. *Acta Orthop Scand* 1983; **54**: 307–11.

Nilsson MH. Bone cementing in the treatment of Colles' fracture. *Opuscula Medica* 1979; **24**: 123–25.

Schmalholz A. Bone cement for redislocated Colles' fracture. A prospective comparison with closed treatment. *Acta Orthop Scand* 1989; **60**: 212–17.

12
Treatment of extra-articular malunions of the distal radius
J Duparc, B Melchior, B Valtin

Extra-articular fractures of the distal radius are considered benign and have a more favourable prognosis than intra-articular fractures. Traditionally, they have been treated by conservative methods. Healing was often obtained with a slight malunion and a fair functional result, allowing normal use for everyday life. Surgical treatment was indicated only for disabling malunions, usually by distal ulnar resection or distal radial alignment osteotomy (Boyd and Stone 1944, Darrach 1915, Merle and Masse 1950).

Malunions are now less common because initial treatment is more precise. Percutaneous pinning, plate or external fixation are more frequently recommended and indicated particularly in high-velocity injuries due to motorbike accidents, which have increased among young people. These injuries result in significant fracture displacement and comminution, and a precise reduction is mandatory. Malunion may cause severe impairment in professional life, particularly for manual workers. In extra-articular malunions, functional alterations are usually linked to distal radio-ulnar joint (DRUJ) disorders (Darrow et al. 1985, Morrissy 1979).

In this chapter, we will present our experience with distal radius osteotomy with realignment and bone graft, which is now preferred to isolated ulnar head resection.

Pathomechanism of extra-articular malunions

The study of malunions of the distal radius enables us to understand the mechanisms of deformity and the cause of functional problems of the wrist. The following aspects have to be considered: the distal radial epiphyseal displacement, the anatomical disorders of the DRUJ and the reaction of the carpus to the radial malunion.

Epiphyseal displacement

Displacement of the distal radial epiphysis reflects the initial fracture displacement. Dorsal tilt results secondary to the dorsal comminution; the distal radial articular surface is dorsally oriented instead of having the normal 15° volar tilt (angulation). A horizontal radial inclination, an epiphyseal translation and, at times, a rotation malalignment may be present. A reverse deformity with an increased volar tilt (Smith's fracture) is less common.

In extra-articular malunions, the distal segment (epiphyseal) displacement does not directly influence the radiocarpal joint but the range of motion (ROM) is modified.

DRUJ disorders

There are two different types of DRUJ disorder: the first is a consequence of a distal radius displacement while the second results from direct injury to the DRUJ.

DRUJ disorders secondary to distal radius displacement

The ulna is the stable element and the radial displacement causes dislocation from the DRUJ. There is a modification in the sigmoid notch orientation. Radial displacement can have several consequences:

- radial shortening, almost always present, leaves a longer ulna;
- lateral displacement of the radius creates a distal radio-ulnar gap;
- dorsal tilt results in incongruency and sometimes a complete dislocation of the DRUJ;
- rotation and displacement of the radius modifies the rotation axis of the two bones which, as a consequence, are no longer concurrent (Fig. 12.1).

The functional consequences depend on the magnitude of distal radius displacement. In significant displacements, combining radial shortening and a complete dislocation of the DRUJ, the articular surfaces lose contact and, surprisingly, pain is mild although the cosmetic deformity is significant. Conversely, when the articular surfaces are in contact but injured, there is a significant functional impairment at the DRUJ with painful pronosupination and loss of joint mobility.

Direct DRUJ injuries

The sigmoid notch can be interrupted by the fracture line in both extra-articular and intra-articular radiocarpal fractures. Ligamentous injuries may be associated with bone displacements. The triangular fibrocartilage (TFC) disruption or ulnar styloid fracture, which can be its equivalent, is associated with distal radio-ulnar volar and dorsal ligament injuries or capsular lesions. The ulnar styloid fracture can result in non-union with a lateral displacement. An ulnar neck fracture may sometimes be associated with a distal radius fracture and can result in a non-union or a malunion if not recognized and treated. The extensor carpi ulnaris tendon can be displaced or dislocated from its sheath. Malunions of the distal radius affecting the DRUJ have been studied recently by several authors (Minami et al. 1987, Morrissy 1979, Watson et al. 1983), who have shown that CT scanning, MRI and perioperative findings allow a better understanding of these injuries.

Carpal consequences of malunions of the distal radius

Carpal instability deformities in distal radial malunions have been described by Taleisnik and Watson (1984). In most cases, it is an 'adaptive carpus' caused by the change of orientation of the distal radius. This secondary carpal instability should be differentiated from that caused by ligament injuries (Oberlin 1990). These secondary instabilities usually produce clinical symptoms of weakness in grip and loss of motion (wrist flexion). Surgical treatment of the radial deformity realigns the carpus (Taleisnik and Watson 1984). However, in a very late malunion, this deformity may cause carpal ligament strain associated with the fracture and this combined injury may be missed initially. When considering treatment of distal radial

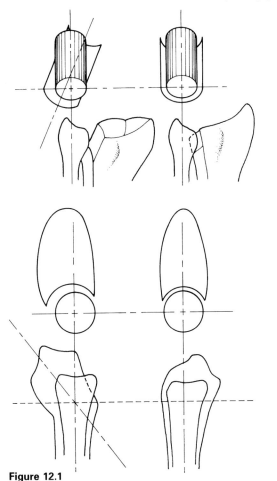

Figure 12.1

Distal radial displacement creates DRUJ incongruency.

malunions, the clinical and radiological signs of carpal instability should be sought because if the two disorders are not treated at the same time, painful sequelae will persist after surgical correction of the malunion.

Examination

Clinical symptoms may be either isolated or associated with other causes of wrist pain or wrist instability. Deformity of the distal radial epiphysis is assessed by a comparative examination of both wrists. In most cases of increased dorsal tilt and loss of radial inclination of the distal epiphysis, the clinical deformity is associated with a dorsal hump in the wrist and dorsal prominence of the distal ulna when the hand is in radial inclination. This cosmetic deformity alone may be a reason for corrective surgery.

Motion should be compared to the opposite side for both the radiocarpal and distal radioulnar joints. A decreased range of motion and modification of the usual planes of motion should be noted. Stiffness, though not common in extra-articular malunions, may be found in certain conditions such as neurosympathetic dystrophy (NSD), long-standing application of external fixation, or infection. A normal ROM (approximately 130–140° flexion–extension) is often preserved but with a predominance of extension. Ulnar deviation may be lost when the loss of radial inclination (increased horizontalization) is significant or when there is an ulnocarpal impingement secondary to loss of radial length. At the DRUJ, the dysfunction of prono-supination is very common and these mechanical disturbances are often associated with painful and clicking motions.

The amount of pain is variable. Mechanical pain usually occurs only when using the wrist, mainly with heavy straining and with prono-supination. Localization of the pain over the ulnar part of the wrist is almost constant. There may be a painful arc of motion, a painful click with ulnar head subluxation, or a painful limitation of the supination. This sudden pain can result in loss of grasp when holding objects. The pain of neurosympathetic dystrophy (NSD) should be considered differently: it is an inflammatory pain, occurs at rest, and is associated with oedema and vasomotor signs. The presence of NSD constitutes a contraindication to surgery.

Decrease of strength is common in malunions. In the absence of pain, this can be the consequence of an alteration in the lever arm of the flexor tendons of the fingers. It should be measured with dynamometers in a comparative and repetitive way. This decrease in strength can be exaggerated by pain.

Combined injuries may be neurological or tendinous (Amadio 1987, Cooney et al. 1980, Duparc and Veltin 1977, Lynch and Lipscomb 1963). Median nerve compression is the most frequent, though still uncommon. The dorsal malalignment of the radius and the deviation of the median nerve as it courses to the carpal tunnel are the usual causes. The initial onset of symptoms should be carefully analysed before assuming that malunion is the cause, since carpal tunnel syndrome is common and the association of these two pathologies can be random.

Chronic compression of the ulnar nerve in Guyon's tunnel is uncommon. The superficial branches of the radial nerve can be injured from the fracture or during percutaneous pinning, and often result in painful neuromas. A longitudinal incision (8–10 mm) incision is proposed by a majority of authors to preserve these branches before inserting percutaneous pins.

Tendinous ruptures from a bone spike or from callus may affect the flexor or extensor tendons of the fingers, but tendon injuries are uncommon. The extensor pollicis longus is the most frequently ruptured within its fibrous sheath, since a compartment syndrome forms from the bony fracture callus.

Radiological assessment

Plain radiographs are necessary to assess the deformity and to make appropriate preoperative planning. On antero-posterior views, radial inclination and the radio-ulnar index are measured. On lateral views, the distal radial dorsal–volar surface orientation is measured (the normal volar angulation being 10°). On standard radiographs, it is not always easy to appreciate DRUJ abnormalities, and slight displacements are not always detected. CT scanning (axial tomography) of the DRUJ in different comparative positions of pronation and supination may point out incongruity. A normal radio-ulnar index does not preclude an incongruency of the DRUJ which may be visible only in the transverse plane. It is well known, as demonstrated by Kapandji (1991) that the DRUJ is unstable in pronation. The distal ulna subluxates dorsally in that position and can be compressed against the dorsal rim of the sigmoid notch. MRI can be of value but is less used. It may be of better value in detecting ligament injuries. The carpal ligament injuries may also be detected on dynamic radiographs (motion views) of the wrist (Oberlin 1990).

Time lapse since injury

Surgical indication also depends on the time which has elapsed since the original injury. Malunion is considered as 'late' after six months. The clinical symptoms will not change and bone calcification is stable by this time and allows for surgical planning.

Conversely, a recent malunion (less than six months) presents with symptoms which can still recede. The bone callus is not totally calcified and osteoporosis is common. Planning surgery is more difficult in these circumstances. Age, sex, occupation, hand dominance and patient needs should always be considered.

Treatment options

The treatment of distal radial malunions has evolved recently. Darrach's procedure (Boyd and Stone 1944, Darrach 1915, Darrow et al. 1985, Linscheid 1985, Minami et al. 1987, Narakas 1977) was first performed for treatment of painful distal radio-ulnar impingement. This procedure takes care of the painful impingement but the distal radial deformity persists. To correct malunion of the distal radius the Darrach procedure was combined with realignment osteotomies to correct the distal radial deformity (Merle and Masse 1950). It became evident that the Darrach procedure may not be indicated (and had complications) and anatomical realignment of the distal radius became the primary aim of surgical treatment (Duparc et al. 1977, Duparc and Veltin 1977 and 1984, Fernandez 1988).

Radial osteotomy without bone graft

Restoration of normal orientation to the distal radial articular surface can be achieved by facet osteotomy, curvilinear osteotomy or plane oblique osteotomy (Sisk 1987, Minami et al. 1987). These techniques are not easy to perform, and correct in only one plane a deformity which exists in three planes. Simple osteotomy (without a graft) does not modify the radial shortening and may worsen the DRUJ incongruity. They often have to be combined with a Darrach procedure (Merle and Masse 1950) (Fig. 12.2) to be successful.

Ulnar shortening has been proposed to restore normal DRUJ anatomy. This is preferred by some authors to radial lengthening (Darrow et al. 1985, Linscheid 1987, Massart and Merloz 1982). Ulnar

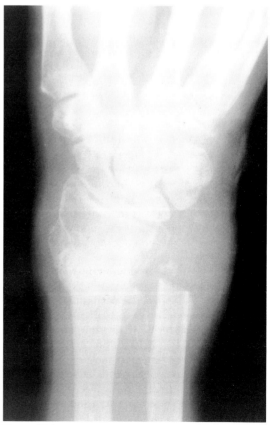

Figure 12.2

Distal radial malunion in an elderly woman, with a radial neck pseudoarthrosis. An ideal indication for a Darrach procedure.

osteotomy is usually performed at the distal third and internal fixation by a compression plate allows early mobilization.

Radial wedge osteotomy with corticocancellous graft was first proposed by Campbell in 1949. The technique was modified by Duparc et al. in 1977 and then used by other authors (Amadio 1987, Cooney et al. 1980, Fernandez 1985, Taleisnik and Watson 1984). It allows reconstruction of the normal anatomy and mechanics of the DRUJ. The aim of the procedure is to obtain an exact correction of the radial malunion by a transverse metaphyseal wedge osteotomy with a corticocancellous graft interposition (Fig. 12.3).

Technique

Using a radiovolar approach, and carefully preserving the superficial branches of the radial nerve, the flexor tendons are exposed and retracted in their sheaths. The distal radius exposed sub-periosteally and proximally to the fibrous sheath after elevating the pronator quadratus. The brachioradialis may be partially elevated from the radial styloid and re-attached at the end of the procedure. The plane of the osteotomy, parallel to the articular surface of the distal radius begins laterally, proximal to the fibrous sheaths, and ends proximal to the sigmoid notch of the radius. For a less severe malunion, the osteotomy should not be complete, but one should keep a cortical hinge at the opposite side of the deformity, volar and medial. It is usually easy to correct the malunion when a simple wedge osteotomy is planned. More often than not, however, there is a significant impaction with radial shortening and an osteotomy with lengthening of the radius should be planned.

A complete osteotomy is necessary with radial lengthening. Once the osteotomy has been done, realignment is performed, inserting a graft in the dorsal–lateral gap. Correction may be more difficult after a complete osteotomy. The wrist should be positioned in traction, using flexion and ulnar deviation with the deformity of the radius corrected, it is then temporarily stabilized with K-wires. The relationship between radius and ulna are then controlled and can be examined. The shape and volume of the bone graft needed can be evaluated. An iliac corticocancellous graft is

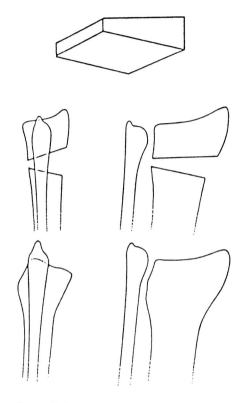

Figure 12.3

Distal radial malunion with shortening. Treatment by radial wedge osteotomy with a corticocancellous graft: osteotomy, shape of the graft, internal fixation by an epiphyso-metaphyseal plate.

harvested and trimmed to the desired size. During graft insertion, care should be taken not to translate the proximal fragment.

Internal fixation is mandatory. K-wire fixation may be used, as it would be in an acute case but plate fixation is preferred because the radial inclination correction can be better controlled and plate fixation is stable (Fig. 12.4). The plate is applied only after temporary K-wire fixation, graft insertion and radiographic examination of the reduction.

Temporary stabilization by external fixation has also been proposed with external fixation. The threaded pins are inserted before the osteotomy, the correction performed using external fixation for traction and the plate applied. The external fixator is removed after plate application. In the great majority of cases, normal anatomical relationships are restored to the radius and the

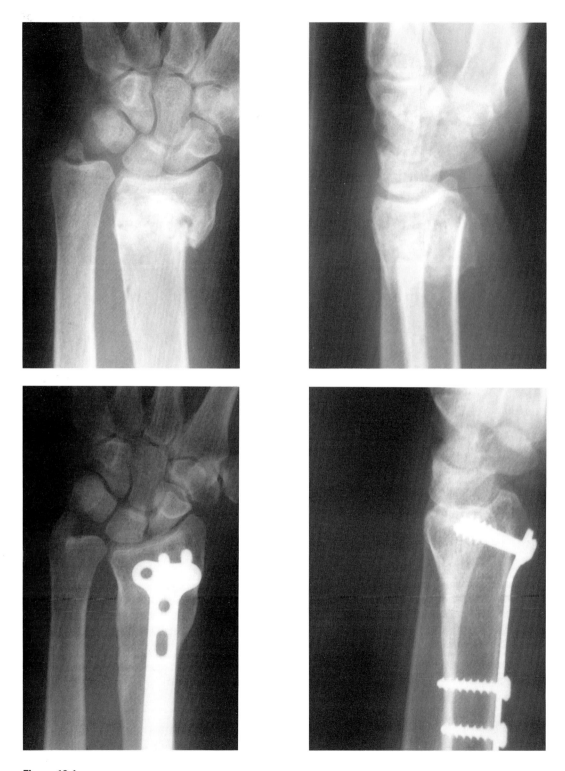

Figure 12.4
Distal radial malunion with a significant displacement. An excellent clinical result was achieved after radial osteotomy.

TREATMENT OF EXTRA-ARTICULAR MALUNIONS OF THE DISTAL RADIUS

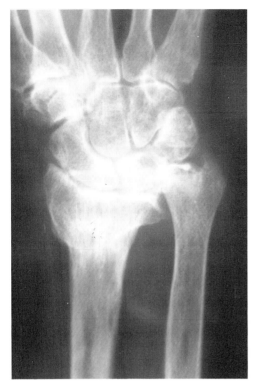

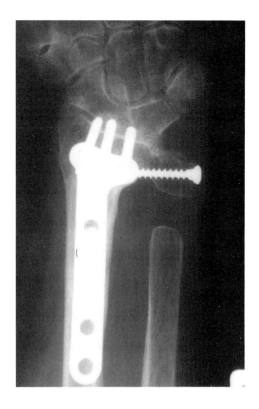

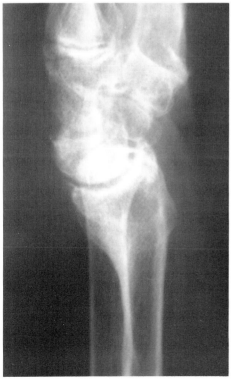

Figure 12.5

Significant distal radial malunion with a DRUJ dislocation. Treatment was by a combined radial osteotomy and Sauvé-Kapandji procedure.

DRUJ. If the perioperative radiographs show persistent malalignment, then an alternative procedure such as ulnar head resection or Sauvé–Kapandji procedure (Fig. 12.5) can be considered to treat malalignment or deformity of the DRUJ.

Postoperative management

After the corrective osteotomy an above-the-elbow cast is applied for five to six weeks. K-wires (if used for fixation) are removed assuming that healing is evident on the radiographs. When normal anatomy has been restored, grip strength recovers to a level that is almost normal.

Indications

Indications for corrective osteotomy of the radius depend on age and the time elapsed since the injury.

In elderly patients, an isolated Darrach procedure may be sufficient if the radial displacement is moderate and disability predominates on the DRUJ. If there is a significant deformity, a radial osteotomy could be performed alone or combined with distal ulnar head resection.

In young and middle-aged patients, normal anatomy should be restored. Wedge osteotomy with an iliac crest bone graft restores radial length, alignment of the radial epiphysis and normal congruency to the DRUJ.

Special cases

1. For recent cases (less than six months) in elderly patients with osteoporotic bone, the corrective osteotomy should be delayed until there is complete bone calcification. For young patients, an osteotomy through the fracture line can be performed earlier (three to four months) with a graft inserted in the fracture line. These cases, however, must be carefully selected.
2. Neurosympathetic dystrophy (NSD) is a case for delaying the procedure until a normal physiological tone is obtained in the skin, nerves and muscle. Recurrence of NSD is quite possible after surgery and can be a devastating complication.
3. Associated carpal tunnel syndrome should be treated at the same time as the corrective osteotomy. An isolated osteotomy will not always improve this syndrome. Preventive opening of the carpal tunnel does not seem necessary in the absence of clinical symptoms.

Conclusion

New imaging techniques have helped the assessment of radial malunions. Treatment has evolved from isolated distal ulnar head resection to the restoration of normal radial anatomy. Metaphyseal radial opening osteotomy with a bone graft is the preferred and an easily performed procedure with predictably good results. Improvement of pain, ROM, and grip strength are regularly obtained. Isolated Darrach procedures are infrequent now. Associated carpal instability from ligamentous strains should always be considered and sought both clinically and radiologically. Additional surgical treatment may be necessary.

References

Amadio PC. Treatment of malunion of the distal radius. *Hands Clinics* 1987; **3**: 4.

Boyd H, Stone M. Resection of the distal end of the ulna. *J Bone Joint Surg* 1944; **26A**: 313–21.

Bowers WH. Distal radioulnar joint arthroplasty; the hemiresection interposition technique. *J Hand Surg* 1985; **10A**: 169–78.

Cooney WP, Dobyns JH, Linscheid RL. Complications of Colles' fractures. *J Bone Joint Surg* 1980; **62A**: 613–19.

Darrach W. Derangements of the inferior radio-ulnar articulation. *Medical records (NY)*, 1915; **85**: 708.

Darrow JC, Linscheid RL, Dobyns JH, Mann JM, Wood MB, Beckenbaugh RD. Distal ulnar resection for disorders of the distal radioulnar joint. *J Hand Surg* 1985; **10A**: 482–91.

Duparc J, Pacault JY, Valtin B. Traitement des cals vicieux du poignet par ostéotomie d'ouverture avec greffe osseuse. *Ann Chir* 1977; **31, 4**: 307–12.

Duparc J, Valtin B. Complications tendinonerveuses des fractures de l'extrémité inférieure du radius. *Ann Chir* 1977; **31**: 335–39.

Duparc J, Valtin B. Les fractures de l'extrémité inférieure du radius. In Tubiana R. *Traité de chirurgie de la main. Tome 2*. Paris: Masson, 1984: 692–722.

Fernandez DL. Radial osteotomy and Bowers arthroplasty for malunited fractures of the distal end of the radius. *J Bone Joint Surg* 1988; **70A**: 1538–51.

Goncalves D. Correction of disorders of the radio-ulnar joint by artificial pseudarthrosis of the ulna. *J Bone Joint Surg* 1974; **56B**: 462–64.

Kapandji AI, Martin-Bouyer Y, Verdeille S. Etude du carpe au scanner à trois dimensions sous contraintes de prono-supination. *Ann Chir Main* 1991; **10, 1**: 36–47.

Lynch AC, Lipscomb PR. The carpal tunnel syndrome and Colles' fractures. *J Am Med Assn* 1963; **185**: 363–66.

Massart P, Merloz P. Raccourcissement segmentaire du cubitus dans certains cals vicieux de l'extrémité inférieure du radius. *Ann Chir Main* 1982; **1**: 65–70.

Merle D'Aubigné R, Masse P. La résection de l'extrémité inférieure du cubitus dans les cals vicieux de l'extrémité inférieure du radius. *Rev Chir Orthop* 1950; **36**: 484.

Minani A, Ogino T, Minami M. Treatment of distal radioulnar disorders. *J Hand Surg* 1987; **12A**: 189–96.

Morrissy RT. Dislocation of the distal radio-ulnar joint: anatomy and clues to prompt diagnosis. *Clin Orthop Rel Res* 1979; **144**: 154–58.

Narakas A. La résection isolée de l'extrémité distale du cubitus dans les séquelles post traumatiques du poignet. *Ann Chir* 1977; **31**: 318–22.

Oberlin C. Les instabilités et désaxations du carpe. Cahiers d'enseignement de la SOCOT, conférences d'enseignement 1990. Paris: Expansion Scientifique Française, 1990: 235–50.

Sauvé L, Kapandji IA. Une nouvelle technique de traitement chirurgical des luxations récidivantes isolées de l'extrémité cubitale inférieure. *J Chir* 1936; **47**: 4.

Sisk TD. Fractures of shoulder girdle and upper extremity. In: Crenshaw AN, ed. *Campbell's Operative Orthopaedics*, 7th edition. St. Louis: C.V. Mosby Company, 1987: 1783–1831.

Taleisnik J, Watson HK. Midcarpal instability caused by malunited fractures of the distal radius. *J Hand Surg* 1984; **9A, 3**: 350–57.

Watson K, Jaiyoung R, Burgess RC. Matched distal ulnar resection. *J Hand Surg* 1986; **11A**: 812–17.

13
Multiplanar osteotomy for treatment of malunions of the distal radius

GA Brunelli, GR Brunelli

Malunions of the distal radius

Distal radial fractures very frequently result in malunions, both from an insufficient reduction and from instability of the reduction which, even if good immediately after the treatment, may deteriorate afterwards (Castaing 1964, DeWulf 1968, Verdan 1975, Chamay 1977, Mansat 1977).

We must distinguish malunions following 'monoblock' (extra-articular) fractures, in which the distal epiphysis remains sound even if displaced, from those occurring after comminuted fractures with involvement of the articular surfaces of the radiocarpal joint (RCJ) and the distal radio-ulnar joint (DRUJ).

In monoblock fractures (Pouteau–Colles' fractures), five different components of the deformity and functional impairment caused by malunion should be considered. The typical postero-lateral tilt of the distal fragment changes the orientation of the articular surface of the radius. The main deformity consists of a dorsal and radial (lateral) deviation of the radial distal epiphysis, which alters the normal angles of the articular surface (Brunelli 1981).

1. In the frontal plane (antero-posterior view), the articular surface normally faces medially (in an ulnar direction), with an average value of 25°. This value must be measured from the styloid of the radius to the volar angle point of the joint surface, since the dorsal tilt present after fracture may alter the dorsal angle point so that it exceeds the volar angle point (Fig. 13.1). This angle may be reduced or even reverted in malunions, thus orientating the wrist in a radial direction (Fig. 13.2).
2. In the sagittal plane (lateral view), the orientation of the articular surface, which normally faces in a volar direction with an angle of 10–12°, changes to face dorsally, thus orientating the carpus in dorsal direction (Fig. 13.3).
3. In malunions following Colles' fractures a rotation in supination of the distal fragment may occur, predisposing the wrist and the hand to more supination and less pronation with post-traumatic stiffness. However, this alteration in the horizontal plane seems to be

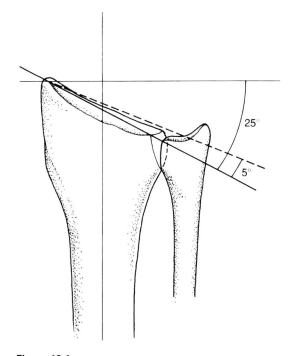

Figure 13.1

Normal distal radius in AP view. The angles are different if measured from the styloid to the dorsal angle point and from the styloid to the volar angle point. The difference is ±5°. The volar angle should be used.

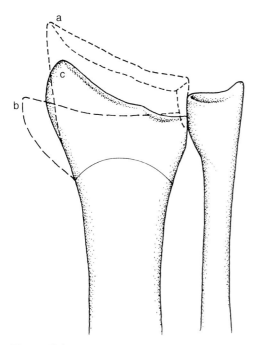

Figure 13.2

The dotted line (a) marks the original shape of the distal epiphysis; the discontinuous line (b) marks the shape of the malunion; the continuous line (c) marks the result after spherical osteotomy. Note the positive variance of the ulna after correction.

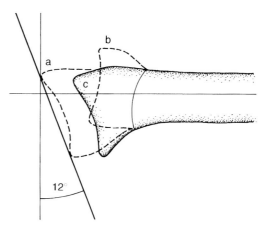

Figure 13.3

Diagram of lateral view of the distal radius: a) the anatomical shape (dotted line); b) shape of the malunion (discontinuous line); c) shape of the radius after osteotomy (continuous line). The angle is restored but the bone is shortened.

of minor importance in the global impairment produced by the malunion.

4. There is a consistent shortening of the radius with equalling or reversal of the distal radio-ulnar difference (DRUD), which is normally 2 mm in favour of the radius (radial styloid to ulnar head). This shortening leads to a relative positive variance of the ulna, with distal dislocation of the caput ulnae, impingement against the carpal condyle and wearing down of the triangular fibrocartilage complex (TFCC). The shortening should also be evaluated by means of comparison with the contralateral wrist (Bell 1985).

   In addition to radial shortening, there is dorsal displacement and backward tilt of the radial ulnar notch such that the axes of rotation of the two articular surfaces no longer coincide.

5. The reversal of the DRUD makes the DRUJ work under poor mechanical conditions, with stretching of DRUJ ligaments and dislocation of the convex ulnar facet from the sigmoid surface of the radius. This causes impairment of prono-supination and pain.

In comminuted fractures with involvement of the articular surfaces, arthritic changes of the RCJ (and DRUJ) may occur even if these changes are less evident, less painful and less impairing than one would expect given the involvement of the articular surface. In a few cases, these changes are severe and very painful, and may demand major surgical treatment such as wrist arthroplasty, wrist arthrodesis or partial arthrodesis.

In malunions of the radius following monoblock fractures (without arthritic changes due to articular involvement), the deformity, besides producing cosmetic changes, often causes painful functional impairment due to abnormal orientation of the wrist in a dorsal direction and to the resulting difference in length of the radius and ulna, which produces conflict between the carpus and the lengthened ulna.

The real damage to wrist function and strength is controversial. Sennwald (1987) wrote that people over 60 (the majority) tolerate the post-traumatic deformity well. Fourrier (1981) stated that the functional impairment is not proportional to the severity of the deformity. The authors believe that, even if there are patients who tolerate the malunion well, there are others who are impaired by it. Indications for surgery must not be restricted to radiographic findings, even if they are very important, but should also consider the clinical impairment and the age and activity of the patient.

It is often the case that painful limitation of pronosupination motion, secondary to stretching of the DRUJ, loss of radial length and/or localized arthritic changes for a fracture line involving the DRUJ, requires corrective osteotomy of the radius or ulna resection.

Even if they are not painful, malunions of monoblock (extra-articular) distal radial fractures do cause marked loss of grip with functional disability that interferes with everyday or professional activity.

Malunion may also cause compression (entrapment) of the median nerve due to the protrusion of the proximal fragment of the radius in a palmar direction.

Other complications which follow distal radial fractures and malunion include painful neurosympathetic dystrophy (sympathetic reflex dystrophy) and frozen shoulder.

In comminuted fractures with arthritic changes secondary to articular surface involvement, the painful impairment may be more severe. Generally this is related to the incongruence of the RCJ and to the stage of secondary arthritic changes. Corrective osteotomy may not be beneficial in these clinical situations.

Treatment options

When facing painful impairment, severe loss of grip or even just a marked cosmetic deformity, surgery is indicated.

A simple treatment, which was used in the past, is resection of the distal end of the ulna. This surgical procedure is certainly able to restore prono-supination to a significant degree and to relieve the pain due to DRUJ alterations. It does not modify the alteration of direction of the RCJ and hand, or improve the loss of grip (Narakas 1977, Cantero 1977).

Osteotomies of the distal end of the radius were first used in the last few decades. The aim of osteotomy is to correct the inclination of the articular surface, to restore the length of the radius and to restore the normal anatomy of the DRUJ (Duparc 1977, Razemon 1977).

The cosmetic deformity and functional impairment due to dorsal and radial deviation, together with median nerve compression, may be overcome by directional osteotomy. DRUJ alterations may need shortening of the ulna (Fig. 13.4) if the joint is stretched owing to loss of radial length. Removal of the caput ulnae (Darrach procedure) or a Sauvé–Kapandji procedure (1936), should be used to treat post-traumatic arthritis (Fig. 13.5).

As the deformity involves the sagittal, frontal and horizontal planes, the cut of the bone in the osteotomy must be multiplanar and must not produce further shortening of the radius. A closing (subtraction) wedge osteotomy will shorten the radius, and further impair function of the DRUJ. This could be a minor drawback but may also be severe as a transverse or oblique osteotomy can correct deformity in only one plane, and the deformity in the other plane will remain.

Opening (addition) wedge osteotomies of the radius involve filling in the opened angle with corticospongious graft. A suitable graft should be withdrawn from the iliac bone, however the

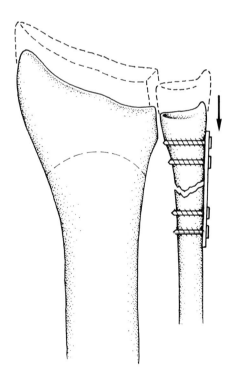

Figure 13.4

The ulna must be shortened if the distal DRUJ is not involved by the fracture line.

Spherical multiplanar osteotomy: the procedure

A linear, 6 cm-long approach is used on the radial aspect of the wrist, volar to the styloid of the radius. The sensory branches of the radial nerve are identified and spared. The periosteum is incised longitudinally, volar to the first wrist compartment. The periosteum is elevated all around the metaphysis at the level of the fracture, together with the tendon insertion of the brachioradialis. Two thin Lowman retractors are passed around the bone. The pronator quadratus may be elevated together with the periosteum or it may be cut at its distal third.

The spherical osteotomy is performed using a spoon-like oscillating saw or a spoon-like gauge. Alternatively, a small curved chisel can be used to make a curved osteotomy.

When the osteotomy is completed, the distal epiphysis of the radius can be adjusted on the spherical convex osteotomy surface of the proximal stump by pulling the hand in various directions. Sometimes the ulna does not allow complete correction and the anticipated treatment of the distal ulna has to be performed immediately (resection osteotomy with shortening or Darrach or Sauvé–Kapandji procedures). The correction

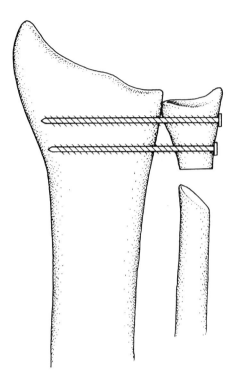

Figure 13.5

If the DRUJ shows fracture or arthritic changes, a Sauvé–Kapandji procedure should be performed, or alternatively, a Darrach procedure (removal of the caput ulnae).

insertion of the graft is never easy and external distraction-fixation may be necessary. An opening osteotomy usually corrects only one plane of deformity easily, while it is able to correct the deformity of the other planes only occasionally and with difficulty. Moreover, it may be difficult to restore the correct alignment and length simultaneously in one plane (Lanz 1977, Fernandez 1982).

It is our opinion that only a spherical osteotomy will allow the distal epiphysis of the radius to rotate over the convex spherical surface of the proximal radius in any direction, thus correcting the deformities and the articular planes without further shortening. The spherical osteotomy may even provide a small amount of lengthening. Of course, as the ulna is too long, it must be shortened, using a Darrach or Sauvé–Kapandji procedure in addition to the spherical osteotomy (Fig. 13.6).

Table 13.1 Reviewed cases

Flexion extension			
very good	good	fair	poor
140°	140–100°	100–60°	≤ 60°
3	10	4	1
Pronosupination			
very good	good	fair	poor
140°	140–100°	100–60°	≤60°
4	9	5	0

Cosmetic result

	evaluation	
	patient	surgeon
very good	15	15
good	2	0
fair	1	3
poor	0	0

Pain

absent			
discontinuous	persistent	continuous	
slight	mild	severe	
15	2	1	0

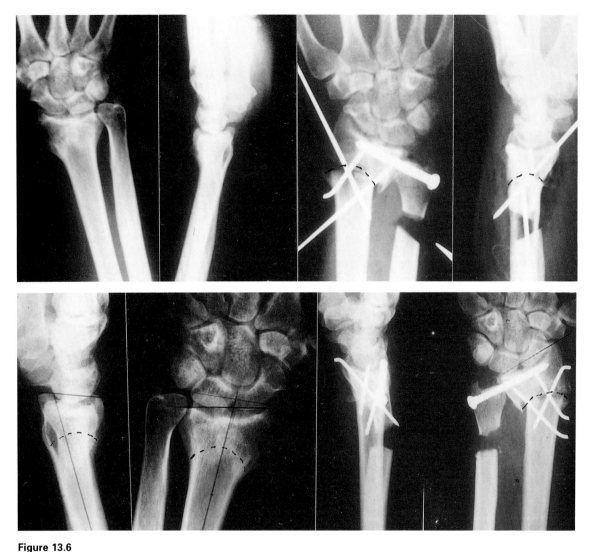

Figure 13.6

Two examples of correction of radial angulation and ulnar variance with Sauvé–Kapandji procedures.

must be temporarily fixed by one K-wire, checked by radiographic examination, and further modified if necessary).

The correction obtained by rotating the distal epiphysis is then maintained by means of two K-wires (a T-shaped miniplate may also be used (Heim 1977). The K-wires are removed when the radiographs demonstrate consolidation.

During the period 1986–1990 20 cases of distal radial malunions have been treated by spherical multiplanar osteotomy. Of these, 18 cases were reviewed at medium and short term (one to six years). Of the 18 cases, 12 had required either a Darrach or a Sauvé–Kapandji procedure and 7 an ulnar shortening. The results of the study are shown in Table 13.1 (Fig. 13.7).

In cases of malunion following articular fracture, providing the arthritic changes are not severe, the same spherical osteotomy used for extra-articular malunions may be enough. If the secondary arthritis is severe, a wrist arthrodesis, especially in young adult males, or a wrist replacement, especially in old adult females, may be necessary.

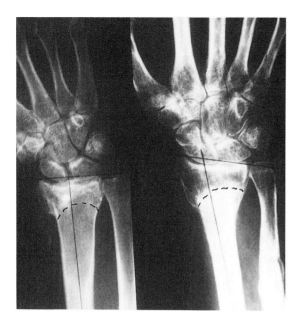

Figure 13.7
Mid-term result after correction by multiplanar osteotomy with shortening of the ulna.

In conclusion, the multiplanar (spherical) osteotomy associated with different types of surgery on the ulna (according to need) has proved to be a very good surgical procedure which can be recommended in the treatment of distal radial malunions.

References

Alcocer L, Irisarri C, Miranda G, Ruiz C. Secuelas oseas de las fracturas de la extremidad distal del radio. In Arisarri ed. *Lesiones de la muneca y carpo*. Madrid: Asepeyo, 1985: 145–9.

Bell MJ, Hill RJ, McMurtry RY. Ulnar impingement syndrome. *J Bone Joint Surg* 1985; **67**A: 126.

Brunelli G, Saffar P. *L'imagerie du poignet*. Paris: Springer-Verlag, 1981: 19.

Cantero J. Raccourcissement du cubitus dans les sequelles de fracture de l'extrémité distale du radius. *Ann Chir* 1977; **31**: 330–4.

Castaing J. Les fractures récents de l'extrémité inférieure du radius chez l'adulte. *Rev Chir Orthop* 1964; **581**: 696.

Chamay A. Considérations sur les limites de tolerance du traitement conservateur des fractures du poignet. *Ann Chir* 1977; **31**: 340–2.

Darrach W, Dwight K. Derangements of the inferior radio-ulnar articulation. *Med Lec (NY)* 1915; **87**: 708.

De Wulf A, Razemon JP. Les sequelles des fractures de l'extrémité inférieure du radius. Leurs causes et leurs traîtements. *Acta Ortho Belgica* 1968; **34**: 11.

Duparc J, Pacault JY, Valtin B. Traitement des cals vicieux de poignet par ostéotomie d'ouverture avec greffe osseuse. *Ann Chir* 1977; **31**: 307–12.

Fernandez D. Correction of post-traumatic wrist deformity in adults by osteotomy, bone grafting and internal fixation. *J Bone Joint Surg* 1982; **64A**: 8.

Fourrier P, Bardy A, Roche G, Cisterne A. Approche d'une définition du cal vicieux du poignet. *Int Orth (Sicot)* 1981; **4**: 229–305.

Heim U. Stabilisation des ostéotomies de l'extrémité inférieure du radius par petit plaque. *Ann Chir* 1977; **31**: 313–14.

Lanz U, Kron W, Greulich M: Ostéotomie d'ouverture avec interposition d'une greffe pour les cals vicieux de l'extrémité inférieure du radius. *Ann Chir* 1977; **31**: 315–17.

Mansat M, Gay R, Mansat Ch. Cal vicieux de l'extrémité inférieure du radius et 'derangements' de l'articulation radio-cubitale inferieure. *Ann Chir* 1977; **31**: 297–301.

Narakas A. La resection isolée de l'extrémité distale du cubitus dans les sequelles post-traumatiques du poignet. *Ann Chir* 1977; **31**: 318–22.

Razemon JP. Les techniques d'ostéotomies des cals vicieux de l'extrémité inférieure du radius. *Ann Chir* 1977; **31**: 302–6.

Razemon JP. Indications thérapeutiques dans les cals vicieux de l'extrémité inférieure du radius. *Ann Chir* 1977; **31**: 343–4.

Sauvé L, Kapandji AI. Une nouvelle technique du traitement chirurgical de luxations recidivantes isolées de l'extrémité cubitale inférieure. *J Chir* 1936; **47**: 3.

Sennwald G. *L'entité radius-carpe*. Berlin: Springer-Verlag, 1987: 235–61.

Verdan Cl. Symposium sur les cals vicieux de l'extrémité inférieure du radius. GEM Paris 28–29 Nov. 1975. *Ann Chir* 1977; **31**: 295–6.

14
Corrective osteotomy for extra-articular malunion of the distal radius

Diego L Fernandez

Historical review

The first attempts to correct post-traumatic wrist deformity began at the end of the last century with the resection of the prominent head of the ulna. Distal ulna resection was attributed to Darrach for his description in 1913, but had been published previously by Desault in 1791 and later by Moore in 1880.

Early reports on surgical correction of radial deformity began in the 1930s. In 1932, Ghormley and Mroz described the results of four osteotomies of the radius in a study of 176 wrist fractures and concluded that radial osteotomy, with or without a bone graft to maintain fragment alignment, could improve the external appearance of a deformed wrist. In 1935, Durman reported good cosmetic and functional results in four patients treated with radial osteotomy. His technique is very similar to the trapezoidal osteotomy published by Watson in 1988, and is worth quoting here. 'An osteotomy through the fracture line is done on the dorsal surface, the ventral portion of the cortex is then fractured subperiostally. Following this a graft of suitable length and breadth is cut longitudinally from the distal end of the upper fragment of the radius and is fitted transversely in the line of osteotomy. The graft holds the distal fragment in normal position. By making one end of the graft slightly broader than the other it is possible to correct the radial deviation of the hand. Resection of the distal ulna has been found unnecessary to secure a good cosmetic result. After the graft is wedged into the line of osteotomy it is practically impossible to displace the lower fragment. In all my cases bone union has been well advanced at the end of three weeks ...' (Durman 1937).

In 1937, Campbell published the first statistically significant article on radial osteotomy. In his technique, the radius is osteotomized transversely about an inch above the radiocarpal joint to give a radial approach between the brachioradialis and extensor pollicis brevis tendons. The graft taken from the prominent medial border of the ulna, with preservation of the distal radio-ulnar joint, is then inserted in the dorsoradial defect of the opening wedge osteotomy. Out of 19 cases treated with this technique, 11 had better functional and cosmetic results than those achieved after simple osteotomy without graft interposition that corrected only the backward angulation of the articular surface of the radius. In 1941, Hobart and Kraft published their results of a similar osteotomy, where the graft is taken from the resected distal ulna or from the proximal fragment of the radius, as in Durman's technique. In the same year Henry Milch described his 'cuff resection of the ulna': a shortening osteotomy of the distal ulna for malunited fractures of the distal radius with severe shortening. Five years before, in 1936, Sauvé and Kapandji reported their technique on distal radio-ulnar arthrodesis with creation of a proximal pseudarthrosis for post-traumatic derangements of the distal radio-ulnar joint. In 1945, Speed and Knight analysed the results of surgical treatment of 60 cases of malunited Colles' fractures. Their basic aims were restoration of anatomy and improvement of wrist function. They recommended the use of an intramedullary bone peg or dual onlay grafts to avoid loss of correction in wrists with severe deformity or osteoporosis. Wrist or finger stiffness represented formal contraindications for surgical treatment. The authors recommended simple osteotomy to correct fractures with dorsal angulation and slight shortening without evident radio-ulnar symptoms. For patients with post-traumatic widening of the wrist, the Campbell operation was indicated.

In the same year, Merle D'Aubigné and Joussemet described a multi-facet curved osteotomy in the sagittal plane (osteotomie à facettes) designed to restore radial length without the need of a graft. The results of this operation, analysed by Merle D'Aubigné and Tubiana (1958) showed satisfactory results in 27 wrists that were treated with this operation: however, the distal ulna had to be resected in 17 cases. By virtue of its form, this osteotomy produces a slight palmar displacement of the distal fragment with respect to the shaft of the radius and permits no correction on the frontal plane. The authors concluded that osteotomy of the radius combined with resection of the distal ulna offered better cosmetic and functional results than a Darrach resection alone. The disadvantage of the operation was the prolonged period of postoperative immobilization in plaster. They also concluded that, although resection of the distal ulna gave satisfactory functional results after a short period of immobilization, the cosmetic correction was insufficient when significant dorsal angulation was present.

A similar osteotomy curved in the sagittal plane was briefly mentioned by Bunnell in 1948 and is known as the Rixford operation.

Following the development of modern internal fixation techniques in the seventies, plate fixation of distal radial fractures to guarantee rigid fixation and early joint rehabilitation is now advocated by various authors (Fernandez et al. 1977, Heim 1977, Lanz 1983, Müller-Färber and Griedel 1979, Reneé and Schmelzeiser 1974). Other use similar techniques, but prefer percutaneous Kirschner wire fixation and plaster immobilization which avoids the necessity of a second operation for removal of hardware (Bora et al. 1984, Duparc et al. 1977, Rodriguez-Meythiaz and Chamay 1988, Watson and Castle, 1988).

The past decade has seen further refinements of surgical techniques, including the concomitant treatment of distal radio-ulnar disorders (Ekenstam et al. 1985, Fernandez 1984, 1987, 1988 and 1989, Jupiter and Masem 1988, Lehner and Sennwald 1989), experimental biomechanical implications of extra-articular radial malunions (Pogue et al. 1990, Short et al. 1987), and the recognition of midcarpal instability associated with malunited fractures of the distal radius (Taleisnik and Watson 1964).

Anatomical and clinical correlation of extra-articular deformity of the distal radius

Following Pouteau–Colles' fractures there is loss of the volar tilt of the joint surface in the sagittal plane, loss of the ulnar inclination in the frontal plane, shortening, and a certain degree of supination deformity of the distal fragment with respect to the diaphysis. In general, there is a strict correlation between the quality of the anatomical result and the residual function of the wrist (Castaing 1964, Cooney et al. 1980, Fernandez 1982, Forgon and Mammel 1983, Fourrier et al. 1981, Martini 1986, McQueen and Caspers 1988, Villar et al. 1987). The most common cause of malunion is progressive loss of initial reduction due to insufficient conservative management. The pathological tilt of the joint surface in the sagittal plane alters the normal mechanics of the radiocarpal joint, producing a dorsal displacement of the flexion-extension arc of motion, which results in limitation of flexion and increased dorsal flexion of the wrist.

From a biomechanical standpoint there is an increase of the axial load supported by the joint surface of the radius and ulna. The dorsal overload of the radial surface has been experimentally shown by Short et al. (1987) and by Pogue et al. (1990). Increased dorsal tilt of the distal radial surface also produces a mechanical imbalance of the carpus. Three types of carpal instability can be seen associated with fractures of the distal radius:

1. radiocarpal instability with dorsal subluxation of the carpus without intercarpal malalignment;
2. a dorsal intercalated segment instability (DISI) deformity as described by Linscheid and collaborators in 1972. These authors concluded that this alteration of carpal alignment is secondary to the radial deformity and not a real carpal instability. This adaptive response

of the carpus to the deformed radius usually disappears if a lateral radiograph of the wrist is taken with the hand in exactly the same amount of dorsiflexion as the malunited distal fragment (Fig. 14.1);
3. extrinsic midcarpal instability as described by Taleisnik and Watson (1984). Certain patients with a malunited distal radius in dorsiflexion reproduce a painful audible subluxation, when actively deviating their wrists in an ulnar direction, with the forearm in a pronated position. In these situations, a lateral radiograph of the wrist shows a dorsal displacement of the long axis of the capitate with respect to the long axis of the radial shaft, and the lunate is rotated dorsally. During active ulnar deviation, the lunate cannot displace palmarly since it is blocked by the dorsally tilted volar lip of the radius. Continuous dynamic overload of the midcarpal joint during active ulnar deviation may lead to synovitis, ligament attenuation, and progressive dynamic midcarpal instability, particularly in wrists with constitutional ligament laxity.

Although radiocarpal subluxation, adaptive dorsal carpal malalignment (Sakai et al. 1991), and dynamic midcarpal instability improve following correction of the radial deformity, DISI deformity that does not improve after restoration of the normal volar tilt has been observed. This is seen mainly in elderly patients, and is probably due to capsular retraction and deep fibrosis following a mild reflex sympathetic dystrophy at the time of initial fracture treatment. For practical purposes, the DISI deformity associated with malunited Pouteau–Colles' fractures may be subdivided as follows: Type I — lax, reducible, dorsal carpal malalignment, that can be improved or totally corrected by radial osteotomy (younger patients, joint laxity, good preoperative range of motion); and a Type II — fixed non-reducible dorsal carpal malalignment, that cannot be improved by radial osteotomy.

Malunited fractures of the distal radius also affect the kinematics of the distal radio-ulnar joint. Dorsal angulation produces incongruency between the head of the ulna and the sigmoid notch in both the sagittal and horizontal planes. Radial shortening leads to impingement of the triangular fibrocartilage complex (TFCC). During physiological forearm rotation, the TFCC 'sweeps' uniformly over the articular surface of the ulnar head. With a positive ulnar variance, the TFCC is tight and relatively blocked in an anterior or posterior position with respect to the ulnar head. This pathological tightness and impingement automatically limits forearm rotation. Significant, long-standing radial shortening leads to ulnocarpal impingement associated with central defects in the triangular fibrocartilage and pathological contact of the ulnar head with the lunate. Early arthritic changes of the radio-ulnar joint may occur following four-part fractures that heal with an incongruity of the sigmoid notch.

Antero-posterior instability of the ulnar head may coexist with malunions of the distal radius due to loss of articular congruity between the ulna and the distal radius and rupture or secondary traumatic elongation of the TFCC. In a study by Castaing (1964) of 440 fractures of the distal radius, a non-union of the ulnar styloid was present in 77.5% of the cases: however, ulnar styloid non-union did not affect the overall results of the series studied. This is explained by the fact that during initial plaster immobilization, the ulnar styloid heals with fibrous union between the ulnar head and the TFCC. The presence of a pseudarthrotic gap does not necessarily imply distal radio-ulnar instability in every case. However, in a recent experimental and clinical article, Shaw et al. (1990) state that ulnar styloid fractures with associated radio-ulnar joint instability, significant displacement, or fractures of the base of the styloid require initial internal fixation to prevent the disability associated with chronic radio-ulnar instability.

Loss of ulnar inclination of the distal radius in the frontal plane produces radial deviation of the carpus and significant loss of grip strength. Radial angulation greater than 20° results in marked limitation of ulnar deviation of the wrist. Malunions following Smith–Goyrand fractures have an increased palmar tilt and a pronational deformity of the distal fragment that favours dorsal subluxation of the ulnar head. Patients with malunited Smith's fractures complain of limitation of active dorsal flexion due to the increased volar tilt, and limitation of supination due to the pronation deformity and the relative subluxation of the distal ulna (Fernandez 1988). In contrast to the Colles' deformity, midcarpal

CORRECTIVE OSTEOTOMY FOR EXTRA-ARTICULAR MALUNION

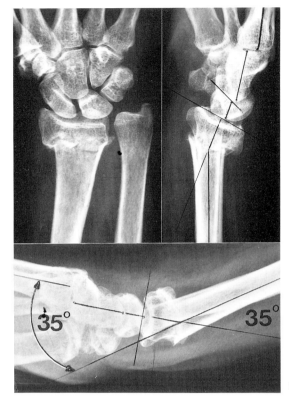

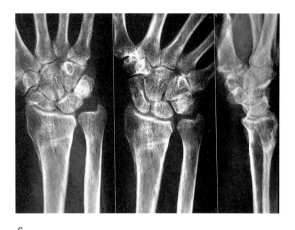

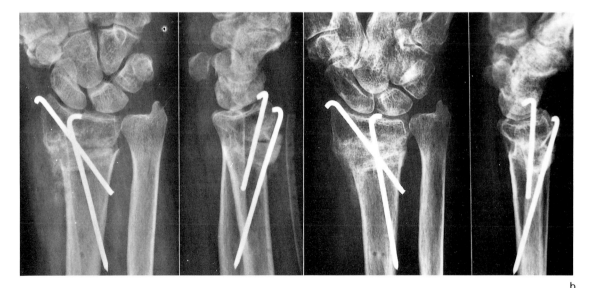

Figure 14.1
a) Malunited Colles' fracture with 35° dorsal tilt and 'adaptive' carpal malalignment. Lateral radiograph with the hand in 35° dorsiflexion reveals normal carpal alignment. b) Radiographs taken immediately after and 6 weeks after corrective osteotomy. c) Follow-up films at 3 years show a well-preserved joint space and normal intercarpal motion in the radial and ulnar deviation views.

instability or carpal malalignment following Smith's fractures have not been reported to date.

Indications for surgical correction of extra-articular malunion of the distal radius

The indication for surgical correction is based on the combined assessment of functional wrist impairment, localization of pain, degree of cosmetic deformity, and the radiographic findings. Careful clinical examination is imperative to determine the localization of pain at the radiocarpal, midcarpal, or distal radio-ulnar joint. Distal radio-ulnar joint (DRUJ) instability should be ruled out. Measurement of grip strength is directly proportional to the amount of pain, the radial deviation, and the shortening, and is a useful parameter for follow-up evaluation. Dorsal tilt and radial deviation of the distal articular surface favours a compensatory spontaneous flexion deformity of the wrist with extensor tendon tightness resulting in slight hyperextension of the PIP joints. Radial deviation produces a radial angulation of the carpal tunnel which decreases the mechanical efficiency of the flexor tendons.

Standardized plain radiographs of both wrists are usually sufficient to assess the need for surgical intervention. Dynamic midcarpal instability can be documented with a lateral radiograph of the wrist in maximal ulnar deviation. Computerized tomography is useful to evaluate post-traumatic incongruence of the DRUJ, subluxation, or rotational malalignment of the distal radius. From a radiological standpoint, there are no fixed parameters to determine the surgical indication for correction. A pathologic displacement of the flexion-extension arc of motion is seen with a sagittal tilt of more than 25°. On the other hand, in patients with a pre-existing potential to develop midcarpal instability, a slight dorsal tilt (10–15°) can resault in symptomatic midcarpal instability.

In a detailed analysis of 64 malunions of the distal radius, Fourrier et al. (1987) correlated functional impairment with the residual deformity of the distal radius. These authors concluded that the lower limit of deformity, at which a malunion of the distal radius becomes symptomatic are a sagittal tilt of 10–20°, a radial deviation of 20–30°, and a radio-ulnar index of 0–2 mm. Furthermore, based on experimental evidence of radial overload of the articular cartilage (Pogue et al. 1990, Short et al. 1987), a dorsal angulation of 20–30° should be considered a prearthrotic condition. Careful radiographic analysis of the DRUJ will inform the surgeon of the necessity of performing a primary procedure at the joint level together with a radial osteotomy. Radial shortening of 10–12 mm without degenerative DRUJ changes can be corrected with a radial osteotomy alone. However, in the presence of severe degenerative DRUJ changes with severe limitation of forearm rotation, an additional procedure on the ulnar side of the wrist is necessary in most cases to guarantee a good functional result.

The indication for radial osteotomy depends on the limitation of function, the severity of pain, the presence of midcarpal instability, the associated DRUJ problems, and a significant deformity on radiographic examination that represents a menace for the future of the wrist. These include the pre-arthrotic deformity, mechanical imbalance of the carpus, and DRUJ incongruence. Contraindications for corrective osteotomy include advanced degenerative changes in the radiocarpal and intercarpal joints, fixed carpal malalignment, or significant trophic disturbances causing limited overall function of the wrist and fingers, or massive osteoporosis. There is no upper age limit for surgical correction, provided that there is adequate bone quality. Ideally, the osteotomy should be performed as soon as the soft tissues show no trophic disturbances, the radiography shows evidence of decreased osteoporosis, and the maximum possible motion of the wrist has been regained with physiotherapy.

Surgical technique

The aims of radial osteotomy are to restore function and improve the appearance of the wrist by correcting the deformity at the level of the old fracture site. The osteotomy should reorientate the joint surface to guarantee normal load distribution, re-establish the mechanical balance of the midcarpal joint, and restore the anatomic relationships of the distal radio-ulnar joint. Since radial shortening is a constant component of the deformity, both in malunited Colles' and Smith's fractures, an opening wedge osteotomy is used, which is transverse in the frontal plane and oblique (parallel to the joint surface) in the sagittal plane to secure lengthening. This osteotomy allows:

1. radial lengthening of up to 10–12 mm;
2. correction of the volar tilt in the sagittal plane;
3. correction of the ulnar tilt in the frontal plane;
4. and correction of the rotational deformity in the horizontal plane.

A corticocancellous bone graft from the iliac crest is cut to fit the bone defect created by the displacement of the distal fragment. If a partial or complete resection of the distal ulna is performed simultaneously, the resected ulnar head can be used to fill the radial defect. Careful preoperative planning and the use of Kirschner wires to mark the angle of deformity are mandatory to guarantee an accurate angular correction, to simplify the procedure, and to diminish the need for intraoperative radiographic control. Radiographs of the uninjured wrist are useful to determine the physiological ulnar variance for each particular patient, and should be used to calculate restoration of radial length (Fig. 14.2).

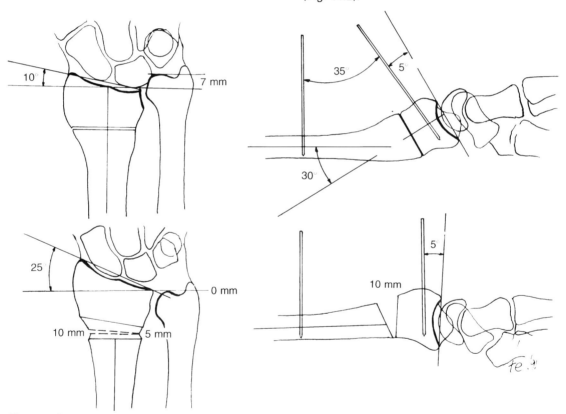

Figure 14.2

Preoperative planning of the osteotomy. Top left: for correction in the frontal plane, the amount of shortening (7 mm in this patient) is measured between the head of the ulna and the ulnar corner of the radius on the antero-posterior radiograph. The lines for the measurement are perpendicular to the long axis of the radius. The ulnar tilt is reduced to 10° in this patient. Bottom left: to restore the ulnar tilt to normal (average 25°), the osteotomy is opened more on the dorsoradial than on the dorso-ulnar side. Top right: for correction in the sagittal plane, the dorsal tilt (30° in this patient) is measured between the perpendicular to the joint surface and the long axis of the radius on the lateral radiograph. The Kirschner wires are introduced so that they subtend the angle that corresponds to the dorsal tilt plus 5° of volar tilt (30° + 5° = 35° in this patient). Bottom right: after opening the osteotomy by the correct amount, the Kirschner wires lie parallel to each other.

Malunited Pouteau–Colles' fractures

A 7 cm long longitudinal dorsoradial incision is used. It begins at a point 2 cm distal to the Lister tubercule and extends 5 cm proximally in the forearm. The radius is exposed between the third and fourth dorsal compartments after mobilizing and carefully retracting the extensor pollicis longus tendon. About 2.5 cm proximal to the wrist joint, the osteotomy site is marked with an osteotome. If T-plate fixation of the osteotomy is planned, Lister's tubercle should be removed with an osteotome to provide a flat surface on which to apply the plate. If Kirschner-wire fixation of the osteotomy is used, Lister's tubercle should be left in place, since it is a useful point of entry for dorsopalmar wire fixation (Rodriguez-Meythiaz 1988).

In order to be sure that the osteotomy, as seen in the sagittal plane, is parallel to the joint surface, a fine Kirschner wire is introduced through the dorsal part of the capsule into the radiocarpal joint and along the articular surface of the radius. In accordance with the preoperative plan two 2.5 mm Kirschner wires with a threaded tip are inserted, subtending the angle of correction in the sagittal plane on both sides of the future osteotomy (Fig. 14.3). These wires not only control the intraoperative angular correction, but also manipulate and maintain the distal radius in the corrected position with a small external fixator bar until the graft is inserted in place.

With careful protection of the volar soft tissues, the osteotomy is performed with an oscillating saw, taking care not to osteotomize the volar cortex completely. The osteotomy is then opened dorsally and radially by manipulating the wrist into flexion, by applying spreader clamps dorsally or by using the 2.5 mm Kirschner wires as lever arms. The osteotomy is opened until both wires are parallel in the sagittal plane.

A 4.0 mm external fixator bar with two clamps is placed between both Kirschner wires to maintain the reduction of the distal fragment. Additional opening of the osteotomy on the radial side can be achieved with a small spreader clamp, allowing the distal fragment to rotate along the long axis of the distal threaded Kirschner wire. Complete tenotomy or Z-lengthening of the brachioradialis tendon is recommended to facilitate lengthening in malunions with severe radial deviation and shortening. For such cases, two

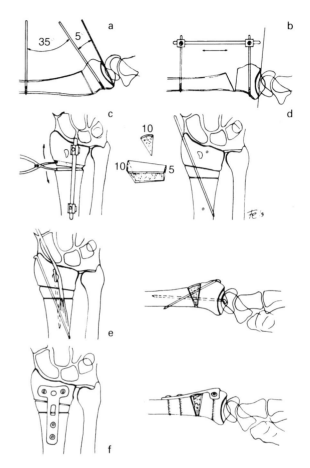

Figure 14.3

Osteotomy technique. a) Threaded wires subtend the angle of correction. The osteotomy is parallel to the joint surface in the sagittal plane. Note the fine Kirschner wire introduced into the radiocarpal joint. b, c) The osteotomy is opened dorsally and radially with a small spreader clamp. A fixator bar maintains the correction. d) An iliac graft shaped to conform to the defect is inserted, and one oblique Kirschner wire is driven through the radial styloid and graft into the radial metaphysis. The fixator is then removed. e, f) Internal fixation with an additional Kirschner wire introduced through Lister's tubercle in oblique dorsopalmar fashion, or with a small-fragment T-plate.

additional Kirschner wires with threaded tips may be used between both fragments to which a distraction device can be applied temporarily.

The iliac bone graft is shaped to conform the dorsoradial bone defect and is inserted, making sure that there is a snug fit. At this point, a 1.6 mm or 2.0 mm Kirschner wire is driven obliquely from the radial styloid across the graft and into the proximal fragment, after which the threaded wires and the external fixator bar may be removed. Then, with the elbow in 90° flexion, intra-operative forearm rotation and wrist motion are checked. Radiographic control with the image intensifier may be advisable at this point to assess the quality of correction and radial lengthening before definitive internal fixation of the osteotomy. For this, a second Kirschner wire can be introduced across Lister's tubercle in an oblique dorsopalmar direction and into the proximal fragment, as suggested by Rodriguez-Meythiaz and Chamay (1988). Rigid T-plate fixation is another option, which allows early unrestricted motion of the wrist (Fernandez 1982, Fernandez et al. 1977). During wound closure, the extensor pollicis longus tendon can be relocated in its groove if Lister's tubercle has been preserved in the cases stabilized with Kirschner wires; otherwise, a proximal transverse retinacular flap should be interposed between the plate and the tendon to prevent attrition tendonitis.

Malunited Smith–Goyrand fractures

These malunions are exposed through the distal part of the classic Henry approach between the flexor carpi radialis and the radial artery, with radial detachment of the pronator quadratus muscle and partial disinsertion of the flexor pollicis longus from the radial shaft. The malunion is approached subperiostally by reflecting the pronator quadratus muscle to the ulnar side, and the soft tissues are protected with Hohmann retractors. Two Kirschner wires are inserted on the volar aspect to mark the angle of correction, as shown in Fig. 14.4. The palmar opening wedge osteotomy, grafting and plating are then carried out as for the Colles' deformity, but in a reversed manner from the volar side. Care must be taken not to overcorrect the physiological palmar tilt of 10° when manipulating the distal fragment into dorsiflexion. The application of a volar T-plate automatically derotates the pronation deformity of the distal fragment by virtue of the flat surface of the plate. Plate fixation is therefore strongly recommended because practically all malunited Smith's fractures have a pronation deformity of the distal fragment and an apparent dorsal subluxation of the distal ulna. Dorsiflexion of the distal fragment and derotation, as well as lengthening, reorients the sigmoid notch of the radius with respect to the ulnar head.

Operations on the ulnar side of the wrist

If the patient's main complaints are localized in the DRUJ (pain associated with limitation of forearm rotation) and the angulation of the joint surface in the sagittal and frontal planes is less than 10°, a reconstructive procedure at the distal radio-ulnar level is indicated, without a radial osteotomy.

For post-traumatic positive ulnar variance and ulnocarpal impingement with acceptable congruency of the sigmoid notch and the ulna, as demonstrated by CT scans, a shortening osteotomy of the ulna is the procedure of choice. Ulnar shortening decompresses the ulnar compartment of the wrist, re-establishes DRUJ congruity, and tightens the TFCC, which exerts a stabilizing effect on the distal ulna. A transverse osteotomy with resection of a bony segment and rigid fixation with a compression plate is recommended.

If plain radiographs or CT scans demonstrate post-traumatic incongruity or degenerative changes of the radio-ulnar joint, a resection arthroplasty or a DRUJ arthrodesis are required to guarantee freedom from pain. The advantages of partial ulnar head resection (Bowers 1985, Watson et al. 1986) over complete resection of the ulnar head, are that the ulnocarpal ligaments and the TFCC remain in continuity with the distal ulnar stump. It must be remembered that partial ulnar resection does not alter the ulnar variance and therefore additional ulnar shortening, either at the styloid level or at the ulnar shaft should be performed to prevent stylocarpal impingement. The disadvantages of the Darrach procedure, such as loss of grip strength, loss of ulnar support of the carpus, and instability of the distal ulnar stump are well known, but the most common cause of failure is due to excessive resection of the distal ulna. The Darrach procedure has still a place in the treatment of distal ulnar derangement or osteoarthritis after a Colles' fracture in the elderly patient, or it can be used as a salvage

112 FRACTURES OF THE DISTAL RADIUS

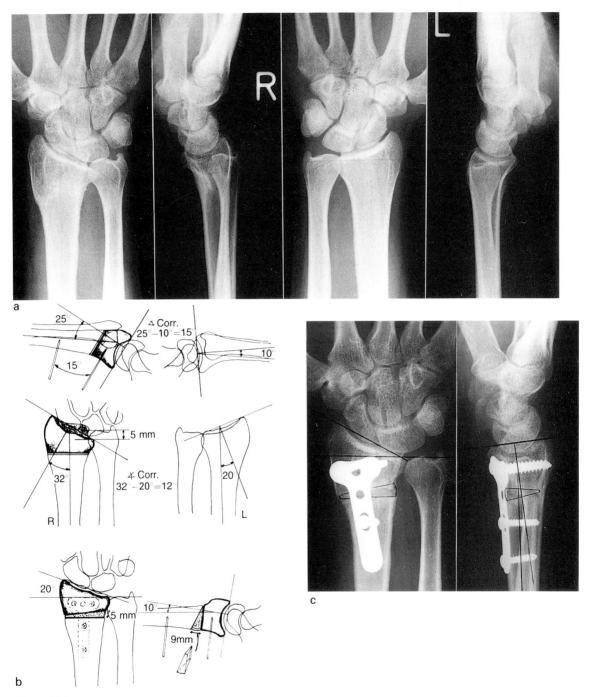

Figure 14.4

a) Malunited Smith's fracture of the right wrist with increased volar tilt, increased ulnar inclination, slight ulnocarpal translation, ulnocarpal impingement, and dorsal subluxation of the ulnar head. b) Preoperative planning: an increased volar tilt of 25° is corrected to 10° of physiological volar tilt with a 15° volar opening wedge osteotomy. An increased ulnar tilt of 32° is corrected to 20° (in the other wrist) with a 12° ulnar opening wedge osteotomy in the frontal plane. c) Late result at 4 years showing anatomical restoration of the radio-ulnar joint and radial angles. The patient has normal forearm rotation and is free of pain.

procedure for failed reconstructive procedures of the radio-ulnar joint.

Finally, DRUJ arthrodesis with the creation of a proximal pseudarthrosis (Sauvé and Kapandji 1936) preserves both the ulnocarpal ligaments and the bony support of the carpus. This operation is extremely useful for restoration of free forearm rotation in cases with fixed DRUJ subluxation following articular fractures of the distal radius with severe destruction of the joint.

Whether or not an associated primary operation on the ulnar side of the wrist should be performed with an osteotomy of the distal radius depends on careful preoperative assessment of the DRUJ. Partial ulnar head resection should be performed as a primary operation in combination with radial osteotomy when the patient's main symptom is painful limitation of forearm rotation due to post-traumatic osteoarthritis of the radio-ulnar joint (Fig. 14.5). Instability and ulnocarpal impingement as a result of shortening, angulation, or malrotation of the distal end of the radius with no degenerative arthritic changes can be corrected by restoration of the radial deformity alone, in an effort to preserve the distal part of the ulna. If the patient still has symptoms after radial osteotomy, ulnar resection arthroplasty or a Sauvé–Kapandji procedure can be performed at a later date.

Post-operative care

The wrist is immobilized in a volar plaster splint until the soft tissues have healed, usually by two weeks after the operation, Early wrist motion is permitted after suture removal in cases where rigid internal fixation can be achieved with plate fixation, that is when there is good bone quality and no osteoporosis. In cases of Kirschner-wire fixation, a forearm cast for four weeks after suture removal is recommended. Heavy manual work is allowed between six to eight weeks after radiographic confirmation of union of the osteotomy. Dorsal plates are usually removed between three and six months after surgery to prevent attrition tendonitis of the extensor pollicis longus. Volar plates, on the other hand, may be left in place.

Discussion

Serious deformities of the wrist can usually be prevented by proper treatment of the original fracture, especially in the unstable types with a strong tendency to redisplace in the plaster cast after adequate initial reduction. Conservative treatment of Colles' fractures in the younger age group leads to satisfactory clinical results in the majority of patients. On the other hand, adequate function of the wrist and absence of pain can be expected, despite radiographic evidence of malunion. These results are mainly due to the fact that these fractures occur predominantly in elderly patients, who no longer engage in strenuous manual activities, and therefore the functional requirements of the wrist are much reduced. Conversely, wrist deformity in the younger, active patient is less well tolerated, especially in heavy manual workers or those who require a normal range of motion of the

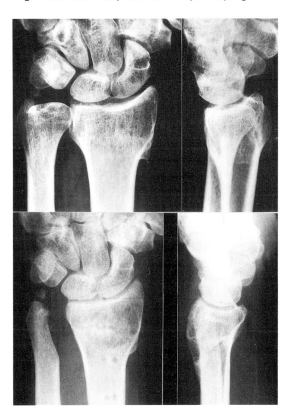

Figure 14.5

Top: malunited Colles' fracture with predominant radio-ulnar pain and severe limitation of forearm rotation. Bottom: result 3 years after radial osteotomy and partial ulnar resection.

wrist. It is mainly for this group that corrective osteotomy to restore function and cosmetic appearance of the wrist should be considered.

Careful analysis of the results of these studies (Fernandez 1982, 1984, 1987 and 1988, Fernandez and Geissler 1989, Fernandez et al. 1977) showed that the best functional results with freedom from pain are obtained in malunions following extra-articular fractures, in which the pre-operative range of motion of the wrist is not less than 70% of normal, when the wrist joint is free of degenerative changes both at the radiocarpal and intercarpal level, and when there is no fixed carpal malalignment. Under these circumstances, and when shortening does not exceed 10 mm, restoration of the normal anatomy of the distal radius and its relationships to the ulna offers highly satisfactory long-term results (Fig. 14.6).

In a more recent review of patients treated in the past ten years, an additional operation on the ulnar side of the wrist had to be performed in about 50% of a total of 79 radial osteotomies (Table 14.1). This substantial increase is mainly a result of having extended the indications for operative treatment of malunions to include those that occur after intra-articular Colles' fractures, malunions after comminuted fractures with severe shortening, and Smith's fractures with subluxation of the DRUJ. Furthermore, preoperative routine assessment of the radio-ulnar joint

Table 14.1

Corrective osteotomies of the distal radius

Malunion after:	
Colles' fractures	36
Smith's fractures	20
Comminuted fractures	15
Reversed Barton's fractures	2
Fractures in children	6
	79

Operations on the ulnar side of the wrist

Darrach procedure	8
Ulnar shortening	3
Partial ulnar head resection	19
Partial ulnar head resection and ulnar shortening	3
Sauvé–Kapandji procedure	3
Epiphysiodesis of distal ulna	2
	38

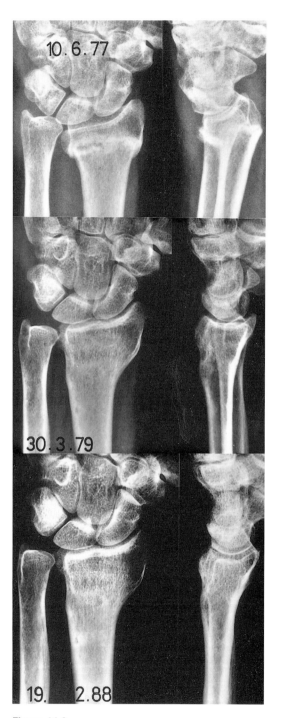

Figure 14.6

Follow-up at 11 years of a malunited Colles' fracture treated by radial osteotomy. Note the well-preserved joint space, the absence of degenerative changes, and the normal carpal alignment.

with CT scans has anticipated the need for an additional operative procedure at this level.

The results have shown that partial resection of the ulnar head is a valuable adjuvant procedure in radial malunion when the symptoms are mainly localized to the radio-ulnar joint. In 15 consecutive patients where both operations were combined (Fernandez 1988), the remaining deficit of pronation was 12% and of supination 14%, compared with the preoperative deficits of 47% and 77% respectively. Lengthening of the radius by osteotomy in turn corrects the ulnar variance, which is imperative to prevent painful stylocarpal impingement after hemiresection arthroplasty. If radial length cannot be obtained with radial osteotomy alone, an additional shortening osteotomy of the ulna has to be performed at the same time.

The overall results of this series are comparable to those of other authors who employ similar techniques (Behrens and Mickley 1987, Bora et al. 1984, Ekenstam et al. 1985, Forgon and Mammel 1983, Jupiter and Masem 1988, Kerboul et al. 1986, Lehner and Sennwald 1989, Rodriguez-Meythiaz and Chamay 1988, Watson and Castle 1988). They show that with careful patient selection, correct indication, and refinements of the surgical technique, over 80% of excellent and good results can be expected. The initial complications and failures were due either to technical errors or to the improper selection of patients who had degenerative changes in the radiocarpal joint following intra-articular fracture or fixed dorsal carpal malalignment that could not be corrected by osteotomy. A mild loss of the initial correction was also observed, probably caused by instability and settling of the interposed graft in cases with inadequate bone quality. However, predictable anatomical results can be expected if the procedure is executed in accordance with a careful preoperative plan based on critical analysis and measurement of the radiographs of both wrists, in an effort to restore the wrist anatomy of each individual patient.

References

Behrens S, Mickley V. Korrekturosteotomien am distalen Unterarm. *Unfallchirurg* 1987; **90**: 6.

Bora FW, Ostermann AL, Zielinski CJ. Osteotomy of the distal radius with a biplanar iliac bone graft for malunion. *Bull Hosp Jt Dis Orthop Inst* 1984; **44**: 122.

Bowers WH. Distal radioulnar joint arthroplasty: The hemiresection-interposition technique. *J Hand Surg* 1985; **10A**:169–78.

Boyd HB, Stone MM. Resection of the distal end of the Ulna. *J Bone Joint Surg* 1944; **26**: 313–21.

Bunnell S. *Surgery of the hand*, 2nd Ed. Philadelphia: JB Lippincott, 1948: 596, 681–82.

Campbell WC. Malunited Colles' fractures. *J Am Med Assn* 1937; **109**: 1105–8.

Castaing J. Les fractures récentes de l'extrémité inférieure du radiuz chez l'adulte. *Rev Chir Orthop* 1964; **50**: 581–696.

Cooney WP, Dobyns JH, Linscheid RL. Complications of Colles fractures. *J Bone Joint Surg* 1980; **62A**: 613.

Darrach W. Partial excision of lower shaft of ulna for deformity following Colles' fracture. *Ann Surg* 1913; **57**: 764–65.

Desault M. Extrait d'un memoire de M. Desault sur la luxation de l'extrémité inférieure du cubitus. *J Chir* 1791; **I**: 78.

Duparc U, Pacault JY, Valtin B. Traîtement des cals vicieux du poignet par ostéotomie d'ouverture avec greffe osseuse. *Ann Chir* 1977; **31**: 307.

Durman CD. An operation for correction of deformities of the wrist following fracture. *J Bone Joint Surg* 1935; **17**: 1014–16.

Durman CD. Malunited Colles' fracture. In abstract of discussion of Dr. Campbell's article. *J Am Med Ass* 1937; **109**: 1105–8.

Ekenstam F, Hagert CG, Engkvist O, Törnvall AH, Wilbrand H. Corrective osteotomy of malunited fractures of the distal end of the radius. *Scand J Plast Reconstr Surg* 1985; **19**: 175.

Fernandez DL. Correction of post-traumatic wrist deformity in adults by osteotomy, bone-grafting, and internal fixation. *J Bone Joint Surg* 1982; **64A**: 1164–78.

Fernandez DL. Osteotomias del antebrazo distal. Indication técnica y resultados. *Acta Ortop Latinoamericana* 1984; **11**: 55–72.

Fernandez DL. Treatment of malunion of the distal radius. Read at the 47th AO Course (advanced) of the Swiss Association for the Study of Internal Fixation, Davos, Switzerland, 1987.

Fernandez DL. Radial osteotomy and Bowers arthroplasty for malunited fractures of the distal end of the radius. *J Bone Joint Surg* 1988; **70A**: 1538–51.

Fernandez DL, Geissler WB. Korrektureingriffe bei Fehlstellungen am distalen Radius. *Z Unfallchir Vers Med Berufskr* 1989; **82**: 34–44.

Fernandez DL, Albrecht HU, Saxer U. Die Korrekturosteotomie am distalen Radius bei posttraumatischer Fehlstellung. *Arch Orthop Unfall Chir* 1977; **90**: 199–211.

Forgon M, Mammel E. Unsere Korrekturosteotomie in Fehlstellung geheilter Frakturen der Speiche an der typischen Stelle. *Unfall Chir* 1983; **9**: 318.

Fourrier P, Bardy A, Roche G, Cisterne JP, Chambon A. Approche d'une définition du cal vicieux du poignet. *Internat Orthop (SICOT)* 1981; **4**: 299–305.

Ghormley RK, Mroz RJ. Fractures of the wrist: a review of 176 cases. *Surg Gynecol Obstet* 1932; **55**: 377–81.

Heim U. Stabilisation des ostéotomies de l'extrémité inférieure du radius par petite plaque en T. *Ann Chir* 1977; **31**: 313.

Hobart MH, Kraft GL. Malunited Colles' fracture. *Am J Surg* 1941; **53**: 55.

Jupiter JB, Masem M. Reconstruction of post-traumatic deformity of the distal radius and ulna. *Hand Clinics* 1988; **4**: 377–90.

Kerboul B, Le Saout J, Plossu JP, Lefevre C, Fabre L, Roblin L, Courtois B. Correction des cals vicieux de l'extrémité inférieure du radius par ostéotomie d'ouverture. *Acta Orthop Belg* 1986; **52**: 134–44.

Lanz U. Correction osteotomy after malunion of distal radius fractures. In Abstract book. Second Congress of the International Federation of Societies for Surgery of the Hand. Boston Mass., 1983.

Lehner M, Sennwald G. Korrekturosteotomie am distalen Vorderarm. *Z Unfallchir Vers Med Berufskr* 1989; **82**: 45–48.

Linscheid RL, Dobyns JH, Beabout JW, Bryan RS. Traumatic instability of the wrist. Diagnosis, classification and pathomechanics. *J Bone Joint Surg* 1972; **54A**: 1612.

Martini AK. Die sekundäre Arthrose des Handgelenkes bei der in Fehlstellung verheilten und nicht korrigierten distalen Radiusfraktur. *Akt Traumatol* 1986; **16**: 143.

McQueen M, Caspers J. Colles' fracture: Does the anatomic result affect the final function? *J Bone Joint Surg* 1988; **70B**: 649.

Merle D'Aubigné R, Joussemet A. A propos du traitement des cals vicieux de l'extrémité inférieure du radius. *Mém Acad Chir* 1945; **71**: 153–7.

Merle D'Aubigné R, Tubiana R. Séquelles de traumatismes du poignet. In: *Traumatismes anciens. Généralités membre supérieur.* Paris: Masson, 1958: 361–76.

Milch H. Cuff resection of the ulna for malunited Colles' Fracture. *J Bone Joint Surg* 1941; **23**: 311–13.

Moore EM. Three cases illustrating luxation of the ulna in connection with Colles' fracture. *Med Rec NY* 1880; **17**: 305–8.

Müller-Färber J, Griedel W. Der sekundäre Korrektureingriff am distalen Radius bei post-traumatischer Fehlstellung. *Unfallheilkunde* 1979; **82**: 23–28.

Pogue DS, Viegas SF, Patterson RM, Peterson PD, Jenkins DK, Sweo TD, Hokanson JA. Effects of distal radius fracture malunion on wrist joint mechanics. *J Hand Surg* 1990; **15A**: 721–27.

Renné J, Schmelzeiser H. Zur operativen Korrektur unter Verkürzung und in Fehlstellung verheilter typischer Radiusfrakturen in Handgelenksnähe. *Mschr Unfallheilk* 1974; **77**: 111.

Rodriguez-Meythiaz AM, Chamay A. Traîtement des cals vicieux extra-articulaires du radius distal par ostéotomie d'ouverture avec interposition d'une greffe. *Med et Hyg* 1988; **46**: 2757–65.

Sakai K, Doi K, Ihara K, Kido K, Kawai S. Carpal alignment after fractures of the distal radius. In Abstract Book of the International Symposium on the Wrist, Nagoya, Japan, 1991: 117.

Sauvé L, Kapandji IA. Une nouvelle technique de traitement chirurgical des luxation récidivantes isolées de l'extrémité cubitale inférieure. *J Chir* 1936; **47**: 4.

Shaw JA, Bruno A, Paul EM. Ulnar styloid fixation in the treatment of post-traumatic instability of the radio-ulnar joint: A biomechanical study with clinical correlation. *J Hand Surg* 1990; **15A**: 712–20.

Short WH, Palmer AK, Werner FW, Murphy DJ. A biomechanical study of distal radial fractures. *J Hand Surg* 1987; **12A**: 529–34.

Speed JS, Knight RA. Treatment of malunited Colles' fractures. *J Bone Joint Surg* 1945; **27**: 361–67.

Taleisnik J, Watson HK. Midcarpal instability caused by malunited fractures of the distal radius. *J Hand Surg* 1984; **9A**: 350–57.

Villar RN, Marsh D, Rushton N, Greatorex RA. Three years after Colles' fractures. *J Bone Joint Surg* 1987; **69B**: 635.

Watson HK, Castle TH. Trapezoidal osteotomy of the distal radius for unacceptable articular angulation after Colles' fracture. *J Hand Surg* 1988; **13A**: 837–43.

Watson HK, Ryu J, Burgess RC. Matched distal ulnar resection. *J Hand Surg* 1986; **11A**: 812–17.

Wermann H, Otto W, Wollenweber HD, Wawro W. Indikation und Wert der Korrekturosteotomie am distalen Radiusende. *Beitr Orthop U Traumatol* 1984; **31**: 453.

15
Open reduction of distal radius fractures: indications, classification and functional assessment

William P Cooney III

Intra-articular fractures of the distal radius represent a specific type of injury of the wrist that is different from the more classical Colles' fracture (Cooney et al. 1979 and 1980). Recent studies (Bradway et al. 1989, Fernandez and Geissler 1991, Melone 1986, Missakian et al. 1992) have emphasized that better methods of identifying and classifying distal radial fractures may direct the treating surgeon to alter treatment and to adapt open reduction of these fractures in the proper circumstances (Axelrod et al. 1988, Bassett 1987, Bradway et al. 1989, Fernandez and Geissler 1991, Melone 1986, Missakian et al. 1992). The purpose of this chapter is to describe the current indications for open reduction of fractures of the distal radius and to bring forth a classification system (Cooney et al. 1990) that will alert the examining physician of the alternatives to consider in determining treatment.

Indications for open reduction

Previous studies by Knirk and Jupiter (1986), Bradway et al. (1989), Bassett (1987) and Melone (1986) have pointed out that traditional cast treatment of intra-articular fractures results in a poor outcome for the patient. Between 28 and 40% of patients will have post-traumatic arthritis. External fixation has improved the results in many comminuted and displaced distal radius fractures (Cooney et al. 1979) but unacceptable results with loss of motion and/or post-traumatic arthritis are still present in 14 to 20% of patients (Cooney et al. 1980, Frykman 1967). A number of cases had incomplete reduction of the joint articular cartilage. It was noted that displacement can occur within the scaphoid fossa or lunate fossa of the distal radius. In addition, the sigmoid fossa of the distal radius, which supports forces across the distal radio-ulnar joint, can be displaced. It may not be possible to use ligamentotaxis to reduce intra-articular fractures since the fracture components may involve simultaneous ligament injury and dorsal ligaments may be ineffective in providing distraction of the fracture components.

Currently, there are guidelines that define unacceptable alignment of distal radial fractures as an articular step-off of more than 2 mm shortening greater than 5 mm (which affects the distal radio-ulnar joint) or dorsal angulation greater than 10° (which can lead to secondary carpal instability), all of which are indications for more sustained treatment. When distal radial fracture reduction does not achieve these goals, closed reduction and pin fixation, or open reduction and internal fixation may be necessary.

The die-punch fracture of the lunate fossa of the distal radius is also a reason to proceed directly to open reduction since our experience has demonstrated that closed reduction is not frequently successful. This fracture often has two components, one dorsal and one volar, that cannot be reduced by longitudinal traction or closed manipulation. We have found that application of external fixation to gain general alignment, followed by limited open reduction to gain anatomic alignment is a worthwhile treatment programme. With more significant fracture involvement of the articular surfaces of the distal radius, traditional open reduction through a dorsal incision, fracture reduction with K-wires, dorsal T-plate stabilization and bone grafting are usually performed. A volar approach is reserved for the occasional volar displaced, intra-articular fractures that would fit into the Smith classification (intra-articular, displaced or volar fracture-dislocation).

Classification of intra-articular fractures

There are a number of different classifications proposed for assessing fractures of the distal radius. Results of treatment of these fractures have been reported previously using the Frykman classification (Cooney et al. 1979 and 1981), the AO classification (Bradway et al. 1989, Muller et al. 1987), and Lidström's classification (1959). Following review of a large series of different types of distal radius fractures and a symposium addressing a practical classification of distal radial fractures (Cooney et al. 1990). The importance of a treatment-based classification system has been recognized, to provide recommendations not only for the more common Colles-type fracture, but, more importantly, for classification of intra-articular fractures. Previous classifications have been primarily descriptive, based either on radiographic findings or the degree of fracture displacement. These systems did not consider other mechanisms of injury or treatment options for the classification of extra-articular versus intra-articular fractures.

The classification of distal radial fractures presented in this chapter is an extension of Gartland's classification (1951), in which general categories of extra-articular and intra-articular fractures were proposed, but without any specific direction or guidance. This new categorization of distal radial fractures is called the universal classification (Table 15.1 and Fig. 15.1). It not only separates extra-articular from intra-articular fractures but further subdivides fractures into stable or unstable, reducible or irreducible. To further direct treatment, the intra-articular fractures are subdivided into four categories which have specific treatment directives (Table 15.2). A

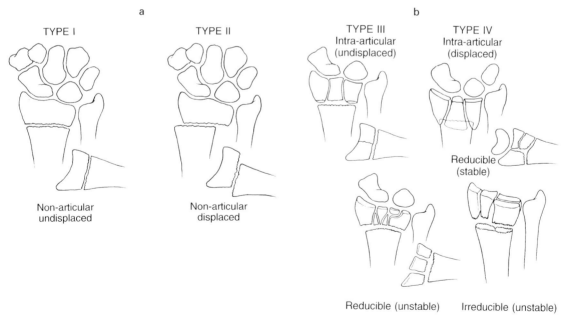

Figure 15.1

Universal classification of distal radius fractures (Cooney et al. 1990). a) Non-articular fractures. Type I: undisplaced; Type II: displaced. b) Articular fractures. Type III: undisplaced; Type IV: displaced. The displaced fractures are subdivided into reducible or irreducible; stable and unstable. Treatment options change with stability, reducibility, and involvement of the articular surface.

Table 15.1 Universal classification of distal radial fractures

Type I	Articular	Undisplaced
Type II	Non-articular A. Reducible* B. Reducible* C. Irreducible	Displaced Stable Unstable
Type III	Articular	Undisplaced
Type IV	Displaced A. Reducible* B. Reducible* C. Irreducible D. Complex	Displaced Stable Unstable Unstable

*(By ligamentotaxis only)

Table 15.2 Universal classification

Treatment indications

Type		Treatment
I	Non-articular	Cast/splint
II	Non-articular	Closed reduction
	Displaced	Percutaneous pins Interfocal pins (External fixation)*
III	Articular	
	Non-Displaced	Cast
		Percutaneous pins
IV	Articular	
	Displaced	Closed reduction
	Reducible, stable	Cast and K-pins External fixation
	Reducible, unstable	External fixation External fixation and K-pins
	Irreducible	Open reduction External fixation Internal fixation Combined external and internal fixation

*External fixation only if stable with ligamentotaxis

nice feature of the universal classification is that several of the newer systems, for example the Melone classification (1986), the Mayo classification (Missakian et al. 1992), and the McMurtry classification (1991) can be adapted into it as further types or subdivisions of the displaced intra-articular fractures (Figs. 15.2–15.4).

The interested reader should also be aware that the Melone (1986) and McMurtry (1991) classifications are based on the number of fracture parts

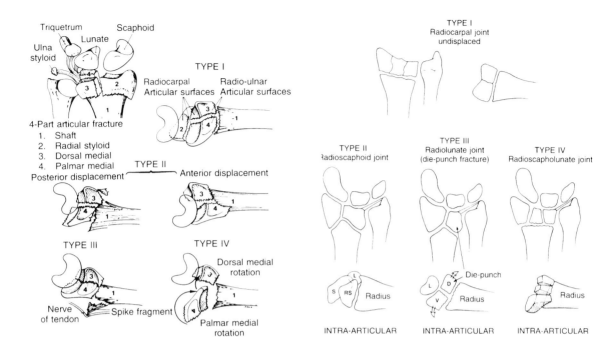

Figure 15.2

Melone classification (1986). Distal radial fracture components are subdivided into four parts: 1) The diaphyseal shaft; 2) radial styloid component; 3) dorsal medial component; 4) volar medial component. A 4-part articular fracture will have displacement of components 2, 3, and 4 from each other and from the diphyseal shaft.

Figure 15.3

Mayo classification (Missakian et al. 1992). The intra-articular fractures are subclassified based on involvement of the radiocarpal joint and distal radio-ulnar joint.
Type I: extra-articular radiocarpal, intra-articular, radio-ulnar joint; Type II: intra-articular scaphoid fossa of distal radius; Type III: intra-articular lunate fossa of distal radius ± sigmoid fossa; Type IV: intra-articular, scaphoid fossa, lunate fossa and sigmoid fossa of the distal radius.
The intent of this classification is to call attention to reduction of each of the 3 articular surfaces of the distal radius.

involved (similar to the Neer classification of two-, three- and four-part fracture dislocations of the shoulder). The proximal radius is part one, the scaphoid fossa component is part two, the lunate fossa components are parts three and/or four, and multiple segment fractures of the radial shaft are part-five fractures. Melone emphasizes the difficulty involved in reducing fractures in which more than three or four components are involved.

A treatment-based classification is therefore currently recommended. The universal classification has incorporated the best of previous classifications (Gartland 1951, Sarmiento 1975, Lidstrom 1959) with treatment alternatives for each of the sub-groups. This system clearly defines the role of open reduction and internal fixation in the overall management of distal radial fractures. It is quite different from the Frykman classification (1967), which is based on the radiographic appearance alone, without reference to treatment alternatives, and the AO classification which is an all-encompassing index of different fracture types but does not direct the treating physician in the management of the patient. The treatment-based universal classification (Table 15.2) separates the extra-articular fractures, which can be treated by cast immobilization, percutaneous pins or a combination of both, from the intra-articular fractures, which generally require external fixation to maintain fracture reduction (stable type) or external and internal fixation to obtain and then hold the reduction (unstable type). The subclassifications of Melone (1986), McMurtry (1991) and Mayo (Missakian 1992) can then be used to identify intra-articular fractures (such as lunate fossa die-

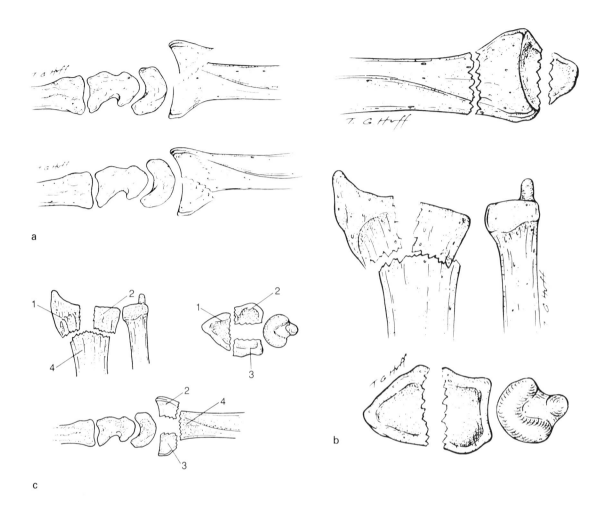

Figure 15.4

McMurtry classification (1991). Intra-articular fractures of the distal radius. a) 2-part fracture involving dorsal or volar intra-articular fracture (top) and metaphysis or shaft of the distal radius (bottom). b) 3-part fracture involving the scaphoid fossa (top), the lunate fossa (middle) and the metaphysis (bottom). c) 4-part fracture involving the scaphoid fossa (1), the dorsal half of the lunate fossa (2), the volar half of the lunate fossa (3) and the metaphysis (4).

punch fractures) which are best treated by open reduction.

In the classification of distal radial fractures, injuries to the distal radio-ulnar joint are not well recognized. When it comes to assessing post-injury problems and complications, however, fractures involving the sigmoid fossa of the distal radius are no less important than those that involve the radiocarpal joint. The universal classification is once again helpful in determining treatment. Fracture types II, III and IV, for example, can be applied to fractures of the distal ulna and distal radio-ulnar joint, with recommendations for cast immobilization (or percutaneous pins) for extra-articular fractures, and closed (or open reduction) with external or internal fixation to maintain the reduction for intra-articular fractures. The distal radio-ulnar joint (DRUJ) is probably the most neglected joint in the management of distal radial fractures, yet this is the area with the highest incidence of post-traumatic arthritis (Cooney et al. 1980).

Functional assessment

A discussion of fractures of the distal radius would not be complete without reference to a method of functional assessment of fracture outcome. The most widely used system of measuring outcome comes from the early work of Gartland and Werley (1951), with additional criteria by Sarmiento (1975) (Table 15.3). This grading or ranking system has been useful previously to compare different methods of treatment for distal radial fractures. It has potential use for future investigations, with the additional advantage of providing an historical reference. Since it includes subjective along with objective evaluations, however, it may be less rigorous than desired for accurate analysis of functional use of the extremity. Any reported series of distal radial fractures should consider the Gartland–Werley classification for comparison.

A second functional assessment system has been proposed by Green and O'Brien (1978). Recent modifications to this system were proposed, which deleted the radiographic component; this is best considered as a separate analysis and should not be included when judging functional outcome criteria. This modified Mayo wrist score (Cooney et al. 1991) is therefore primarily an objective assessment of pain, motion, strength and the ability to return to daily activities (Table 15.4). With a maximum grade of 100 (25 points for each category), it provides a wide range for functional assessment. It is suggested as an alternative test of wrist function to the Gartland–Werley system (1951) and as an excellent method of comparison of different forms of treatment of distal radial fractures. From our own analysis of open reduction of displaced intra-articular fractures of the distal radius (Bradway et al. 1989, Missakian et al. 1992), the Mayo wrist scoring system proved a more stringent test of hand and wrist function after fractures of the distal radius than the Gartland–Werley system.

Table 15.3 Demerit point system used to evaluate end results of healed Colles' fracture (after Gartland and Werley 1951 and Sarmiento et al. 1975)

	Points
Residual Deformity	
Prominent ulnar styloid	1
Residual dorsal tilt	2
Radial elevation of hand	2–3
Point range	0–6
Subjective Evaluation	
Excellent: no pain, disability, or limitation of motion	0
Good: occasional pain, slight limitation of motion; no disability	2
Fair: occasional pain, limitation of motion, feeling of weakness, activities slightly restricted	4
Poor: pain, limitation of motion, disability, activities more or less restricted	6
Objective Evaluation*	
Loss of dorsiflexion	5
Loss of ulnar deviation	3
Loss of supination	2
Loss of pronation	2
Loss of palmar flexion	1
Loss of radial deviation	1
Loss of circumduction	1
Pain in distal radio-ulnar joint	1
Grip strength — 60% or less of opposite side	1
Complications	
Arthritic Change	
Minimum	1
Minimum with pain	2
Moderate	3
Moderate with pain	4
Severe	4
Severe with pain	5
Nerve complications	1–3
Loss of finger motion	1–3
Point range	0–10
End Result Point Range	
Excellent	0–2
Good	3–8
Fair	9–20
Poor	21 and above

*Objective evaluation is based on range of motion. The minimum required for normal function: dorsiflexion 45 degrees, palmar flexion 30 degrees, radial deviation 15 degrees, ulnar deviation 15 degrees, pronation 50 degrees, supination 50 degrees.

Summary

In summary, the universal classification is recommended for the analysis and treatment of fractures of the distal radius. This classification, based on original concepts by Gartland and Werley (1951), provides treatment guidelines based on the extra-articular and intra-articular nature of the injury. It is relatively easy to remember and apply.

Table 15.4 Modified clinical-scoring system of Green and O'Brien

Category	Score (Points)	Findings
Pain (25 points)	25	None
	20	Mild, occasional
	25	Moderate, tolerable
	0	Severe or intolerable
Functional status (25 points)	25	Returned to regular employment
	20	Restricted employment
	15	Able to work but unemployed
	0	Unable to work because of pain
Range of motion (25 points)		Percentage of normal
	25	100
	15	75–99
	10	50–74
	5	25–49
	0	0–24
		Dorsiflexion-plantar flexion arc (injured hand only)
	25	120° or more
	15	91°–119°
	10	61°–90°
	5	31°–60°
	0	30° or less
Grip strength (25 points)		Percentage of normal
	25	100
	15	75–99
	10	50–74
	5	25–49
	0	0–24
Final result		
Excellent	90–100	
Good	80–89	
Fair	65–79	
Poor	<65	

References

Axelrod T, Poley D, Green J, McMurtry RY. Limited open reduction of the lunate facet in comminuted intra-articular fractures of the distal radius. *J Hand Surg* 1988; **13A**: 372–77.

Bacorn RW, Kurtzke JF. Colles' fractures: a study of two thousand cases from the New York State Workmen's Compensation Board. *J Bone Joint Surg* 1953; **35A**: 643–48.

Bassett RL. Displaced intraarticular fractures of the distal radius. *Clin Orthop* 1987; **214**: 148–52.

Bradway JK, Amadio PC, Cooney WP. Open reduction and internal fixation of the displaced, comminuted intra-articular fractures of the distal end of the radius. *J Bone Joint Surg* 1989; **71A(6)**: 839–47.

Cassebaum WH. Colles' fractures: a study of end results. *JAMA* 1950; **143**: 963–65.

Cooney WP, Linscheid RL, Dobyns JH. External pin fixation for unstable Colles' fractures. *J Bone Joint Surg* 1979; **61A**: 840–45.

Cooney WP, Rayhack J, Agee J, Melone C, Hastings N. Managing intra-articular fractures of the distal radius. *Contemporary Orthopedics* 1990; **21(1)**: 71–104.

Cooney WP, Linscheid RL, Dobyns JH. Complications of Colles' fractures. *J Bone Joint Surg* 1980; **62A**: 613–19.

Cooney WP, Bussey R, Dobyns JH, Linscheid RL. Difficult wrist fractures. Perilunate fracture-dislocations of wrist: classification and analysis. *Clin Orthop* 1981; **214**: 136–47.

Frykman G. Fractures of the distal radius including sequelae. *Acta Orthop Scand* 1967; **108 (Suppl)**: 1–153.

Gartland JJ, Werley CW. Evaluation of healed Colles' fractures. *J Bone Joint Surg* 1951; **33A**: 895–907.

Green DP, O'Brien ET. Open reduction of carpal dislocations. *J Hand Surg* 1978; **3**: 250–65.

Fernandez DL, Geissler WB. Treatment of displaced articular fractures of the radius. *J Hand Surg (Am)* 1991; **16A**: 375–84.

Knirk JL, Jupiter JB. Intraarticular fractures of the distal end of the radius in young adults. *J Bone Joint Surg* 1980; **68A**: 647–59.

Jupiter JB. Fractures of the distal end of the radius. *J Bone Joint Surg* 1991; **73A**: 461–67.

Kristiansen A, Gjersoe E. Colles' fractures: operative treatment, indications and results. *Acta Orthop Scand* 1968; **39**: 33–46.

Lidström, A. Fractures of the distal end of the radius. *Acta Orthop Scand* 1959; **41(Suppl)**: 1–118.

Melone Jr CP. Open treatment for displaced articular fractures of the distal radius. *Clin Orthop* 1986; **202**: 103–11.

McMurtry RV, Jupiter JB. Fractures of the distal radius. In Browner B, Jupiter J, Levine A, Trafton P, eds. *Skeletal* trauma. Philadelphia: WB Saunders: Vol 2, 1063–94: 1991.

Missakian M, Cooney WP, Glidewell H. Open reduction and internal fixation of distal radius fractures. *J Hand Surg* 1992; **17A**: 745–55.

Müller ME, Nazarian S, Koch P. *AO classification of fractures*. Berlin: Springer-Verlag, 1987.

Sarmiento A, Pratt GW, Berry NC, Sinclair WF. Colles' fracture. Functional bracing in supination. *J Bone Joint Surg* 1975; **57A**: 311–17.

Seitz WH, Putnam MD, Dick HM. Limited open surgical approach for external fixation of distal radius fractures. *J Hand Surg* 1990; **15A**: 288–93.

Solgaard S. Classification of distal radius fractures. *Acta Orthop Scand* 1985; **56(6)**: 249–52.

Weber SC, Szabo RM. Severely comminuted distal radius fractures as an unsolved problem. Complications associated with external fixation and pins and plaster. *J Hand Surg* 1986; **11A**: 157–65.

16
Classification of intra-articular fractures of the distal radius

Ch Mathoulin, E Letrosne, Ph Saffar

Introduction

As Castaing mentioned in 1964, fractures of the distal end of the radius traditionally have a bad reputation.

Articular fractures, which are usually due to violent trauma, are the main cause of these unsatisfactory results. This chapter is an analysis of articular fractures with a view to choosing the best therapy. In fact, anatomical reduction is necessary in these cases because the incongruence of the articular surfaces often results in a more or less long-term arthrosis. This chapter also describes a classification system for articular fractures which takes into account the potential instability that results from different fracture patterns.

Historical background

Fractures of the distal extremity of the radius were treated in ancient civilizations, as indicated by a splint which was found on the wrist of a Pharaoh of the ninth dynasty. However, it was the Frenchman, Claude Pouteau who provided the first description of fractures of the distal radius. The Irish surgeon Abraham Colles described this fracture in more detail in 1814. Since then, many authors have worked on the description and comprehension of the mechanism of these fractures. Cauchoix and Duparc made the distinction between anterior marginal and bimarginal fractures in 1960. Castaing, in his exceptional study for the SOFCOT symposium in 1964, analysed the many types of displacement of these fractures. His classification is based on the mechanisms of fracture, which are differentiated by the type of displacement:

1. Fractures by extension-compression or posterior (dorsal) fractures which can be divided into:
   - extra-articular fractures (classic Colles' fractures);
   - articular fractures (with posterior (dorsal) internal fragment displacement or complex fractures).

2. Fractures by flexion-compression or anterior fractures, which can be further divided into:
   - the extra-articular fractures (Goyrand–Smith);
   - articular fractures (anterior marginal, simple and complex);
   - unclassable fractures.

Frykman (1967) provided a classification for these fractures, which is the basic reference for many English papers on the subject. In this system, there are two types of extra-articular and six types of intra-articular fractures, which differentiate into radiocarpal and radio-ulnar articular involvement and which may or may not be associated with an ulnar fracture. The Melone (1984) classification subdivides fractures according to four fracture components (diaphysis, radial styloid, internal dorsal fragment, internal palmar fragment) and their displacement. Cooney (1983) described a classification which differentiates the articular surfaces involved: the inferior radio-ulnar, the scaphoid, and the lunar.

All of these systems focus on articular fractures, the fragments involved, the mechanisms of fracture and the type of displacement which occurs.

Classification according to potential instability

As it is difficult to evaluate the potential instability of articular fractures, this system of classification (Mathoulin 1990) takes the instability into account, but also evaluates the relative ease with which the fracture can be kept stable by well managed treatment.

This classification is the result of a multicentre, radiological-anatomical study which included 137 articular fractures in young adults, with at least a two-year follow-up. It divides intra-articular fractures into four types according to the association of the fracture lines. Fragment analysis was based on radiographic assessment after orthopaedic reduction in the operating suite. The initial radiographs were usually uninterpretable, since only the amount of displacement could be determined; this sometimes resulted in incorrect classification of simple fractures as comminuted fractures.

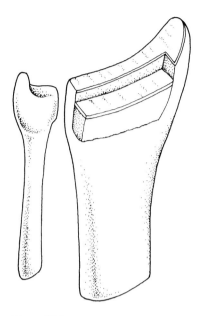

Figure 16.1

Articular fracture of the distal radius type I (illustration by S. Zakine).

Type 1

Fractures with a single articular fracture line in the frontal plane (Fig. 16.1). This fracture can be observed on a lateral radiograph and can be subdivided into two types:

- classic anterior marginal simple fractures;
- and, less commonly, posterior marginal fractures (1 out of 1500 in a study of a ten year series).

These fractures are easier to stabilize after reduction, and treatment is usually surgical.

Type 2

Type 2 fractures have an articular fracture line in the sagittal plane (Fig. 16.2). This fracture may be observed in antero-posterior radiographs and the line joins a dorsal cortical lateral fracture with the articular surface fracture.

The following types of fracture were observed, depending on the slant of the fracture line and the surface affected:

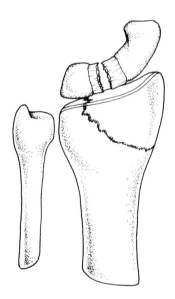

Figure 16.2

Articular fracture of the distal radius type II, showing rupture of the scapholunate ligament (illustration by S. Zakine).

- type 2 scaphoid — the fracture line extends into the scaphoid fossa;
- type 2 lunar — the fracture line extends into the lunar fossa;

- type 2 radio-ulnar — the fracture line extends into the distal radio-ulnar articulation.

The indications for treatment and results following treatment for the first two subtypes of fracture are nearly identical.

Generally, these fractures are the result of a movement that involves dorsal flexion and supination, often from an attempt to break a fall backwards. Thus, the fractures result from radial extension and dorsal angulation. In fact, the greater the radial angulation of the hand, the more the fracture pattern will extend internally, thus determining these three subtypes.

It should also be emphasized that type 2 scaphoid and type 2 lunar fractures are often associated with a tear of the intraosseous scapholunate ligament. This injury, which is an intrinsic source of carpal instability, must be diagnosed and treated.

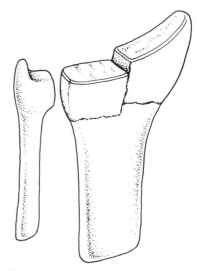

Figure 16.3

Articular fracture of the distal radius type III (illustration by S. Zakine).

Type 3

This type includes two subtypes of fracture pattern (Fig. 16.3):

- a horizontal, extra-articular line;
- and an articular line which involves either the lunate or the scaphoid surfaces.

These are, of course, the patterns observed most often in these types of fracture. Other fracture lines are possible, however, especially when dorsal comminution is present in the fracture pattern.

The T-fractures described by Castaing are included in the type 3 group of this classification, in particular the 'die-punch' fracture, which is associated with a horizontal fracture line and a vertical articular line. This fracture is the result of a depression in the lunate surface by the lunate compression load. It is difficult to diagnose and reduce, and often requires surgery like the other type 3 fractures. It is important to note that these fractures can also be associated with scapholunate instability.

Type 4

This type of fracture is the most interesting, but also the most difficult to analyse. It is associated with three fracture patterns (Fig. 16.4):

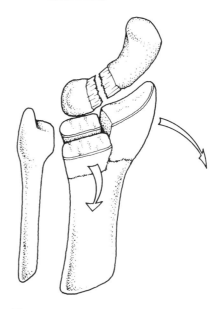

Figure 16.4

Articular fracture of the distal radius type IV (illustration by S. Zakine).

- a horizontal extra-articular fracture line;
- a frontal articular fracture line
- a sagittal articular fracture line

The simplest form of this type is a fracture with a posterior (dorsal) intra-articular fragment, which is, in fact, only partially type 4. Most type 4 fractures, however, which have been well described by Melone (1984), involve the entire articular surface. They include the sagittal and frontal T-fractures described by Castaing, as well as X- and bimarginal fractures.

In this series, type 4 fractures with slight displacement were found which had been misdiagnosed as external articular fractures, causing unsatisfactory results with secondary displacement of the internal fragments. This misdiagnosis occurred because only part of the problem had been identified and treated. On the other hand, certain type 4 fractures with marked displacement were unfortunately diagnosed as 'comminuted', although it is nearly always possible to analyse the different fragments and provide appropriate treatment when the patient is examined in the operating room after reduction.

Complications

Aggravating osteoarticular lesions

Associated lesions worsen prognosis, increase instability in most cases and are a clear indication for surgery.

Lesions involving the fracture

Displacement

Displacement can be absent, slight or marked. We have a tendency to use more aggressive techniques in fractures due to violent trauma with significant displacement, because these cases often include injury to the intrinsic carpal ligament system, which increases instability.

Posterior comminution (bone loss)

Frequently associated with these fractures, this complication causes significant secondary displacement and instability. In these cases, bone grafts after reduction should be considered, usually combined with external fixation.

Associated lesions

Distal ulnar injury

Ulnar styloid fractures are a frequent occurrence (59% of cases). Fractures at the end of the ulnar styloid which are not managed surgically must be distinguished from fractures at the base, where the entire styloid is detached and often includes the insertion of the articular disc of the inferior radio-ulnar joint. Cases which have a fracture of the base of the ulnar styloid should be managed with osteosynthesis.

Fractures of the ulnar head. These are not common and include injury to radio-ulnar articulation.

Fractures of the ulnar neck are also unusual (3%) and significantly increase instability. Surgical treatment is recommended.

Scapholunate ligament instability

This injury can occur in all types of articular fracture involving the distal radius. It is seen especially in type 2 scaphoid and types 2, 3 and 4 lunate fossa fractures. In fact, scapholunate ligament tears should be investigated in all cases presenting with a vertical fracture line which extends into the scapholunate interspace.

This observation is always an indication for surgery. When present, it must be recognized and treated (Fig. 16.5).

Conclusions

In conclusion, this simple classification provides an easy method of identification of different types of articular fractures, according to the fracture patterns. Thus, it is possible to develop a well planned surgical treatment programme, which

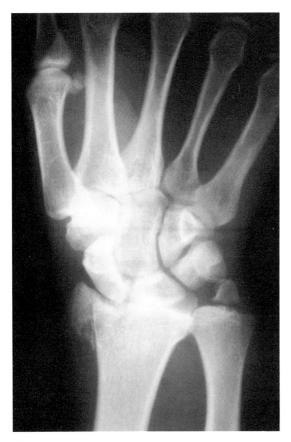

Figure 16.5

Type 4 articular fracture of the distal radius showing a vertical fracture line which extends into the scapholunate space

avoids the drawbacks of closed reduction, and allows correct stabilization of the different fracture fragments.

References

Castaing J, 'Le club des dix'. Les fractures récentes de l'extrémité inférieure du radius chez l'adulte. *Rev Chir Orthop* 1964; **50**: 581–96.

Cauchoix J, Duparc J, Postel M. Les fractures luxations marginales antérieures. *Rev Chir Orthop* 1960; **46**: 233.

Colles A. On the fracture of the carpal extremity of the radius. *Edin Med Surg J* 1814; **10**: 182–6.

Cooney WP. External fixation of distal radial fractures. *Clin Orthop* 1983; **180**: 44.

Frykman G. Fracture of distal radius including sequelae. Shoulder, hand, finger syndrome, disturbance in the distal radio-ulnar joint and impairment of nerve function. A clinical experimental study. *Acta Orthop Scand* 1967; **108 (Suppl)**: 1–153.

Mathoulin C. *Fractures articulaires du radius chez l'adulte*. Expansion scientifique Fr., Cahier d'enseignement de la Société Française de Chirurgie de la Main. Tome 2, 1990.

Melone Jr CP. Articular fractures of the distal radius. *J Bone Joint Surg* 1984; **15**: 217–36.

Pouteau C. *Œuvres posthumes*, Paris, 1783.

17
Classification and treatment of intra-articular fractures of the distal radius

H Saito

A wide variety of classification systems for fractures of the distal end of the radius have been published. Those systems using numbers or letters seem to be more confusing than those that use eponyms, although neither system refers directly to the site or type of fracture. The eponymous systems are easier to remember, and also allow classical eponyms to be incorporated into new concepts as they arise.

There is, however, some confusion regarding the definition of each eponymous fracture because a long time has elapsed since the publication of the orginal papers and new definitions are being published continuously. This chapter will describe a new classification system based on review of classical articles (Böhler 1930, Cotton 1900, Fitzsimons 1938, Peltier 1953 and 1959), including those of Colles (1814), Smith (1847) and Barton (1836), as well as the radiological analysis of 1083 fractures.

Definitions of eponymous and non-eponymous fractures

Colles' fracture is a fracture across the distal end of the radius with its distal fragment displaced dorsally. Abraham Colles described this injury in 1814 and described the location of the fracture as being an inch and a half proximal to the articular surface but later Smith, his student, corrected this measurement to an inch proximal to the articular surface. This fracture is also known as Pouteau's fracture (Decoulx and Razemon 1976).

Smith's fracture occurs at the same level on the distal radius as a Colles' fracture, with the distal fragment displaced in a palmar direction. There is some confusion regarding the definition of this fracture. Watson-Jones (1985) included Smith's fracture in his discussion of anterior marginal fracture of the radius with subluxation of the wrist. Thomas (1957) included all fractures of the distal end of the radius with palmar displacement of the carpus under the category of Smith's fracture. Type 2 fracture in Thomas's classification is an intra-articular fracture through the anterior margin of the distal radius with palmar displacement of the carpus. This fracture type is also identified as the Barton's fracture. These are some of the reasons for the confusion that exists. Smith's original description, however, is clear. This fracture is an extra-articular fracture. An intra-articular fracture, such as type 2 of Thomas's classification, should be excluded from this category. The French eponym for this fracture is the Goyrand fracture (Decoulx and Razemon 1976).

Dorsal Barton's fracture is an intra-articular fracture involving the dorsal margin of the distal end of the radius associated with dorsal dislocation or subluxation of the proximal carpal bones.

Palmar Barton's fracture is an intra-articular fracture involving the palmar margin of the distal end of the radius associated with palmar dislocation or subluxation of the proximal carpal bones. In 1838, John Barton described 'A subluxation of the wrist consequent to a fracture through the articular surface of the carpal extremity of the radius. The fragment may be, and usually is, quite small and is broken from the end of the radius on the dorsal side'. According to this description, Barton's fracture should be limited to a fracture involving the dorsal margin of the distal radius. However, a palmar marginal fracture was also mentioned at the end of his article. For this reason, a fracture involving the palmar margin is occasionally called a reverse Barton's fracture (Aufranc et al. 1966). Ellis (1965) stated that a dorsal marginal fracture was a rare injury and that Barton's dorsal fracture-dislocation was probably a Colles' fracture. He advocated that a palmar fracture-dislocation of the wrist should be known as Barton's fracture. Therefore, the use of the word 'reverse' may be confusing (Thompson and Grant 1977). It seems wise to use the terms 'dorsal Barton' and 'palmar Barton'.

Chauffeur's fracture is defined as an intra-articular fracture involving the radial styloid according to Cautilli's description (1974). This is also known as Hutchinson's fracture. The radial styloid is cleaved in a sagittal plane and the fragment is displaced proximally, allowing the scaphoid to come into contact with the malaligned articular surface of the radius. Fitzsimons (1938) stated that this fracture generally differs from the common type of Colles' fracture only in its aetiology. He, however, mentioned that isolated fractures of the radial styloid process were fairly common from a direct blow, for example from a starting handle of a car. Therefore, it is reasonable to call this injury chauffeur's fracture.

Medial cuneiform fracture (lunate fossa) is an intra-articular fracture through the ulnar corner of the distal end of the radius (Scheck 1962, Decoulx and Razemon 1976). It is caused by an impact of the lunate on the lunate facet of the distal radius.

Comminuted Colles' (or Frykman) fracture is defined as a Colles-type fracture with a comminuted distal fragment and fracture lines extending into the radiocarpal joint according to Gartland's description (1951). Comminution in this case refers to shattering of the distal fragment but not comminuted fracture between the distal fragment and the main proximal fragment. Groups II and III of Gartland's classification are included in this category. The new classification system described in this chapter divides comminuted Colles' fracture into five subtypes from the standpoint of treatment; this will be discussed later.

Comminuted Smith's fracture is defined as a Smith-type fracture with a comminuted distal fragment and fracture lines extending into the radiocarpal joint.

New types of intra-articular fracture

Through radiographic review of 1083 fractures (Saito and Shibata 1983), two types of fracture were found which do not fit into any of the basic types mentioned previously. These do not have a high incidence but are quite characteristic, and should be distinguished from other types of fracture from the standpoint of treatment.

Combined dorsal Barton's and chauffeur's fracture resembles a chauffeur's fracture in the AP view but a dorsal Barton's in the lateral view (Fig. 17.1). It consists of fractures at two sites on

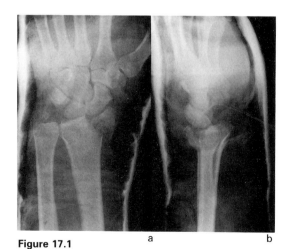

Figure 17.1   a   b

Combine dorsal Barton's and chauffeur's fracture. a) AP view; b) lateral view.

the distal end of the radius, one through the radial styloid and the other through the dorsal margin. The proximal carpal bones subluxate dorsally with the fracture fragments. There are two subtypes distinguished by the direction of displacement, which can be ulnodorsal or radiodorsal (see Fig. 17.3). The former is stable because the ulnar styloid is not broken and the triangular fibrocartilage complex (TFCC) is preserved intact. The latter is quite unstable because the ulnar styloid is fractured and the TFCC is torn.

Combined palmar Barton's and chauffeur's fracture resembles a chauffeur's fracture in the AP view but a palmar Barton's in the lateral view (Fig. 17.2). Fractures occur through the radial styloid and the palmar margin, and the proximal carpal bones displace in a palmar direction together with the fracture fragments. This type of fracture is also divided into two subtypes, ulnopalmar and radiopalmar (Fig. 17.3). The former is stable while the latter is unstable.

The author's classification

This classification consists of two extra-articular and eight intra-articular fractures (Table 17.1). The latter are divided into two groups — simple and comminuted (Fig. 17.4). Those with a fracture at one site, producing a single free intra-articular fragment are included in the simple category. Fractures at two or more sites producing multiple intra-articular free fragments are included in the comminuted category. Many varieties of fractures of the distal radius fulfil the definition of the comminuted Colles' fracture and so these are divided into five subtypes from the standpoint of treatment (Fig. 17.5). The name of each subtype was coined with reference to Hohl's classification (1967) of fractures of the tibial condyle. Comminuted Smith's fractures can be subdivided in a similar way.

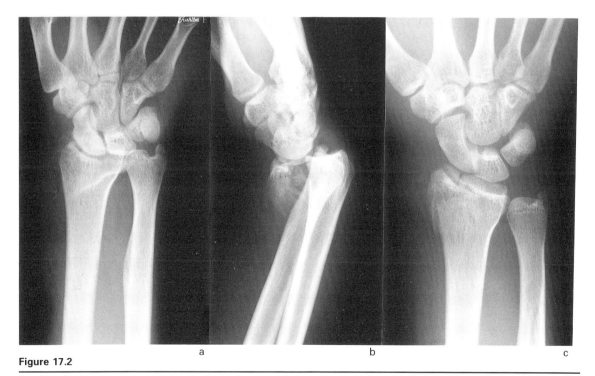

Figure 17.2

Combined palmar Barton's and chauffeur's fracture. a) AP view; b) lateral view; c) AP view taken under traction, showing fracture fragments of the radial styloid and the palmar margin.

Table 17.1 The author's classification of distal radial fractures

Extra-articular fractures
  1) Colles' fracture
  2) Smith's fracture

Intra-articular fractures
  a. Simple intra-articular fractures
  1) Chauffeur's fracture
  2) Medial cuneiform fracture
  3) Dorsal Barton's fracture
  4) Palmar Barton's fracture
  b. Comminuted intra-articular fractures
  5) Comminuted Colles
      subtype I: undisplaced
      subtype II: ulnar split
      subtype III: ulnodorsal split
      subtype IV: dorsal split-depression
      subtype V: central depression
  6) Comminuted Smith's fracture
  7) Combined dorsal Barton's and chauffeur's fracture
  8) Combined palmar Barton's and chauffeur's fracture

Comminuted Colles' fractures

Subtype I (undisplaced)

The displacement of the intra-articular fragments is minimal at the articular surface of the distal end of the radius, regardless of the degree of displacement at the fracture through the metaphysis.

Subtype II (ulnar split)

The ulnar intra-articular fragment containing the sigmoid notch is separated off from the radial fragment and displaced proximally. Displacement of more than 2 mm seems to be significant. This subtype corresponds to type II of Melone's classification (1984).

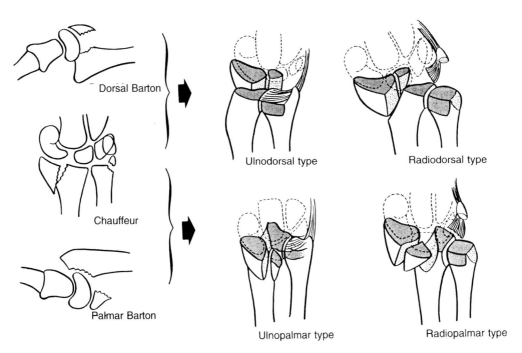

Figure 17.3

Subtyping of combined Barton's and chauffeur's fractures. Top: ulnodorsal and radiodorsal subtypes of combined dorsal Barton's and chauffeur's fracture. Bottom: ulnopalmar and radiopalmar subtypes of combined palmar Barton's and chauffeur's fracture.

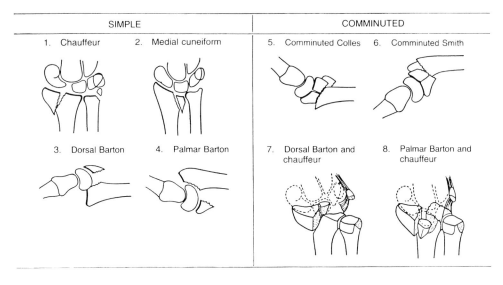

Figure 17.4

The author's classification of intra-articular fractures of the distal radius.

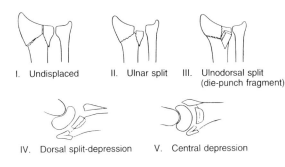

Figure 17.5

Subtypes of comminuted Colles' fractures.

Subtype III (ulnodorsal split)

The dorsal portion of the ulnar corner of the distal radius is broken off by the compressive force of the lunate and displaced proximally. The fracture line enters into the distal radio-ulnar joint as well as the radiocarpal joint. This split fragment is identical to the 'die-punch fragment' described by Scheck (1962).

Subtype IV (dorsal split-depression)

The articular surface is depressed into the intramedullary space by the compressive force of the carpus applied in a dorsal and proximal direction, while the dorsal cortex is sprung off. The palmar portion of the articular surface is occasionally displaced in a palmar direction and rotates through more than 90°. This subtype corresponds to Melone's type IV.

Subtype V (central depression)

The central portion of the articular surface is depressed into the intramedullary space by a compressive force of the carpus applied along the longitudinal axis of the radius. The dorsal and palmar cortices are intact or minimally displaced and so this fracture is quite stable. The 'scaphoid impression fracture' described by Bennett and Bowers (1983) is a mild form of this type.

Incidence of fracture types

The incidence of each type of fracture was analysed by classifying 400 consecutive distal radial fractures treated at two hospitals — one a trauma hospital, taking care of patients injured in road traffic and industrial accidents, and the second an orthopaedic hospital treating the same kind of patient plus elderly patients.

As shown in Table 17.2, about half of the fractures are extra-articular and one-third are intra-articular. Comminuted Colles' fractures compose two-thirds of the intra-articular group. The incidence of dorsal or palmar Barton's fracture is very low, as is that of combined dorsal or palmar Barton's and chauffeur's fracture.

Table 17.2 Incidence of each type of fracture at the distal end of radius: 400 cases treated at Niigata Chuo Hospital (1976–1984) and Tominaga-Kusano Hospital (1981–1984)

A. Extra-articular	
Colles	50.0%
Smith	2.8%
B. Intra-articular	
Comminuted Colles	23.8%
Chauffeur	6.3%
Comminuted Smith	2.5%
Palmar Barton	1.3%
Combined dorsal Barton and chauffeur	1.3%
Dorsal Barton	0.5%
Combined palmar Barton and chauffeur	0.3%
C. Undisplaced	11.5%

Treatment of intra-articular fractures

Simple intra-articular fractures

Chauffeur's fracture

Closed reduction is carried out by bringing the wrist into ulnar deviation, and letting the lunate on the remaining articular surface of the radius work as the fulcrum, so that the radial collateral ligament is tightened and the proximally displaced radial styloid is reduced. A long arm thumb spica cast is applied with the elbow in 90° flexion and the wrist in ulnar deviation. When the radial styloid tends to redisplace in the case, it is better to fix it by percutaneous pinning. A post-reduction radiograph should be checked to see if there is scapholunate dissociation. When it exists, open reduction and pinning of the scapholunate articulation, as well as fixation of the radial styloid, should be performed.

Medial cuneiform fracture (lunate fossa)

Simple distal traction of the hand usually fails to reduce a lunate fossa fragment because there is no tight ligament between the lunate and capitate to transmit traction force to the lunate and the fragment. Thus, open reduction and internal fixation are usually indicated. Scapholunate dissociation can be caused by this injury too.

Dorsal Barton's fracture

Closed reduction is carried out, as proposed by King (1980), by bringing the wrist into dorsiflexion while distal traction is applied, reducing the carpus into a pocket formed by the remaining palmar portion of the articular cartilage of the radius and the palmar radiocarpal ligament (Fig. 16.6). A short arm plaster cast is applied with the wrist in slight dorsiflexion.

Palmar Barton's fracture

Closed reduction of this fracture-dislocation can also be accomplished by bringing the wrist into palmar flexion while distal traction is applied, as King (1980) proposed. The fragment, however, usually displaces palmarward, together with the carpus, despite the cast because the articular surface tilts palmarward. It is practical to carry out open reduction and internal fixation with a T-shaped buttress plate or a small screw.

Comminuted intra-articular fracture

Comminuted Colles' fracture

Subtype I. Closed reduction and casting is indicated, unless there is comminution along the main fracture line across the metaphysis. In these cases, pins and plaster or external fixator is indicated.

Subtype II. The ulnar fragment is usually not reduced by traction. Osteotaxis using an external fixator and supplementary open reduction of the ulnar fragment, with or without internal fixation,

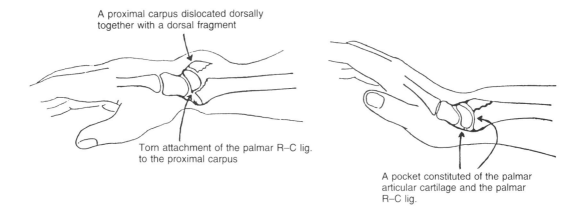

Figure 17.6

King's method of closed reduction of a dorsal Barton's fracture: a) before reduction; b) after reduction.

are indicated. This supplementary open reduction can also be achieved by applying pins and plaster and making a large window in the cast.

Subtype III. An ulnodorsal die-punch fragment cannot be reduced by closed reduction. Treatment similar to that applied for subtype II is indicated (i.e. osteotaxis and supplementary open reduction) (Fig. 17.7).

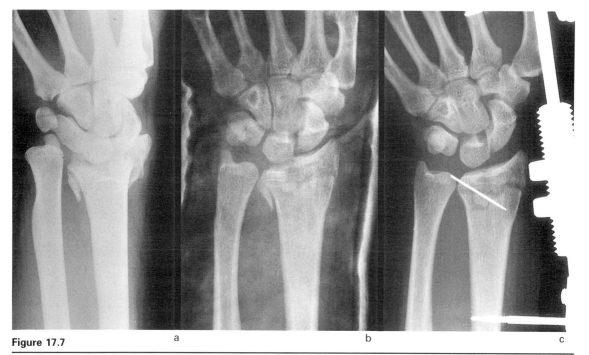

Figure 17.7

Case 1. A 35-year-old women, with a subtype III comminuted Colles' fracture. a) AP view taken just after being involved in a car collision; b) AP view after closed reduction and casting, showing an unreduced ulnodorsal fragment; c) after osteotaxis and supplementary open reduction and pinning of the fragment.

Subtype IV. Osteotaxis and supplementary open reduction combined with bone graft are indicated. Gross alignment of the fragments is adjusted with an external fixator and then unreduced depressed articular fragments are elevated through a dorsal approach and stabilized with pieces of iliac bone, grafted into a cavity made underneath the fragments (Fig. 17.8).

Subtype V. For cases with a mild degree of depression, immobilization with a short arm splint for 7–10 days is sufficient. When the articular fragment is markedly depressed, open reduction and bone grafting are indicated. The radial cortex is usually intact or stable. If it is fractured, windowing either the dorsal or the palmar cortex is occasionally necessary to elevate the depressed fragment.

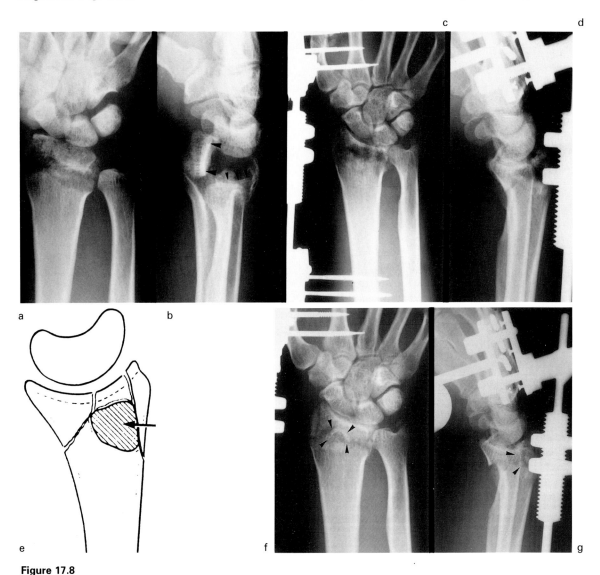

Figure 17.8

Case 2. A 39-year-old man, with a subtype IV comminuted Colles' fracture. a,b) AP and lateral views (under skeletal traction), showing a rotated articular fragment (large arrowheads) and a depressed articular fragment (small arrowheads). c,d) AP and lateral views taken during application of Hoffmann's external fixator and supplementary open reduction of the unreduced articular fragments. e) diagram showing placement of an iliac bone graft (arrow) underneath the reduced articular fragment. f,g) AP and lateral views taken after completion of all procedures, demonstrating bone graft (arrowheads).

Comminuted Smith's fracture

Each case is classified in the same way as the subtypes of comminuted Colles' fractures and treated in a similar fashion.

Combined dorsal Barton's and chauffeur's fracture

Closed reduction and casting is indicated for the ulnodorsal type (Fig. 17.9). After distal traction, the wrist is brought into slight radial deviation and dorsiflexion to place the carpus into a saucer formed by the remaining ulnar portion of the articular surface and the TFCC. A long arm cast is applied with the elbow in 90° flexion and the wrist in slight radial deviation and dorsiflexion. The radiodorsal type is so unstable that either open reduction and internal fixation, or immobilization with an external fixator or pins and plaster is needed (Fig. 17.10).

Combined palmar Barton's and chauffeur's fracture

The ulnopalmar type is stable and treated with closed reduction and casting. The carpus is reduced into a saucer, formed from the remaining dorso-ulnar portion of the articular surface of the radius and the TFCC, by bringing the wrist into slight radial deviation and palmar flexion after distal traction. A long arm cast is applied with the elbow in 90° flexion and the wrist in the position mentioned above. The radiopalmar type is so unstable that open reduction and internal fixation are necessary. Osteotaxis with an external fixator and supplementary open reduction, with or without a bone graft, are also indicated (Fig. 17.11).

Discussion

Most of the classification systems published previously use various risk factors as the criteria of classification which might affect the functional prognosis unfavorably. Nissen-Lie took several factors into account in his classification, including the site of the fracture in relation to the joint surface, the degree of joint involvement, and the direction and the degree of displacement (Lidström 1959). Gartland and Werley (1951) divided Colles-type fractures into three types based on whether fracture line entered the radiocarpal joint and the degree of displacement of the articular

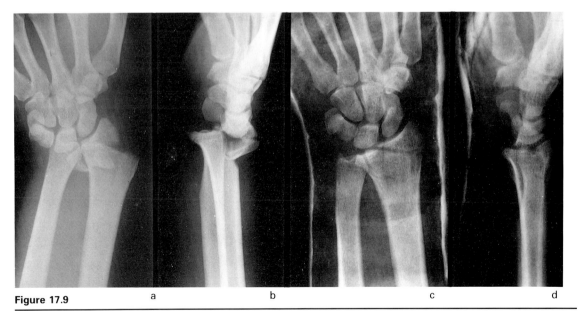

Figure 17.9 a b c d

Case 3. A 30-year-old man, with an ulnodorsal combined dorsal Barton's and chauffeur's fracture. a,b) AP and lateral views taken before reduction; c,d) after closed reduction and casting.

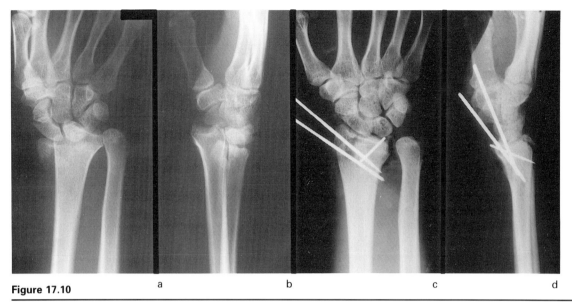

Figure 17.10

Case 4. A 19-year-old boy, with a radiodorsal combined dorsal Barton's and chauffeur's fracture. a,b) AP and lateral views taken after falling down while motorcycling; c,d) after open reduction and pinning.

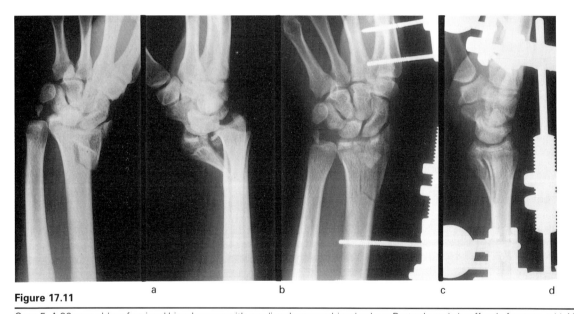

Figure 17.11

Case 5. A 36-year-old professional bicycle racer with a radiopalmar combined palmar Barton's and chauffeur's fracture. a,b) AP and laterial views taken just after sustaining an injury on falling down during a race; c,d) after osteotaxis and supplementary open reduction combined with iliac bone graft.

surface. Taylor and Parson used the presence or absence of injury to the triangular fibrocartilage as the criterion of classification (Lidström 1959). Frykman (1967) divided fractures of the distal end of the radius into seven types according to the presence or absence of involvement of the radiocarpal and/or distal radio-ulnar joint, and of fracture of the distal ulna. This classification is often referred to but is not so useful in planning the treatment of an individual fracture because the direction and the degree of displacement are not taken into account. Melone (1984) described four principal patterns of intra-articular fractures. His classification is very useful in understanding the mechanism and displacement pattern of comminuted fractures involving the distal end of the radius. However, an individual case cannot always be classified into one of these four types. In that sense, it is not quite practical.

The new types of fracture proposed in this chapter, the combined dorsal or palmar Barton's and chauffeur's fractures, seem to have been classified as Barton's fracture in some studies. De Oliveira (1973) stated that there is some variation in the fragment size or the degree of comminution in palmar Barton's fractures. He described a case with a fracture through the radial styloid, as well as the palmar margin, as a palmar Barton's fracture and treated it by fixing the palmar fragment with a buttress plate and the radial styloid with percutaneous pinning of the radial styloid. Such a case undoubtedly has two fragments and definitely differs from the Barton-type fracture. According to the AO classification, these fractures are classified under the categories of 'B2 partial articular fracture, of the radius, dorsal rim (Barton)' and 'B3 partial articular fracture, of the radius, volar rim (reverse Barton)' (Müller et al. 1990). B2-2 is a combined dorsal Barton's and chauffeur's fracture and B3-3 a combined palmar Barton's and chauffeur's fracture. In the illustrations of each type (Müller et al. 1990), two articular fragments are drawn. These two types of fracture cannot be treated nonoperatively by King's method, and so they too should be distinguished from a dorsal or palmar Barton fracture.

The author (Saito 1989) has tried to establish a treatment plan aimed at anatomical reduction by classifying a wide variety of distal radial fractures in detail and clarifying the characteristics of each type of fracture. This treatment plan is summarized as follows.

In the simple intra-articular fracture group, chauffeur and dorsal Barton types can be treated conservatively, while most cases of lunate fossa and palmar Barton's fractures need open reduction and internal fixation. In the comminuted intra-articular fracture group, osteotaxis using an external fixator or pins and plaster is needed in almost all cases except those of the subtype I comminuted Colles' fracture, the ulnodorsal type of combined dorsal Barton's and chauffeur's fracture, and the ulnopalmar type of combined palmar Barton's and chauffeur's fracture, which require different treatment. Supplementary open reduction, with or without a bone graft, is added when the articular fragment is not reduced simply by osteotaxis.

The results of 48 cases treated according to this treatment plan were evaluated as excellent or good in all but one patient.

This classification might seem to be complex but it is very useful because any fracture of this region can be categorized into one of the types and its treatment plan then follows automatically.

References

Aufranc OE, Jones WN, Turner RH. Anterior marginal articular fracture of distal radius. *JAMA* 1966; **196**: 788–91.

Barton JR. Views and treatment of an important injury of the wrist. *Med Exam* 1838; **1**: 365–68.

Bennett JT, Bowers WH. Scaphoid impression fracture; A case report. *J Hand Surg* 1983; **8B: 205–6.**

Böhler L. Verrenkungen der Handgelenke. *Acta Chir Scand* 1930; **67**: 154–77.

Cautilli RA. Classifications of fractures of the distal radius. *Clin Orthop* 1974; **103**: 163–66.

Colles A. On the fracture of the carpal extremity of the radius. *Edinburgh Med Surg J* 1814; **10**: 182. Quoted from Fallon, M. *Abraham Colles*. Oxford: William Heinemann Medical Books Ltd, 1972, 181–85.

Cotton, FJ. The pathology of fracture of the lower extremity of the radius. *Ann Surg* 1900; **32**: 194–218.

Decoulx P, Razemon JP. *Traumatologie clinique séméiologie chirurgicale de l'appareil moteur de l'adulte*. 3rd Ed. Paris: Masson, 1976.

De Oliveira JC. Barton's fractures. *J Bone Joint Surg* 1973; **55A**: 586–94.

Ellis J. Smith's and Barton's fractures; A method of treatment. *J Bone Joint Surg* 1965; **47B**: 724–27.

Fitzsimons RA. Colles' fractures and chauffeur's fracture. *Br Med J* 1938; **2**: 357–60.

Frykman G. Fracture of the distal radius including sequelae, shoulder-hand syndrome, disturbance in the distal radio-ulnar joint and impairment of nerve function; A clinical and experimental study. *Acta Orthop Scand* 1967; **108 (Suppl)**: 1–153.

Gartland JJ, Werley CW. Evaluation of healed Colles' fractures. *J Bone Joint Surg* 1951; **33A**: 895–907.

Hohl M. Tibial condylar fractures. *J Bone Joint Surg* 1967; **49A**: 1455–67.

King RE. Barton's fracture-dislocation of the wrist. In Ahstrom JP et al., eds. *Current Practice in Orthopaedic Surgery*, Vol. 6. St Louis: CV Mosby, 1980: 133–44.

Lidström A. Fractures of the distal end of the radius. *Acta Orthop Scand* 1959; **41(Suppl)**: 1–118.

Melone CP Jr. Articular fractures of the distal radius. *Orthop Clin North Amer* 1984; **15**: 217–36.

Müller ME, Nazarian S, Koch P, Schatzker J. *The Comprehensive Classification of Fractures of Long Bones*. Berlin–Heidelberg: Springer-Verlag, 1990: 106–14.

Peltier LF. Eponymic fractures; John Rhea Barton and Barton's fractures. *Surgery* 1953; **34**: 960–70.

Peltier LF. Eponymic fractures; Robert William Smith and Smith's fracture. *Surgery* 1959; **45**: 1035–42.

Saito H, Shibata M. Classification of fractures at the distal end of the radius with reference to treatment of comminuted fractures. In Boswick JA, ed. *Current Concepts in Hand Surgery*. Philadelphia: Lea and Febiger, 1983: 129–45.

Saito H. Fractures of the distal end of the radius; Anatomical characteristics, classification and treatment (in Japanese). *Orthop Surg Traumatol* 1989; **32**: 237–48.

Scheck M. Long-term follow-up of comminuted fractures of the distal end of the radius by transfixation with Kirschner wires and cast. *J Bone Joint Surg* 1962; **44A**: 337–51.

Smith RW. *A Treatise on Fractures in the Vicinity of Joints and on Certain Forms of Accidental and Congenital Dislocations*. Dublin: Hodges and Smith, 1847.

Thomas FB. Reduction of Smith's fracture. *J Bone Joint Surg* 1957: **39B**: 463–70.

Thompson GH, Grant TT. Barton's fractures — reverse Barton's fractures; Confusing eponyms. *Clin Orthop* 1977; **122**: 210–21.

Watson-Jones R. *Fractures and Joint Injuries*, 4th Ed. Edinburgh: Churchill Livingstone, 1955.

18
Evaluation of comminuted intra-articular distal radial fractures with computerized tomography

Richard M Singer, Guy Pierret

Introduction

Proper treatment of displaced intra-articular distal radial fractures depends on accurate radiographic evaluation. The frequency of post-traumatic arthritis of the wrist after this injury has been reported to be as high as 40% in some series (Cooney et al. 1979 and 1980, De Palma 1952, Dobyns and Linscheid 1978, Dowling and Sawyer 1961, Gartland and Werley 1951, Green 1975, Smaill 1986). In 1986, Knirk and Jupiter showed that anatomic articular restoration is the most critical factor in achieving a successful result. At a mean follow-up of 6.7 years, they reported radiographic evidence of post-traumatic arthritis in 91% of the fractures that had healed with any degree of articular step-off. All wrists with articular incongruity of 2 mm or more developed arthritis; however, they noted only an 11% incidence of arthritis in fractures that healed with a congruous radiocarpal joint. Melone (1984, 1986) stated that maximum recovery requires precise correction of the articular disruption. Previous reports (Patel 1985) have demonstrated the capacity of computerized tomography to display fractures through casts (Fig. 18.1). In some cases, patients presented late, having had closed reduction and cast application, or closed reduction and percutaneous pinning, or closed reduction and external fixation, thus complicating the plain film evaluation. Because of the uniformly poor results with articular incongruity and the occasional difficulty in evaluating the distal radius with conventional radiography, a study was undertaken to evaluate more accurately the articular surface of the distal radius using computerized tomography.

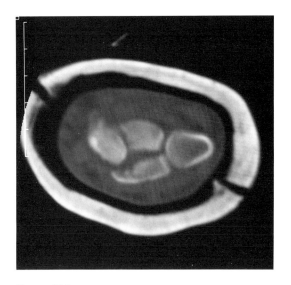

Figure 18.1

CT scan through a heavy cast.

Patients and methods

Over a two-year period, 22 fractures in 22 patients were treated operatively. Of these patients, 18 were evaluated with computerized tomography that included transverse axial sections with coronal and sagittal reconstruction. The age range was 15–64 years, with an average age of 38.6 years. The dominant limb was involved in 15 cases. Fourteen of the fractures occurred as the result of a fall, four were the result of motor vehicle accidents and four occurred during recreational activities. Associated injuries included scaphoid fracture, scapholunate dissociation, dislocated distal radio-ulnar joint, carpal tunnel syndrome, and an acetabular fracture. There were no open fractures. All fractures were classified as type VII or VIII according to the Frykman classification of 1967.

The patients presented at 5–29 days (mean: 15.3 days) after closed reduction. All patients had had closed reductions; three patients had undergone previous operative procedures.

Computerized tomography was performed at several hospitals using different scanners; 1.5 mm slices were requested (Fig. 18.2). The specific technique used was determined by the radiology personnel involved. Axial and coronal sections of each case were taken. Occasionally, coronal or sagittal reconstructions were utilized when additional information was needed. On obtaining the images, those sections corresponding to the articular surface were reviewed qualitatively and quantitatively. Displacement in millimetres was calculated using a ratio of the measured displacement on the scan to a measured 5 cm bar. Fracture displacement can also be calculated by internal programming on certain scanners.

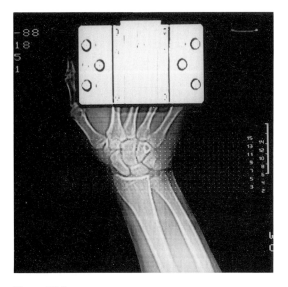

Figure 18.2

CT scout film with slice reference lines and 5 cm reference bar.

Results

Following CT evaluation, 18 patients underwent surgical intervention. Fifteen patients who had been scheduled for operative treatment did undergo open reduction. Three of these patients had had previous operative intervention and underwent a second operation to correct disruption of the articular surface (Fig. 18.3). In addition, three patients who were thought to be candidates for non-operative treatment underwent open reduction and internal fixation after computerized tomography (Figure 18.4). Surgical intervention was deemed necessary if displacement measured greater than 1.5 mm.

Conclusions

Conventional radiographs may be inadequate to thoroughly evaluate the fractured distal radius. Treatment methods are dependent on the degree of displacement of the fracture and perceived stability. Computerized tomography provides the means to evaluate the number, the size, and the position of the fracture fragments. Transaxial sections can be obtained by placing the extremity in the scanner at 90° to its axis. Coronal sections can also be obtained directly. This gives an accurate measurement of displacement when compared to coronal reconstructions. Despite this, coronal and sagittal reconstructions were utilized in this study in cases of severe comminution, where extra information was needed for correlation.

Conventional radiographs are sufficient to evaluate the majority of patients with comminuted intra-articular fractures of the distal radius. Tomography can also be utilized when comminution is great; however, at times these views are difficult to interpret and have one-dimensional limitations. Arthroscopy can also be used to evaluate acute comminuted intra-articular fractures of the distal radius, but it is expensive and invasive. Computerized tomography provides significant additional information for the evaluation of comminuted fractures that often appear to have acceptable alignment on conventional radiographs. Often, it will reveal unacceptable displacement, which is then verified at the time of open

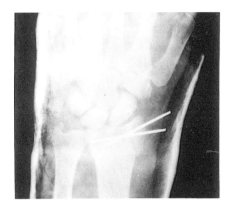
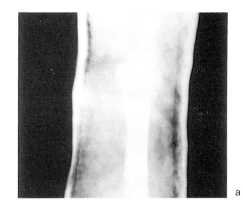
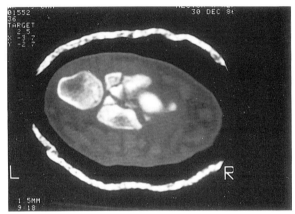
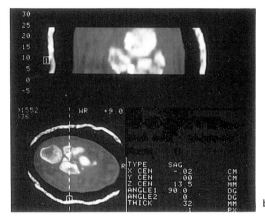
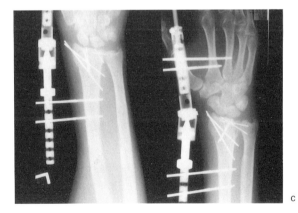

Figure 18.3

a) A 23-year-old patient, 4 weeks after closed reduction and percutaneous pinning. b) Transaxial sections with sagittal reconstruction. c) Postoperative radiographs with external fixator in place.

reduction and internal fixation. Computerized tomography is extremely useful in evaluating patients who have been treated previously by closed reduction, with or without percutaneous pinning, and with or without external fixation, and often demonstrates the inadequacy of this treatment. It is also helpful in evaluating patients who present late with subacute fractures. Computer-

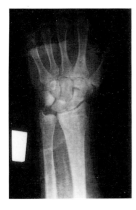
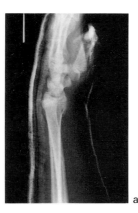
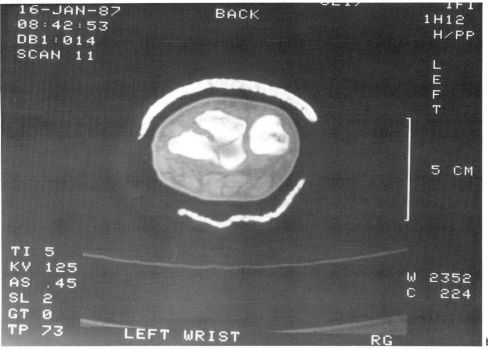

Figure 18.4

a) A 15-year-old patient with closed reduction and a short arm cast. b) Transaxial computerized tomography.

ized tomography is useful in preoperative planning, as it correlates well with the distorted anatomy that is encountered intra-operatively. In the study described in this chapter, computerized tomography altered previously determined treatment plans in 14% of the cases, and provided detailed, quantitative information regarding the articular congruity of these complex distal radial fractures.

Summary

Anatomic articular restoration has been reported to be the most critical factor in achieving a successful result in comminuted intra-articular distal radius fractures. Because of the uniformly poor results reported in the literature, and with less than adequate treatment and the additional difficulty in evaluating the fracture pattern, a prospective study of 18 patients with displaced fractures were evaluated with conventional PA, lateral, and oblique radiographs. In addition, computerized tomography with transaxial, coronal and sagittal sections were obtained. The average age of the patient population was 38.6 years (range 15–64 years). The average time from injury to presentation was 15.3 days (range 5–29 days). All the patients had had a previous closed reduction, and three had had previous operative procedures.

No patient scheduled for open reduction and internal fixation was treated non-operatively after obtaining computerized tomography. Three patients scheduled for closed treatment subsequently underwent open reduction and internal fixation after the computerized tomography had been performed. The cross-sectional display and superior resolution of computerized tomography made it an important adjunct in radiological evaluation of these fractures.

References

Cooney WP, Dobyns JH, Linscheid RL. Complications of Colles' fractures. *J Bone Joint Surg* 1980; **62A**: 613–19.

Cooney WP, Linscheid RL, Dobyns JH. External pin fixation for unstable Colles' fractures. *J Bone Joint Surg* 1979; **61A**: 840–45.

De Palma AF. Comminuted fractures of the distal end of the radius treated by ulnar pinning. *J Bone Joint Surg* 1952; **34A**: 651–62.

Dobyns JH, Linscheid RL. Complications of treatment of fractures and dislocations of the wrist. In Epps DH Jr. *Complications in Orthopaedic Surgery*, Vol. 1. Philadelphia: JB Lippincott, 1978: 271–352.

Dowling JJ, Sawyer B Jr. Comminuted Colles fractures. Evaluation of a method of treatment. *J Bone Joint Surg* 1961; **43A**: 657–68.

Frykman G. Fracture of the distal radius including sequelae — shoulder-hand-finger syndrome, disturbance in the distal radio-ulnar joint and impairment of nerve function. A clinical and experimental study. *Acta Orthop Scand* 1967; **198(Suppl)**: 1–153.

Gartland JJ, Werley CW. Evaluation of healed Colles' fractures. *J Bone Joint Surg* 1951; **33A**: 895–907.

Green DP. Pins and plaster treatment of comminuted fractures of the distal end of the radius. *J Bone Joint Surg* 1975; **57A**: 304–10.

Knirk JL, Jupiter JB. Intra-articular fractures of the distal end of the radius in young adults. *J Bone Joint Surg* 1986; **61A**: 657–59.

Melone CP Jr. Articular fractures of the distal radius. *Orthop Clin Nth Am* 1984; **15(2)**: 217–36.

Melone CP Jr. Open treatment for displaced articular fractures of the distal radius. *Clin Orthop* 1986; **202**: 103–11.

Patel RB. Evaluation of complex carpal trauma: Thin section direct longitudinal computed tomography scanning through a plaster cast. *J Computer Asst Tomography* 1985; 9: 107–9.

Smaill GB. Open treatment for displaced articular fractures of the distal radius. *Clin Orthop* 1986; **202**: 103–11.

19
Treatment by plates of anteriorly displaced distal radial fractures

Ph Ducloyer

Distal radial fractures with anterior displacement are relatively rare: in a large series, Castaing (1964) found anterior rim fractures in only 4.5% of the cases studied, Cauchoix et al. (1960) reported isolated or complex fractures of this type in 3%.

Treatment has been controversial. As early as 1907, Lambotte recommended internal fixation but conservative treatment was the rule until the 1960s (Castaing 1964). Since then, some authors have reported the results of short series treated by K-wires, screws or different types of plates (Auffray and Comtet 1968, Dionis du Séjour et al. 1966, Largier and Dupuis 1976). These fractures have two principal features: they are intra-articular and unstable. The goals and the potential difficulties with treatment depend on these two factors.

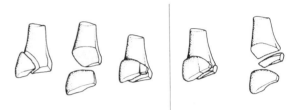

Figure 19.1

Classification of anterior rim fractures (Cauchoix et al. 1960). Type I (left): isolated anterior or anterolateral fracture; Type II (right): complex rim fracture with anterior and simple or complex posterior fragments.

Classification

The mechanism of flexion-compression of distal radial fractures leads to extra-articular Smith fractures, and anterior rim isolated or complex intra-articular fractures. In 1838, Letenneur had already described the isolated anterior rim fracture. In 1957, Thomas described three types of anteriorly displaced fractures, type III being Smith's extra-articular fracture. In 1960, Cauchoix et al. described two types of anterior fracture-dislocations (Fig. 19.1).

The isolated anterior rim fracture (Cauchoix type I and Thomas type II), has a detached anterior fragment with an oblique fracture line dorsally and distally. A radial styloid fragment is also present with a volar and lateral fracture. This fragment may be smaller or bigger than the anterior fragment and can be intact or split.

The complex anterior rim fracture (Cauchoix type II and Thomas type I) is associated with a posterior rim fracture, displaced or not, intact or split, producing an epiphyseal-metaphyseal dissociation. The associated fragments are often difficult to visualize and careful examination of the lateral peri-operative radiographs is necessary (Fig. 19.2).

Whatever the type of the fracture a radial styloid fragment can be detached by a sagittal line of fracture.

Mechanism

Two mechanisms can explain these fractures:

1. Fall on a hyperextended wrist can place axial pressure on the volar aspect of the distal

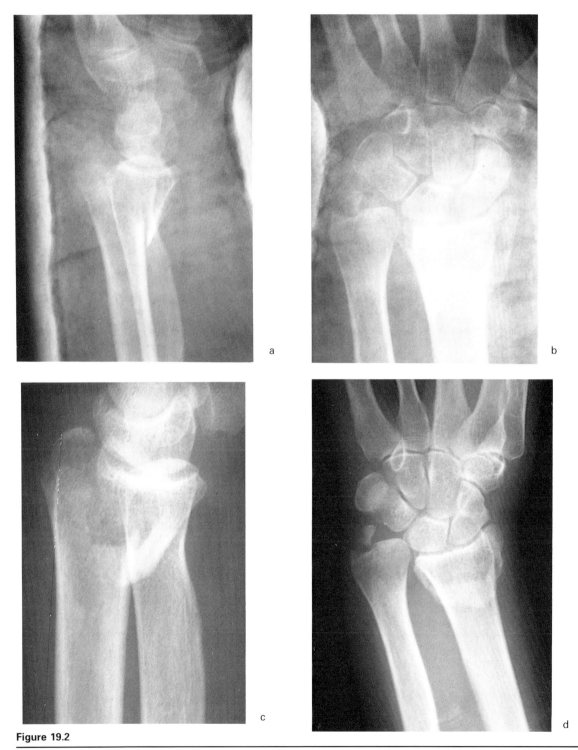

Figure 19.2

A complex fracture, operated on after failure of conservative treatment. a,b) Control radiographs of an anterior rim fracture with cast at the 8th day: there is significant displacement. c,d) AP and lateral radiographs after cast removal. A posterior fragment is suspected. e,f) Good reduction on AP and laterial views. On the lateral view, the posterior fragment is seen partly fixed by an epiphyseal screw. g,h) Excellent clinical and radiological result at 5 year follow-up.

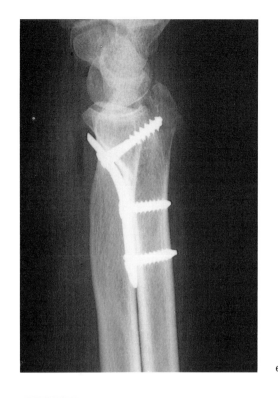

e

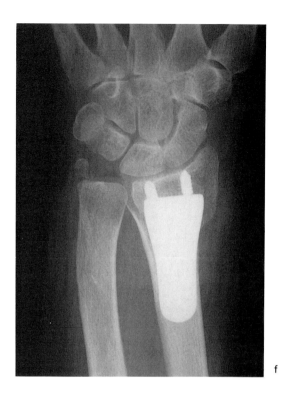

f

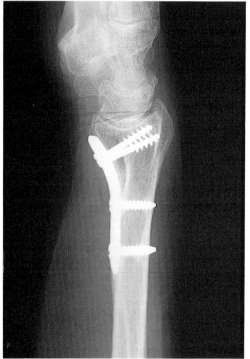

g

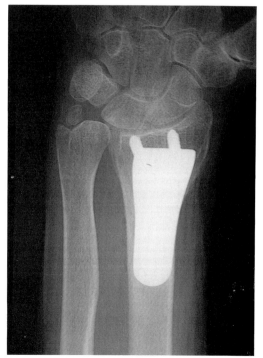

h

radius and traction forces on the dorsal aspect (Castaing 1964).

2. An injury to the wrist in forced flexion can also result in pressure on the volar aspect and traction on the dorsal aspect of the distal radius.

In the study described below (Ducloyer and Kerboull 1990) both mechanisms of injury are implicated.

Patients and methods

Perfect reduction and stabilization are mandatory for these displaced and unstable intra-articular fractures. It was proved by Castaing (1964) that immobilization by cast in any position was not able to stabilize or maintain the reduction of these types of fractures. In previous studies, conservative treatment led to unsatisfactory results in over 50% of the cases (Castaing 1964, Cauchoix et al. 1960, Dionis de Séjour et al. 1966).

In this study (Ducloyer and Kerboull 1990), of 58 fractures treated surgically, 38% were early failures of conservative treatments due to inadequate initial reduction or secondary displacement of an initially good reduction (Fig. 19.2). The mean age of the patients was 44 years old (age range 18–81 years). There were 32 male and 26 female patients. Fracture classification showed that 23 were type I, 30 were type II and 5 were type III fractures of the Thomas classification.

These fractures should be treated surgically. Percutaneous pinning of volar or laterovolar fractures seems very dangerous because of the numerous vulnerable vascular, nervous, and tendinous structures. In addition, K-wire fixation can lead to a position of imperfect reduction.

Open reduction and internal fixation by a special plate is the preferred choice. Different types of plates are available: straight, curved, and T- or V-shaped. Most plates are straight when observed from the side and have to be curved to fit exactly the concave volar aspect of the distal radius. The Kerboull plate is large enough to cover the volar aspect of the distal radius and has a sagittal curvature that exactly reproduced the anatomical curve of the distal radius. Six different lengths are available and the distal enlarged part has two holes where screws can fix the epiphysis.

The technique of plate fixation has been reported extensively in previous papers (Angereau et al. 1983, Ducloyer and Kerboull 1990) and only the pertinent details will be discussed here. For the surgical approach a longitudinal incision is made lateral to the flexor carpi radialis, extending up to the wrist crease, then following this crease ulnarward to turn at the wrist crease to extend longitudinally in the axis of the hand. The carpal tunnel is then opened. The pronator quadratus is elevated to expose the volar aspect of the radius. The wrist capsule is opened if the joint surface needs to be examined.

The reduction is assessed by checking the alignment of the lateral and medial cortices, and by viewing the joint if necessary. Temporary pinning can be useful before plate fixation. When a radial styloid fragment is detached, percutaneous pinning, entering at the radial styloid tip, is always recommended.

After the initial reduction, plate fixation to the metaphyseal region of the distal radius by screws is performed first, with the plate in good alignment. Screws are placed in the distal fragment through the plate, engaging the anterior and posterior fragment configuration to provide solid fixation. The buttress action of the plate is often not sufficient.

Cast immobilization is not always necessary but a splint should be worn, usually for one or two weeks and occasionally for up to four weeks to protect the internal fixation.

Results

This operation was performed on 58 consecutive cases from 1972 to 1986 (Ducloyer and Kerboull 1990). Complications were mostly due to technical failures:

- Six carpal tunnel syndromes were observed when the volar retinaculum (transverse carpal ligament) was not released.
- One extensor tendon rupture occurred over a long screw.
- Eleven secondary displacements occurred in cases with distal fracture fragments, which were not internally fixed due to an insufficient

buttressing by the plate, and radial styloid fragments. A better understanding of the mechanism of these failures will prevent mistakes in technique.
- Seven neurodystrophic phenomena (sympathetic dystrophias) were observed in elderly patients when a cast was maintained for too long a period of time.

The functional results were excellent or good in 76.1% of the cases, fair in 21.7% and poor in 2.2%. Radiological results were good in 67.4% of the cases, fair in 8.7% and poor in 23.9%. Two out of three bad results were observed in type II cases with a posterior rim fragment. These occurred either because the posterior rim fragment was unrecognized or underestimated, or because it was inadequately fixed in elderly patients who had osteoporotic bone. The secondary proximal migration of a detached, unfixed radial styloid fragment was the cause of poor results in both simple and several complex fractures.

A good anatomical reduction almost always leads to a good clinical result. However some anatomical shortcomings were more acceptable than others (Castaing 1964, Chamay 1977).

Failure to restore radial length to correct rotational displacement or to restore normal dorsal-volar tilt of the distal radius can be associated with poorer results. This series confirms that good surgical technique results in good anatomical and functional results and prevents complications in complex fractures with posterior fragments. Intrafocal pinning, using Kapandji's technique (1987), can be performed to stabilize the posterior aspect in reduced position. External fixation is reserved for comminuted fractures, in which the anterior fragment is only part of the problem.

Conclusion

Anteriorly displaced distal radial fractures are fairly rare. The initial radiographic analysis should not let a posterior fragment go unnoticed because secondary displacement is possible. Internal fixation by plate is the treatment of choice. The technique is difficult, but when performed precisely a stable and anatomical reduction will result.

References

Auffray Y, Comtet JJ. Place de l'ostéosynthèse par voie antéreiure dans les fractures de l'extrémité inférieure du radius. *Lyon Méd* 1968; **31**: 193–98.

Augereau B, Lance D, Kerboull M. L'ostéosynthèse par plaque des fractures instables du poignet à déplacement antérieur. *Inter Orthop* (SICOT) 1983; **7**: 55–59.

Thomas FB. Reduction of Smith's fracture. *J Bone Joint Surg* 1957; **39B**: 463–70.

Castaing J, le Club des Dix. Les fractures récentes de l'extrémité inférieure du radius chez l'adulte. *Rev Chir Orthop* 1964; **50**: 581–96.

Cauchoix J, Duparc J, Postel M. Les fractures luxations marginales antérieures du radius. *Rev Chir Orthop* 1960; **46**: 233–45.

Chamay A. Considération sur les limites de la tolérance du traitement conservateur des fractures du poignet. *Ann Chir* 1977; **31**: 340–42.

Dionis du Séjour H, Basset J, Apoil A. Fractures marginales antérieures de l'épiphyse radiale inférieure. *Ann Chir* 1966; **31**: 238–45.

Ducloyer Ph, Kerboull M. L'ostéosynthèse par plaque dans les fractures de l'extrémité inférieure du radius à déplacement antérieur. *Rev Chir Orthop* 1990; **76**: 451–59.

Ducloyer Ph, Kerboull M. Fractures of the lower end of the radius anteriorly displaced treated by plating. *French J Orthop Surg* 1990; **4**: 3–12.

Kapandji A. L'embrochage intra-focal des fractures de l'extrémité inférieure du radius dix ans après. *Ann Chir Main* 1987; **6**: 57–63.

Lambotte A. Intervention dans les fractures marginales antérieures du radius. In *Chirurgie opératoire des fractures*. Paris: Masson, 1907.

Largier A, Dupuis JF. Fractures marginales antérieures du radius chez l'adulte. In *Actualités de Chirurgie à Garches*. Paris: Masson, 1976: 183–96.

20
The postero-medial fragment in distal radial fractures: description and treatment

JP Mortier, S Baux

The constant presence of a postero-medial fragment (PMF) in intra-articular fractures of the distal radius was reported by Castaing et al. at the SOFCOT meeting in 1964. They called it 'the potential fracture', that is, the initial fragment around which the other lines of fracture develop as the energy of the injury increases.

In 1976, Uhl pointed out a positive statistical relationship between, on the one hand, the dorsal tilt and the radio-ulnar variance index (normal = 2mm, Burdin 1979) and, on the other, the decrease of flexor tendon strength and the residual pain of the ulnar head.

This fragment (PMF) plays an important functional role in intra-articular fractures and is also important in the radiographic assessment of these fractures.

In their study of 175 cases, Mortier and Baux (1983) confirmed that when normal anatomy is restored, functional impairment exists in one out of six cases, versus one out of two cases with malunion: a dorsal tilt exceeding 20° and a positive ulnar variance are significant in determining the sequelae. In this study, poor results were obtained after isolated radial styloid pinning due to residual displacement in 16% of the cases and due to secondary displacements in 48%. This led the authors to propose specific pin fixation of the postero-medial fragment. In 1986, they reviewed 70 intra-articular fractures treated by double pin fixation (one in the radial styloid and one in the PMF). A normal or near normal anatomy was restored in 95.7% of the cases, thus showing the value of a correct diagnosis and specific treatment of the PMF in intra-articular fractures of the distal radius.

Pathomechanics of the PMF

It was impossible to reproduce a standard pattern intra-articular fracture in cadavers, so the pathomechanism was investigated by performing an osteotomy on the bone and then studying the displacement, reduction and the fixation while taking radiographs. The usual radiological measurements were taken: radial tilt, dorsal tilt, radial translation and ulnar variance (Table 20.1), as recommended by Castaing (1964).

The PMF is part of the radiocarpal and radio-ulnar joint. Radiographic examination in the sagittal plane shows that the volume of the PMF is due to the relative position of the radial arch and carpal dome at the time of the injury. Two elements have to be considered:

1. the resultant of two force vectors. The first is vertial due to gravity, and the second is hortizontal due to the forward projection of the body on the revolving hand;
2. the more or less extended position of the wrist at the time of the fall.

The more the wrist is extended and the more horizontal the resultant force is, the more the surface of the radial facet extends forward as it is displaced by the carpal dome. This explains the variability of the PMF shape, from the very rare fracture of the dorsal rim to a fragment including the complete lunar facet with the anterior cortex (T-fracture, Burdin 1979).

Radiographic examination in the transverse plane shows that wrist deviation at the moment of impact determines the extent of the fragment. The 'potential fracture' of Castaing is not always

Table 20.1 Radiological measurements.

Measurement	Normal value	Grading	
Radial tilt	25°	0 + ++ +++	≥ 23° 19–22° 15–18° < 15°
Ulnar variance	+2 mm	0 + ++ +++	> +2 +2 – −2 −2 – −5 ≤ −6
Dorsal tilt	+10°	0 + ++ +++	3–10 2 – −5 −6 – −18 ≤ −19
Radial translation	< 12 mm	0 + ++ +++	< 8 8–10 11–13 > 13

present. The lunate bone is always the proximal point of the carpal dome in the sagittal plane. In the coronal plane, however, the contact area of the lunate, and thus the pressure exerted on it, decreases as radial deviation increases. In forced radial deviation, the force is transmitted through the scaphoid bone rather than the lunate, which is in contact with the triangular fibrocartilage complex (TFCC). This explains the pathomechanism of the isolated radial styloid fracture.

Conversely, in ulnar deviation, the force transmission shifts ulnarward and the lunate is in contact with the radius.

Radiographic examination in the vertical plane shows that the PMF height is almost constant and its proximal border is at the level of the posterior tubercle of the radial sigmoid notch. However, extension up to the top of the birfucation of the medial border of the radius is possible, producing a proximal cortical split. Two important features should be noted:

1. the distal insertion of the wrist volar and dorsal capsule and ligaments on the radial epiphysis, means that the horizontal line of fracture is always extra-articular. This distal fragment (fractured epiphysis) with the carpus can always be reduced by axial traction;
2. the distal radio-ulnar ligament insertion on the dorsal tubercle of the radius explains the PMF displacement during wrist pronation; this motion must be prevented when fixing the fracture.

Finally, TFCC tears can explain a number of the poor functional results: these tears result from posterior and radial translation combined with proximal migration of the PMF. The complex can also become slack when the ulnar styloid is fractured. A central tear allows the head of the ulnar to impinge on the lunate. If the PMF is not reduced, this impingement persists. Malunion of the PMF causes progressive worsening of these lesions. There is a statistically significant relationship between PMF malunion, decrease of strength and pain at the ulnar head (Tables 20.2 and 20.3). The impingement of the ulnar head on the lunate is confirmed by conventional radiographs, CT scans and peroperative findings, where matched cartilage erosions are seen on the lunate and ulnar head (Figs 20.1 and 20.2). Radial translation of the carpus can prevent this impingement.

Diagnosis

Antero-posterior and lateral radiographs do not allow visualization of the PMF. Different studies have reported a wide range of incidence of a PMF in distal radial fractures. In 1976, Uhl found this fragment in 25% of distal radial fractures. Castaing (1964) reported an incidence of 35%, Rogers (1944) found the fragment in 56% of cases and Gartland and Werley (1951) in 86% of the cases. Only inadequate radiographic views can explain these discrepancies. The PMF is seen on an AP view as an enhanced density of the volar cortex; in the lateral view, it is superimposed on the dorsally displaced distal epiphysis and is frequently missed. Even the radio-ulnar index (Boabigbi 1988) gives a poor reflection of it. The natural

Table 20.2 Statistical correlations between ulnar variance and strength of flexor.

Measurement	Average values		Type	t-Test	P
	Reduced	Normal			
Ulnar variance (mm)	−3.5	+1	3	3.8	$< 10^{-4}$
Dorsal tilt	−12°	−4.5°	11.8	2.8	< 0.01
Radial tilt	20°	19°	6.5	0.3	NS
Radial translation (mm)	7.8	7.9	3	0.3	NS

Table 20.3 Statistical correlations between ulnar variance and ulnar pain.

Measurement	Average values		Type	t-Test	P
	Pain+	Pain−			
Ulnar variance (mm)	−2.2	+1	3	2.09	< 0.05
Dorsal tilt	−6.7°	−5.6°	11	0.3	NS
Radial tilt	19.1°	18°	6.5	0.3	NS
Radial translation (mm)	8.4	7.9	3	0.6	NS

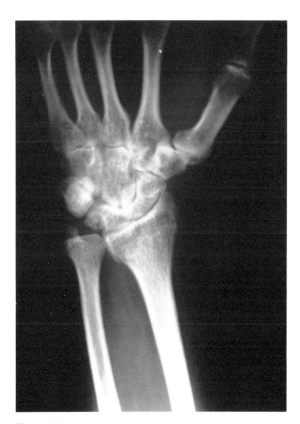

Figure 20.1

Ulnolunate impingement with secondary cyst changes.

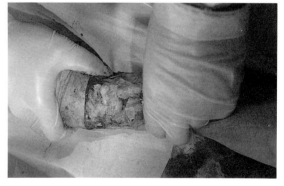

Figure 20.2

Ulnolunate impingement and malunion found in a cadaver. There is cartilage erosion of the lunate.

angulation of the distal radius means that volar and dorsal oblique views are necessary to visualize this fragment (Mortier et al. 1983). In the author's study (1986), these radiographic views detected the PMF in 91% of cases. These oblique views have since been included systematically in our practice. Without them, unstable intra-articular fractures can be mistaken for Colles' fractures with inevitably poor results.

Treatment

Specific reduction of the PMF should be included in the treatment of intra-articular distal radial fractures. In this study, the effectiveness of the reduction by external manoeuvres was studied in cadavers, in which the fracture lines were reproduced, whilst keeping the capsule attached and the tendons present.

An axial traction force is applied to reduce the fragment which is proximally displaced and impacted. Whatever the wrist deviation, the ligamentotaxis exerted by the dorsal radiocarpal ligaments pulls the fragment distally but displacement tends to recur if the axial traction stops. Furthermore, if the wrist is in ulnar deviation, the fragment redisplaces. Only osteosynthesis can prevent redisplacement and maintain the reduction. A fragment that is completely detached from all capsular and ligamentous connections cannot be reduced by external manoeuvres: open reduction or percutaneous reduction under fluoroscopy should be performed. When feasible the dorsal displacement is reduced by direct compression, with wrist flexion of up to 45°, which provides pressure from the extensor tendons. This is possible only after traction and disimpaction. If there is a crushing injury of the PMF, it is impossible to reduce this displacement.

Prevention of pronation and supination by immobilization is necessary but this alone will not prevent secondary displacement of the fragment.

Fixation is performed on a perfectly reduced fracture. The aim is to fix both the radial styloid fragment and the PMF independently. The latter can be fixed to the head of the ulna with a horizontal K-wire when there is associated injury to the TFCC.

Percutaneous fixation of the radial styloid fragment is performed first. The surgeon pulls on the thumb, producing ulnar deviation. A 1.8 mm or 2 mm K-wire is inserted into the radius bone, volar to the styloid but dorsal to the first compartment, and is directed at a 45° angle through the dorsal cortex. This pin does not go through the PMF, but must be inserted radial to it (Fig. 20.3).

Traction is exerted on the third and fourth rays by an assistant, or with finger trap traction, while the surgeon uses one hand to maintain reduction

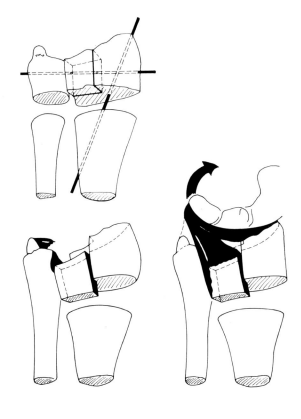

Figure 20.3

The PMF with its capsuloligamentous attachments showing placement of the radial styloid pin.

of the PMF and the other to introduce a K-wire. This K-wire (2 mm) is inserted into the ulnar head, proximal to the ulnar styloid, entering at a distal to proximal angle of 20° with a slight dorso-volar direction towards the radial styloid without perforating it. If too distal, the K-wire is felt to penetrate too easily into the radiocarpal joint; if too proximal, it goes through the fracture line. When properly inserted, this type of fixation ensures good stability: the pins cross each other in all planes and prono-supination is blocked (Fig. 20.4). The K-wires are cut and an above-the-elbow cast is applied, allowing the MP joints to flex. Antero-posterior lateral, and posterior oblique radiographs are taken on the third and tenth days after operation (Figs 20.5 and 20.6). The cast and K-wires are removed after four weeks and rehabilitation is initiated.

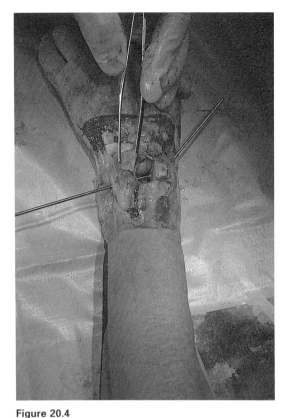 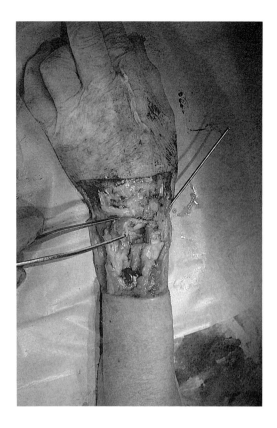

Figure 20.4

Ulnoradial K-wire seen from the PMF.

Results

Four radiological measurements were assessed and four stages of radiological classification were used to assess the results. For function, three features were assessed including pain, motion, and strength. The average follow-up was eight months (range 45 days to 6 years). It should be noted that 45 days is a short follow-up and patients usually improve with time.

Of the 68 patients reviewed, 2 had a bilateral injury. Their ages ranged from 20 to 93 years. There were 58 female patients and 10 male patients; 41 fractures were left-sided and 29 right-sided. Only two of the patients were seen following a delay; the remainder were seen immediately after injury.

Anatomical results

Normal anatomy was restored in 95.7% of the cases. Of the three residual deformities, two were caused by inadequate initial reduction, and one by secondary displacement when the K-wire was inserted too proximally.

A good initial reduction of comminuted fractures is achieved with this technique. Uhl noted in 1976 an inadequate initial reduction in only 16% of cases. Only a small number of secondary displacements occurred in this study, compared with the 60% reported by Garland and Werley (1951), 37–41% reported by Castaing (1964), 14% reported by Judet et al. (1968), and 100% reported by Ledoux et al. (1973). Such a restoration of normal anatomy is very valuable, especially since the double pin fixation has only been used on unstable fractures.

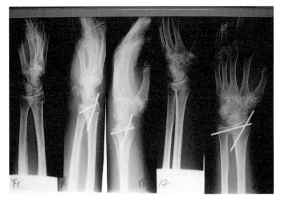

Figure 20.5

Pinning of a T-fracture. Oblique radiographs taken before and after the procedure.

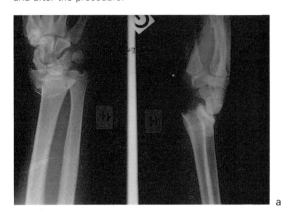

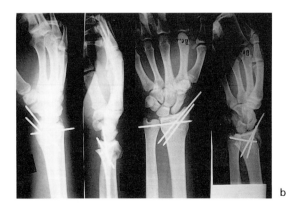

Figure 20.6

Comminuted fracture a) before and b) after pinning.

Functional results

Poor results were due to:

- unacceptable anatomical results (4.3%);
- a loss of wrist motion (6%) without anatomical deformities;
- carpal tunnel syndrome (3%) in a fracture with significant displacement;
- neurosympathetic dystrophy (15.7%) recovering in two to three months, except in one case that lasted for a year;
- residual loss of motion in prono-supination (this being less than after DRUJ malunion or subluxation) in four cases (Pequignot et al. 1985).

Conclusions

Fractures involving the postero-medial fragment of the distal radius are not benign fractures. Workers' compensation cases have shown functional impairment ranging from 10.8% (Judet et al. 1968) to 17% (Uhl 1976). Oblique radiographic views are necessary to assess this type of fracture thoroughly. The treatment we propose is directed at restoring a normal ulnar variance, correcting dorsal displacement, and avoiding ulnolunate impingement. Isolated radial styloid pinning cannot achieve these goals.

Statistical results show that horizontal pinning, which maintains the radial sigmoid notch at its proper level by going through the ulna, is a simple, harmless and effective method (Uhl 1976). Other studies have confirmed this view (Lortat-Jacob et al. 1982, Pequignot et al. 1985). Furthermore this technique stabilizes the distal radio-ulnar pain and helps with ligamentous cicatrization when a subluxation is associated (Kuhlmann 1985).

References

Boabigbi A, Kuhlmann JN, Guérin-Surville H. L'indice radio-lunaire sagittal. *J Radiol* 1988; **69**: 227–28.

Burdin Ph. Fracture récente de l'extrémité inférieure du radius. Cahier d'enseignement de la SOFCOT 1979; **10**: 93–109.

Castaing J, le Club des Dix. Fracture récente de l'extrémité inférieure du radius chez l'adulte. *Rev Chir Orthop* 1968; **50**: 581–696.

Gartland JJ, Werley CW. Evaluation of Colles' fractures. *J Bone Joint Surg* 1951: **38**: 895.

Judet J, Judet R, Leconte P, Plumerault J. Les fractures sus articulaires de l'extrémité inférieure du radius. *Rev Prat* 1968; **18**: 1953–67.

Kuhmann JN, Fahrer M, Kapandji AI, Tubiana R. Stability of the normal wrist. In Tubiana R, ed. *The hand*. Philadelphia: WB Saunders, 1985.

Ledoux A, Rauis A, Vanderghinst M. L'embrochage des fractures inférieures du radius. *Rev Chir Orthop* 1973; **59**: 427–38.

Lortat-Jacob A, Franck A, De Bonduwe A, Beaufils Ph. Le borchage en Y dans le traitement des fractures à déplacement postérieur de l'extrémité inférieure du radius. *Acta Orthop Belg* 1982; **48**: 936–46.

Mortier JP, Baux S, Uhl JF, Mimoun M, Mole B. Importance de fragment postéro-interne et son brochage spécifique dans les fractures de l'extrémité inférieure du radius. *Ann Chir Main* 1983; **2**: 219–29.

Mortier JP, Kuhlmann JN, Richet C, Baux S. Brochage horizontal cubito-radial dans les fractures de l'extrémité inférieure du radius comportant un fragment postéro-interne. *Rev Chir Orthop* 1986; **72,8**: 567–71.

Pequignot JP, Giboin P, Argenson C, Allieu Y. Les atteintes de la radio-cubitale inférieure dans les traumatismes du poignet. *Ann Chir Main* 1985; **4**: 273–85.

Rogers SC. An analysis of Colles's fracture. *Br Med J* 1944; **1**: 807–9.

Uhl JF. Etude des facteurs influençant le résultat fonctionnel des fractures de l'extrémité du radius. Thèse médecine, Paris, 1976.

21
Treatment of articular distal radial fractures by intrafocal pinning with arum pins

Al Kapandji

Distal radial fractures are the most common type of upper extremity fracture, and among them, articular fractures are the most frequent. The use of intrafocal pinning to treat non-articular fractures of the distal radius has already been discussed in chapter 10. This explained the principle of intrafocal pinning, which is not complicated by secondary displacement thanks to the immediate abutment of the distal fragment onto the pins. The reader is referred to chapter 10 for a description of 'arum' pins, which prevent secondary pin displacement and damage to the skin and tendons. This chapter will focus on the use of intrafocal arum pinning for the treatment of intra-articular fractures.

Indications

Arum pins can be used in articular fractures to provide the same benefits as those conferred to non-articular fractures.

The extremely frequent postero-medial fragment (Fig. 21.1) constitutes the simplest type of articular fracture (Fig. 21.2a). This fracture involves the articular surface of both the radius and the sigmoid notch. It is very important to use a third pin to control this postero-medial fragment, because the distal radio-ulnar joint (DRUJ) function may be restricted or even completely blocked if it is not reduced in the correct anatomic position. The postero-medial fragment may be combined with a T-shaped, sagittal plane fracture (Fig. 21.2b): in this case, posterior blocking of the distal fragments is better achieved with two posterior pins (Fig. 21.3).

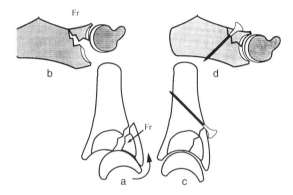

Figure 21.1

The postero-medial fragment. a) Medial view: the postero-medial fragment (Fr) crosses the sigmoid notch and the glena with a posterior dislocation. b) Coronal cut: the displacement of the postero-medial fragment (Fr) produces a posterior dislocation of the DRUJ. c) Medial view: the pinning of the postero-medial fragment reconstructs the glena. d) Coronal cut: the pinning of the postero-medial fragment reconstructs the sigmoid notch.

Fractures with anterior tilt are less common, but it is possible to insert anterior pins (Fig. 21.4) through two anterior approaches:

1. the antero-lateral approach, proposed by Hoël (1991);
2. the antero-medial, proposed by the author (Hoël and Kapandji, in press).

When correctly inserted, the arum pins are well tolerated by the flexor tendons and by the nerves and arteries. Thus, fractures with anterior tilt (Fig. 21.5) may be controlled as effectively by pinning as they would be by an anterior plate. In the same

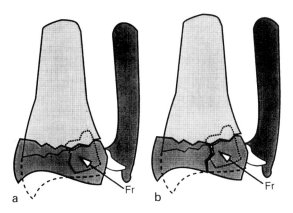

Figure 21.2

Distal radial fracture with a postero-medial fragment (Fr). a) Typically, this fragment is difficult to visualize on an AP radiograph. b) Fracture with a postero-medial fragment and a sagittal split, which is often not obvious when the two main fragments are displaced together.

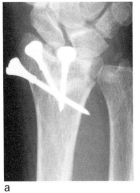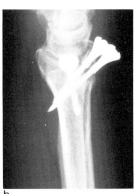

Figure 21.3

Arum pins in a fracture with a postero-medial fragment. a) AP view: the postero-medial fragment is close to the ulnar head. b) Lateral view: 2 posterior arum pins have been used to reconstruct the glena.

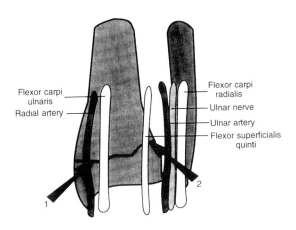

Figure 21.4

The two anterior approaches for arum pinning. 1) The antero-lateral approach: between the tendon of the flexor carpi radialis and the radial artery. 2) The antero-medial approach: between the tendons of the flexor digiti, especially the flexor quinti, and the ulnar nerve and artery flanked by the tendon of the flexor carpi ulnaris.

way, it is possible to control fractures of the anterior border of the radius (Fig. 21.6) after obtaining good anatomic reduction (Fig. 21.7). With posterior and anterior pins, a fracture involving two articular borders of the radius (Fig. 21.8) may be perfectly reduced with a reconstruction of the articular surface.

In some cases, fractures of the distal radius with posterior tilt can be combined with a fracture of the radial styloid process (Fig. 21.9): these are anatomically reduced with three pins. However, in this type of radial styloid process fracture, be aware that a scapholunate dislocation can be present (Figure 21.10): if a dorsal intercalated segment instability (DISI) deformity is visible on the lateral radiograph, an antero-posterior view must be taken with traction on the thumb to emphasize the gap between the scaphoid and the lunate. If there is an associated anterior border fracture, look carefully for carpal instability. Fixation will require three (or four) pins, with an obligatory lateral one, and the scapholunate dislocation must be pinned with a special pin-screw after reducing the lunate DISI deformity (Fig. 21.11).

On the ulnar side of the wrist, a fracture of the ulnar styloid process is very common. This causes rupture of the triangular fibrocartilage complex (TFCC), which is quite obvious when the ulnar styloid is fractured, but often not visible when the styloid process is intact (Fig. 21.12). This TFCC dislocation may compromise DRUJ function; this explains why it is so important to fix the ulnar styloid process in its proper place with a special pin-screw. This complex fracture of both radius and ulna (Fig. 21.13) illustrates several means of fixation. A concave plate is used to fix the ulnar fracture, an anterior plate with two arum pins (one posterior and one anterior) are needed to fix the

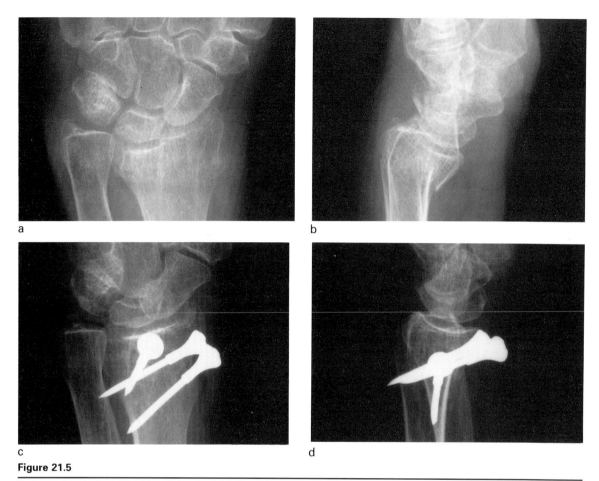

Figure 21.5

Radiographs of a fracture with anterior tilt. a) AP view: there is a small antero-medial fragment. b) Lateral view: the anterior tilt is obvious. c) AP view with arum pins: the antero-medial fragment is reduced and the anterior border is realigned. d) Lateral view with arum pins; the two anterior pins restore the normal orientation of the glena.

radius and a special pin-screw is used to fix the ulnar styloid process.

Finally, and contrary to what might be expected, multifragment fractures can be controlled with three or four pins. When such a fracture is seen, most surgeons will think first of external fixation. In this situation, it is worth first trying to insert one or two intrafocal pins, beginning with the lateral one which often confers good stabilization. Then, if the 'puzzle' is simplified, a second pin (posterior or anterior) may be set and in a short time, one can see the radial epiphysis being reconstructed. Secondary displacement is frequent in this type of fracture, but the functional result may be unexpectedly good, because the operation is not too invasive and allows early rehabilitation.

Evaluation of results

The results were evaluated following the same principles as those applied to the non-articular fractures. For radiographic evaluation, the use of objective criteria, measured in degrees and millimeters (as explained in chapter 10) was indispensable.

Results

Globally, the results are the same as those of the non-articular fractures (see chapter 10). However, due to the number of fragments and the articular

INTRAFOCAL PINNING WITH ARUM PINS   163

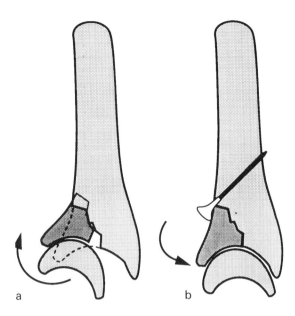

Figure 21.6

Setting an anterior arum pin on a fracture of the anterior border. a) The displaced fragment of the anterior border. b) Fixing the anterior fragment with an arum pin.

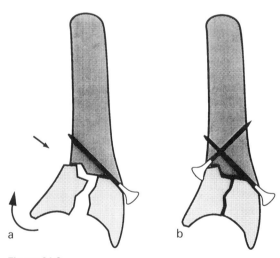

Figure 21.8

Fracture of both glenoid borders. The two borders of the radial glena are fractured with a frontal split. a) First, the posterior fragment is fixed with an arum pin. b) The same procedure is performed on the anterior fragment: the glena is rebuilt.

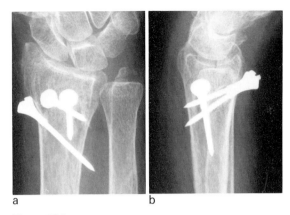

Figure 21.7

Fracture of the anterior border of the glena. a) AP view: the anterior border fracture is not seen. b) Lateral view: the anterior border fracture is obvious and the glena is reconstructed.

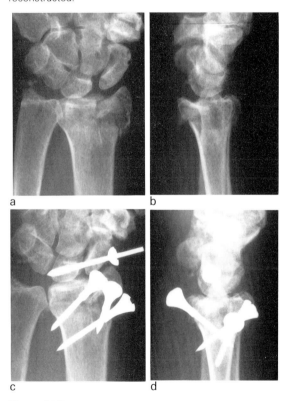

Figure 21.9

Fracture of the radial styloid process. a) AP view: in the main distal fragment, there is a split separating the radial styloid process. b) Lateral view: the posterior tilt is obvious but there is no DISI of the lunate. c) AP view with 3 arum pins, 2 posterior and 1 lateral, which controls the radial styloid process fracture. d) Lateral view: the 2 posterior pins correct the posterior tilt; there is no lunate DISI.

164 FRACTURES OF THE DISTAL RADIUS

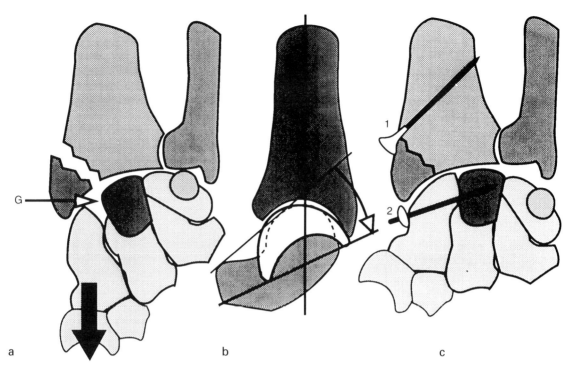

Figure 21.10
Scapholunate dislocation associated with a radial styloid process fracture. a) AP radiograph taken with thumb traction displaying the associated scapholunate dissociation (G). b) Lateral view showing the lunate DISI and the anterior border fracture, frequently associated with a radial styloid process fracture. c) AP view after pinning showing (1) fixation of the radial styloid process with an arum pin and (2) fixation of the scapholunate dislocation with a special pin-screw, after reduction of the DISI.

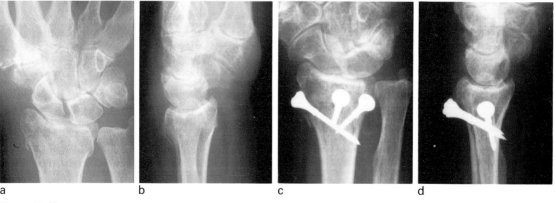

Figure 21.11
A complex radial styloid process fracture. a) AP view displaying the radial styloid process fracture and the scapholunate dislocation. b) Lateral view showing the associated fracture of the anterior border and the lunate DISI. c) AP view with 3 arum pins, 1 controlling the radial styloid process fracture; the scapholunate dislocation has been fixed with a special pin-screw. d) Lateral view: the anterior arum pin fixes the fracture of the anterior border, the posterior one controls the posterior tilt and the special pin-screw keeps the lunate in the correct position.

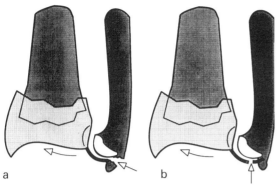

Figure 21.12

TFCC dislocation. a) Fracture of the ulnar styloid process is very common in Colles' fractures. The associated TFCC dislocation jeopardizes the stability of the DRUJ. b) When the ulnar styloid process is not broken, there is often a tear to the TFCC with the same result as the styloid process fracture.

surface involvement, results may not be so good. Secondary displacements were more frequent, but if an early rehabilitation is undertaken, the results were unexpectedly better than those achieved after complicated and invasive techniques.

The restriction of mobility is not too troublesome in flexion–extension, but in pronation–supination, due to DRUJ dislocation, it is not so good. In these cases, secondary operations may be needed. These include simple shortening of the ulna (Milch 1926), or reposition arthrodesis of the ulnar head combined with a short resection of the ulnar shaft (Sauvé–Kapandji procedure).

Conclusions

The results of treatment of distal radial articular fractures have been greatly improved by the arum pinning procedure. This technique allows immediate rehabilitation thanks to a precise and firm fixation, which does not need a wide approach and is easy to perform. The results are not as good as those of non-articular fractures, but are unexpectedly better than those obtained following invasive techniques, because of the early rehabilitation. The most common problem is poor prono-supination, due to DRUJ dislocation; this can be solved with secondary operations to correct DRUJ instability without having to correct the radial malunion.

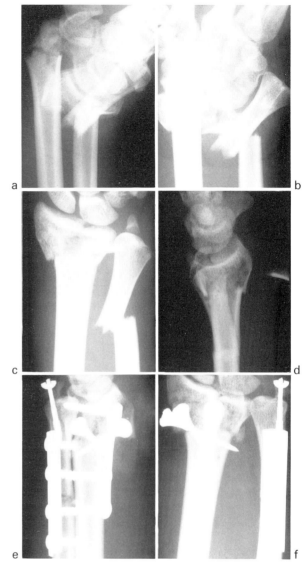

Figure 21.13

A complex fracture of the extremities of the two bones. a) AP view. b) Lateral view. c) AP view after an approximate reduction under general anaesthesia: there are two fractures of the ulna, at the styloid process and the lower shaft; on the radius, there is a multifragment fracture. d) Lateral view of the same case: among the numerous fragments of the radial epiphysis, one is seen far in front and distal from the radius; this fragment was very important for the anterior stability. e,f) AP and lateral views showing the material used to fix this complex fracture. There is a plate on the ulnar shaft and a special pin-screw on the ulnar styloid process; an anterior plate and 2 arum pins have been used to fix the radial epiphysis. Note that the glena is reconstructed in AP and lateral views and that the ulnar variance is only slightly positive.

References

Hoël G. La voie antero-externe pour le brochage intrafocal des fracture de l'extrémité inférieure du radius à déplacement antérieur. Communication at The International Symposium on the Wrist, Nagoya, March 1991.

Hoël G, Kapandji AI. Osteosynthèse par broches intrafocales des fractures à déplacement antérieur de l'épiphyse radiale inférieure. *Ann Chir Main* (in press).

Kapandji AI. Operation de Kapandi M et Sauvé L. Techniques et indications dans les affections non-rhumatismales. *Ann Chir Main* 1986; **5**: 181–5.

Milch H. Dislocation of the inferior end of the ulna: suggestion of a new operative procedure. *Am J Surg* 1926; **7**: 141.

Sauvé L, Kapandji, M. Nouvelle techniques de traitement chirurgical des luxations récidivantes isolées de l'extrémité inférieure du cubitus. *J Chir* 1936; **47**: 589–94.

22
Management of comminuted distal radial fractures

Jesse B Jupiter, Craig S Williams

Introduction

Fractures of the distal end of the radius are common. As such, most practising surgeons will have had experience of managing these injuries. While these fractures are traditionally identified by eponymic descriptions, for example, 'Colles' ', 'Smith's', or 'Barton's' fractures, they in fact represent a heterogeneous group of injuries — some with very different prognostic features than others. A lack of agreement on the precise definition of these fractures has resulted in both confusion and difficulty in management and evaluation of outcome.

Given that the distal end of the radius supports two important yet distinct articulations — the radiocarpal and radio-ulnar joints — it is the multifragmented (comminuted) fractures that have the greatest possibility of causing long-term functional disability, and it is this subgroup of fractures that this chapter will address.

Evaluation

Evaluation of the patient with a comminuted fracture of the distal radius should give consideration to the individual patient's functional needs, local factors which involve both skeletal and associated soft tissue structures, and the specific fracture pattern.

A thorough history and physical examination will reveal important factors regarding the patient's physiologic age and overall health status, handedness, occupation, avocation, lifestyle, compliance, and expectations. Appreciation of these patient factors will allow the surgeon to begin to tailor the treatment to help meet the goals and expectations of the individual patient. It goes without saying that the functional requirements of a young active adult with a comminuted fracture of his or her dominant distal radius are likely to be very different from those of a sedentary, elderly nursing-home patient with a similar fracture pattern.

Furthermore, an appreciation of the mechanism of injury will contribute to the assessment of the severity of the traumatic event. Severe soft tissue swelling, median nerve dysfunction, and even the presence of a forearm compartment syndrome, all occur more frequently with comminuted fractures, to a large degree due to a higher velocity of impact (Bickerstaff and Bell 1989, Knirk and Jupiter 1986, Melone 1984).

Radiographic evaluation should include, at a minimum, good quality antero-posterior, oblique, and lateral views of the distal radius. Assessment of the extra-articular displacement of the distal radius can be obtained by measurement of the radial alignment on the horizontal, frontal, and sagittal views. These include the measurement of volar tilt, radial inclination, radial length (or ulnar variance), and radial width (Dowling and Sawyer 1952, Gartland and Werley 1951, Rubinovich and Rennie 1983, Van der Linden and Ericson 1981). Trispiral tomography is extremely valuable in the preoperative planning of intra-articular fractures. This will shed light on the direction and degree of displacement of the articular fracture fragments (Fig. 22.1). Generally, computerized tomography of the distal radius is not as valuable as trispiral tomography in assessing the anatomic configuration of the fracture.

Evaluation of four interdependent local variables:

1. the degree of comminution;
2. the bone quality;

168 FRACTURES OF THE DISTAL RADIUS

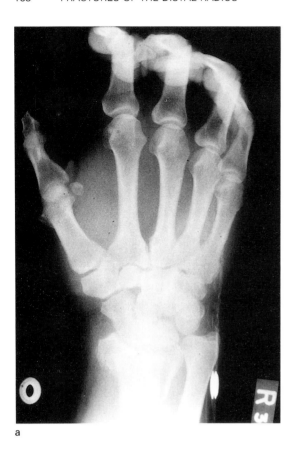

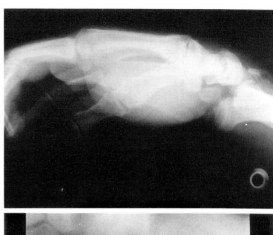

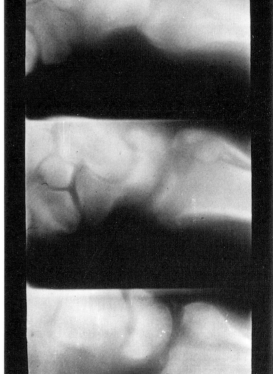

Figure 22.1
Comminuted intra-carticular fracture of the distal radius with dorsal subluxation of the carpus. a) AP view. b) Lateral view. c) Lateral tomography demonstrates displacement of the dorsal half of the lunate facet and the carpus, as well as the presence of impacted articular fragments.

3. the energy of an injury; and
4. the degree of displacement

will contribute greatly to the surgeon's appreciation of the severity of the injury (Axelrod and McMurtry 1990). These factors, when considered together, form the basis of decision making, as they reflect the degree of inherent stability or instability of the fracture, the ability to obtain, if necessary, stable internal fixation, and the extent of soft tissue injury.

Classification

The true value of any classification system lies in its ability to help direct treatment and group similar types of injuries together for the evaluation of outcome. However, in order to be of practical use in approaching clinical problems, such classification systems must be of manageable size and applicable to most practising physicians.

In 1967, Frykman proposed a classification which divides these fractures into eight groups, based on the presence or absence of intra-articular involvement of the radiocarpal and/or distal radio-ulnar joints, as well as the presence or absence of ulnar styloid involvement. Unfortunately, this classification is not helpful in management considerations, as it fails to offer insight into the extent or direction of displacement or associated soft tissue injury.

A useful insight into the pattern of intra-articular involvement in fractures of the distal radius was offered by Charles Melone who, in 1984, divided the distal end of the radius into four parts, suggesting that the direction of displacement and rotation of articular fracture fragments tended to follow a pattern, and that treatment could be more accurately determined on the basis of these patterns.

A more thorough and comprehensive classification of fractures of the distal end of the radius has been proposed by AO/ASIF (Müller 1991), which has identified specific fracture patterns of both the intra- and extra-articular aspects of the end of the radius and classified them by degrees of severity (Fig. 22.2).

Lastly, a useful and manageable classification of these fractures has been proposed by McMurtry and Jupiter (1992). This system divides fractures of the distal end of the radius into extra- and intra-articular types. Intra-articular fractures are defined as those that extend into the radiocarpal or distal radio-ulnar joint with more than 2 mm displacement. The intra-articular fractures are further subdivided based on the number of parts present. A part is defined as a fragment of bone with more than 2 mm displacement, which is of sufficient size to be functionally significant and to be manipulated and/or internally fixed (McMurtry and Jupiter, 1992).

Two-part intra-articular fractures are typically associated with radiocarpal subluxation and/or dislocation. There are four variants of these fractures, including volar and dorsal Barton's fractures, fracture of the radial styloid (chauffeur's fracture), and the die-punch fracture. The

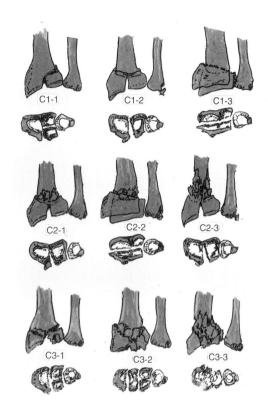

Figure 22.2

AO classification of complete articular distal radial fractures. Modified from McMurtry and Jupiter 1992.

unifying concept in this group is that there is an isolated, displaced articular fragment, with the remainder of the articular surface in continuity with the distal radial metaphysis (Figs 22.3a and 22.4).

Three-part fractures constitute those lesions in which the articular surface consists of two fragments, each of which is displaced from the distal radial metaphysis. This typically involves the scaphoid and lunate facets as the major fragments, which are separated from the radial metaphysis (Figs 22.3b and 22.5).

Four-part fractures comprise those injuries in which a third fracture line is found. This typically occurs in a coronal plane and serves to divide the lunate facet fragment into anterior and dorsal components (Figs 22.3c and 22.6).

The remainder of intra-articular fractures classified by McMurtry consists of highly-comminuted

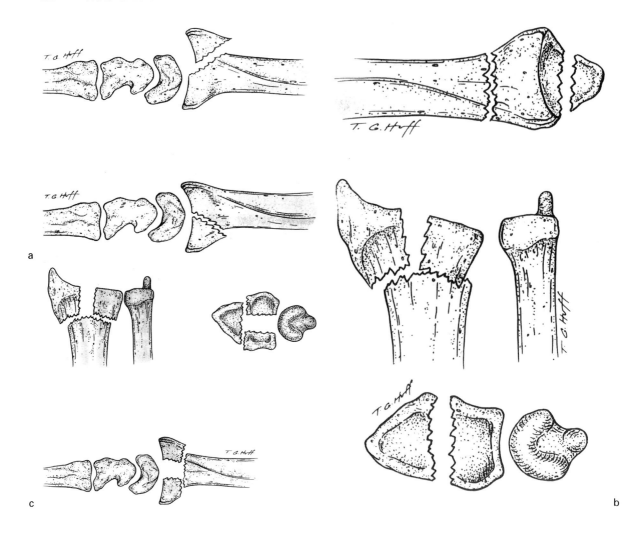

Figure 22.3

McMurtry a) two-part, b) three-part and c) four-part articular fractures.

injuries which are often the sequelae of more severe trauma or underlying osteoporosis. These are considered, as a group, as fractures with five or more parts. The degree of comminution may preclude methods of direct manipulation and stabilization (Fig. 22.7).

Treatment

The approach to fractures of the distal radius in general and, specifically, comminuted intra-articular fractures, must be individualized. Many factors must be carefully considered prior to selection of a specific form of treatment for a given individual. The anatomic type of the fracture should not be the sole determinant of the treatment method selected. The importance of patient and local factors cannot be overemphasized. Additionally, the surgeon must critically assess his or her own personal experience and abilities and level of comfort with each of the various treatment options. The goal of treatment should be to achieve a maximal functional outcome that will meet an individual

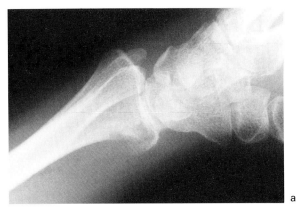
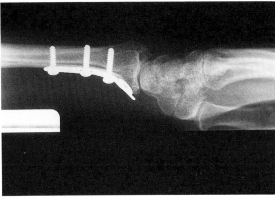
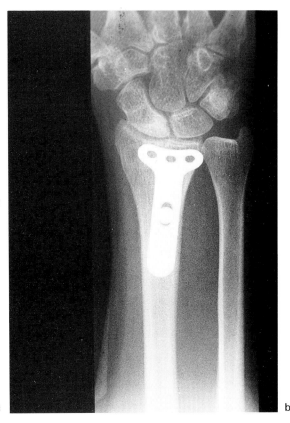

Figure 22.4

A 28-year-old female with an anterior fracture-dislocation. a) The lateral radiograph demonstrates an unstable shearing 2-part fracture-dislocation. b,c) AP and lateral views following open reduction and internal fixation through an anterior approach.

patient's needs and expectations while, at the same time, exposing the patient to a minimal risk of morbidity (Axelrod and McMurtry 1990).

Closed reduction and cast immobilization alone will rarely control comminuted fractures of the distal radius. Even in the setting of an anatomic reduction, there is a strong tendency for the fracture to redisplace to its original position during the course of cast immobilization. This may occur despite frequent cast changes and remanipulations (Collert and Isaacs 1978, McQueen and Caspers 1988). For this reason cast treatment alone should generally be reserved for those patients whose functional demands are extremely low and in whom a restoration and maintenance of normal anatomy is not a significant consideration. This holds true for both comminuted extra- as well as intra-articular lesions.

Percutaneous pinning

The use of percutaneous pins may facilitate the conversion of an unstable, comminuted fracture to a relatively stable configuration. This is especially the case for comminuted extra-articular fractures, in which the use of one or two pins across the fracture site into the proximal metaphysis and diaphysis will frequently prevent a loss of reduction during the treatment course (Clancey 1984). This method is ordinarily combined with cast immobilization, although external fixation

172 FRACTURES OF THE DISTAL RADIUS

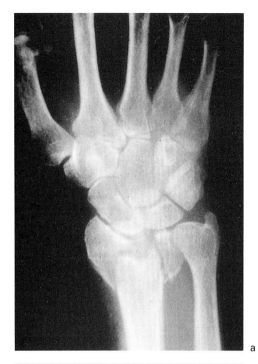
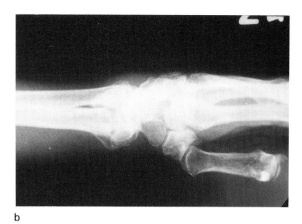
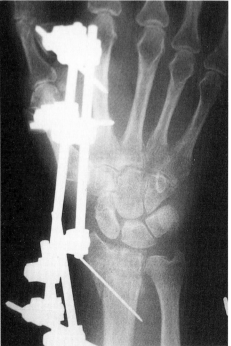
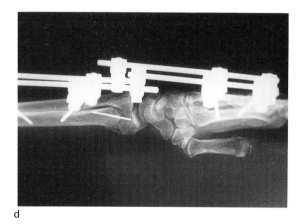

Figure 22.5

A 62-year-old female with a complex 3-part intra-articular fracture. a,b) AP and lateral radiographs demonstrating the fracture. c,d) AP and lateral views following closed reduction, percutaneous pinning and external fixation. e,f) External fixation facilitates early postoperative soft tissue mobilization. g,h) AP and lateral radiographs 3 months post injury.

MANAGEMENT OF COMMINUTED DISTAL RADIAL FRACTURES 173

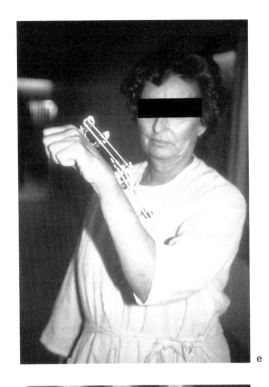

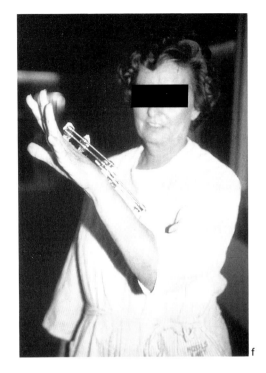

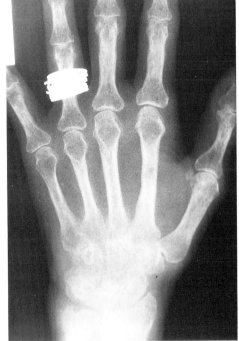

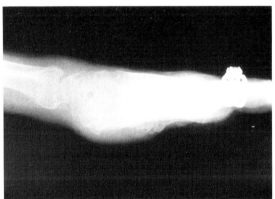

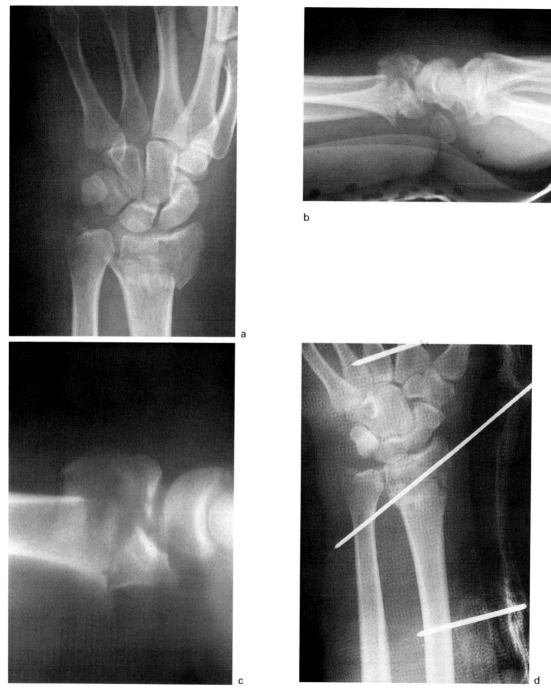

Figure 22.6

A 39-year-old male with a comminuted 4-part intra-articular distal radial fracture with dorsal subluxation of the carpus. a,b) AP and lateral radiographs. c) Lateral tomogram demonstrating anterior and dorsal fragments at the lunate facet and dorsal subluxation of the carpus. d,e) 3 weeks after closed reduction and stabilization with percutaneous pins, as well as pins and plaster. Note: the styloid pin does not have solid purchase in the proximal radius, and the reduction is lost. f,g) AP and lateral radiographs following open reduction and internal fixation through a dorsal approach.

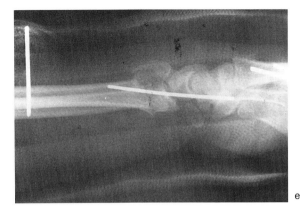
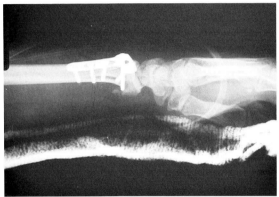
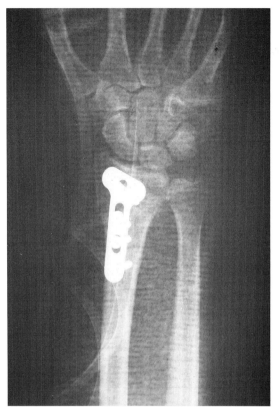

e

g

f

may be advisable in the presence of associated soft tissue swelling. The intrafocal technique of Kapandji (1991) can be accomplished without circular immobilization, although it has proven less effective with comminuted fracture patterns.

Clancey's technique (1984), based upon one or two percutaneous pins in conjunction with plaster immobilization is recommended. Following manipulative reduction, the hand and wrist are placed on a radiolucent table, with the wrist flexed over a soft 'bump'. Once the manipulative reduction has been achieved, stabilization of the fracture begins with a smooth pin placed from the radial styloid into the intact proximal radial shaft. As the styloid lies anterior to the mid-axis, this pin must be placed in a volar-radial to dorso-ulnar direction in a retrograde fashion. It is essential that firm purchase be obtained in the cortex of the proximal radius to prevent later fracture displacement. This may be supplemented by a second pin placed through the radial styloid pin in a similar fashion (Fig. 22.8). The surgeon must take heed to avoid injury to branches of the superficial radial nerve. The use of either a protective drill guide or an oscillating attachment to the wire driver will reduce the risk of injury to the underlying soft tissue structures.

An additional wire may then be placed, starting from the dorso-ulnar aspect of the radius into the proximal volar aspect of the radial shaft. In some three-part fractures the lunate facet may still require additional reduction. This may be accomplished using a percutaneously placed wire to help manipulate the fragment. It is preferable to cut the wires off just beneath the level of the skin. Immobilization can be accomplished with a short arm volar splint in the presence of soft tissue swelling and/or external fixation. A short arm cast may be considered if there is no swelling or following three weeks of external fixation. The cast can be removed after six weeks, and the pins are generally removed two weeks following this.

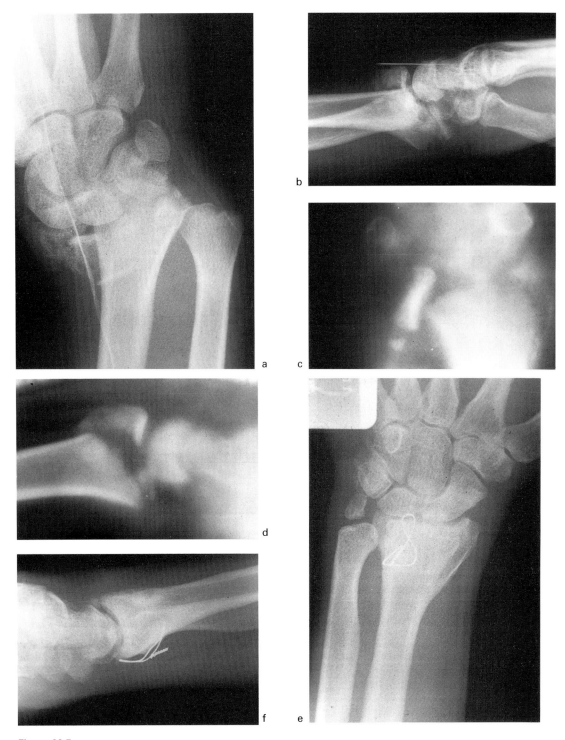

Figure 22.7

A 23-year-old male with a severely comminuted 5(+)-part fracture of the distal radius. a,b) AP and lateral radiographs. c,d) AP and lateral tomography demonstrate the extensive articular disruption. e,f) The fracture was treated through anterior and dorsal incisions with Kirschner wires, interosseous wiring, bone grafting, and external fixation. These AP and lateral radiographs, taken at 3-year follow-up reveal mild joint space narrowing. The functional outcome was good.

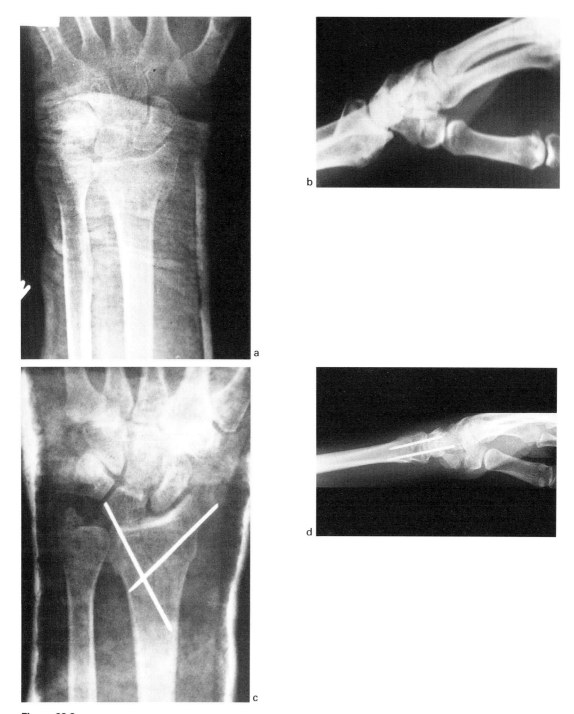

Figure 22.8

Unstable distal radial fracture in a 33-year-old patient. a,b) AP and lateral radiographs show significant radial shortening. c,d) AP and lateral view of fracture reduction and percutaneous pinning with two crossed pins. Note: the restoration of radial length and radial tilt. e,f) AP and lateral radiographs showing the healed position of fracture. Note: there is no loss of reduction after percutaneous pinning.

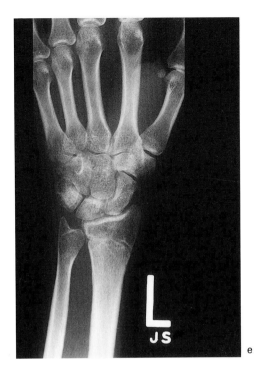

e

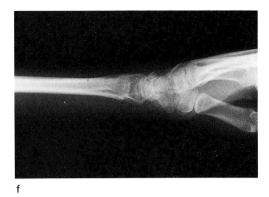

f

Figure 22.8

(continued)

External skeletal fixation

The indications, types of external frames, and purported complications of external fixation for complex distal radial fractures has remained controversial. The authors believe that external fixation is most effective in maintaining the axial length of the reduced multifragmented distal radial fracture, while permitting early functional rehabilitation of associated soft tissue injury (Howard et al. 1989). In most instances, it is advisable to add percutaneous pins, or even utilize external fixation in conjunction with internal bone grafting and/or internal stable fixation (Leung et al. 1990, Seitz et al. 1990).

While a number of types and applications of external fixation exist for distal radial fractures, when used in conjunction with pins and/or internal bone grafting, simple frames can be applied along the radial aspect of the hand and forearm (Fig. 22.9). Positioning the hand and wrist in neutral permits a more functional position for digital motion and restoration of strength.

Open reduction and internal fixation

Operative management of complex fractures of the distal radius has a definite role. This is particularly the case for some intra-articular fractures which cannot be reduced by traction or manipulative manoeuvres. This approach is the procedure of choice for two-part intra-articular fractures with volar or dorsal displaced fragments, as these fractures generally represent radiocarpal fracture-dislocations and are more commonly seen as a result of high-energy trauma in young, active patients with healthy bone (de Oliveira 1973, Ellis 1965, Pattee and Thompson 1988, Thompson and Grant 1977).

A second indication involves those intra-articular fractures with a displaced and rotated anterior fragment of the lunate facet of the distal radius. This is particularly the case when this fracture is associated with soft tissue swelling and the possibility of compromised median nerve function (Axelrod et al. 1988).

Finally, a third indication is found in those fractures which displace late in treatment, or present beyond 3–4 weeks of injury with severe displacement. In these cases, early operative

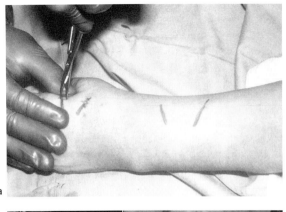
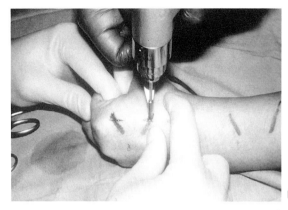
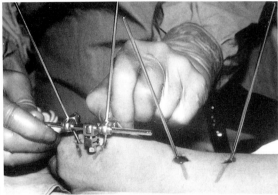
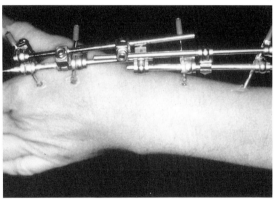

Figure 22.9

Placement of external fixator. a) With fluoroscopic guidance, the skin is marked for the approximate direction of the pins. Longitudinal incisions are made, and the bony cortex is accessed using blunt spreading technique. b) Pins are placed under power while the soft tissues are protected. c,d) Once the fracture is reduced and all pins are placed, the frame is assembled.

intervention is preferential to later osteotomy (see Fig. 22.6).

Operative technique

Pre-operative planning may be essential in determining the extent and direction of the fracture fragment displacement. As a general rule, the placement of the surgical incision is based on the direction of displacement of the major fragments. The use of intra-operative distraction with temporarily applied external fixators is often exceptionally useful in aiding both reduction and the ability to gain surgical access for the placement of definitive internal fixation.

Anterior approach

An incision based along the ulnar aspect of the palmaris longus, coursing across the wrist crease and into the palm in line with the ring finger, has proven to be both extensile and less likely to cause injury to crossing sensory nerves. The palmar fascia is divided in line with the incision and the transverse retinaculum; this can be performed in a zig-zag fashion for later loose approximation. The antebrachial fascia is likewise divided in line with the cutaneous incision.

The approach to the radius can be through two directions: either radial or ulnar to the median nerve. On the radial side the approach is between the radial artery and the flexor carpi radialis, while an ulnar-based approach has the median nerve protected by all of the flexor tendons, which are

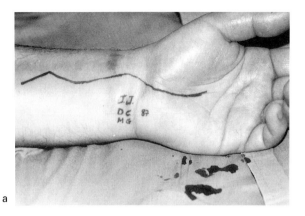 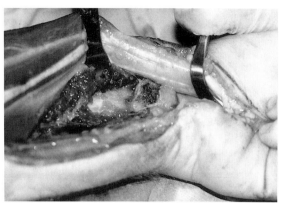

Figure 22.10

a) The incision for an anterior surgical approach is outlined. b) The distal radius can be easily approached by retracting radially the flexor tendons, the median nerve and the radial artery.

retracted radially. The pronator quadratus is approached and elevated on one side for later reapproximation over the definitive internal fixation (Fig. 22.10).

Fluoroscopy can be extremely useful in assessing the position of the fracture fragments at this point. In those cases of comminuted articular fragments, however, direct vision may be required. This is best accomplished through a dorsal approach to the wrist rather than overzealous mobilization of the volar carpal ligaments which may lead to the development of a dissociative form of intracarpal instability. A second incision on the dorsal aspect of the wrist will provide for accurate visualization of the articular surface.

Once satisfactory reduction has been achieved, temporary stabilization is accomplished with Kirschner wires. A bone graft, either local or from the iliac crest, is an important part of the procedure, as its placement beneath the elevated articular fragments will help prevent subsidence of these reduced fragments.

The small, angled 3.5 mm T-plates are ordinarily used to serve as a buttress for the reduced articular fragment. At times, this may not be possible due to the extensive comminution. Additional support, either with a cerclage fashion or Kirschner wires, may be necessary (Fig. 22.11).

The pronator quadratus is sutured back over the implant to serve as a protective layer.

Open reduction: dorsal approach

The dorsal approach is performed through a longitudinal midline incision centered over the distal radius and carpus. The radius is approached between the second and third extensor retinacular compartments. The retinaculum is elevated subperiosteally both in a radial and ulnar direction, without opening additional retinacular compartments. Direct visualization of the end of the radius is accomplished quite easily. The articular surface can be visualized through a longitudinal dorsal capsulotomy of the wrist. Here, too, a plate applied dorsally, to act as a buttress, has proven to be most effective. As with the anterior approach, autogenous bone graft is recommended for support of the articular fragments.

Once the fracture has been anatomically reduced and internal fixation applied, the retinaculum should be closed over the plate. It is preferable to leave the extensor pollicis longus out of the retinacular closure to avoid potential constriction and subsequent ischemic rupture of the tendon.

Functional outcome

Despite a significant degree of intra-articular or extra-articular comminution, an accurate

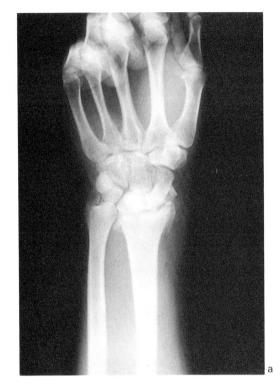
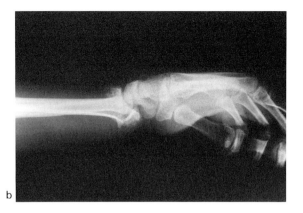
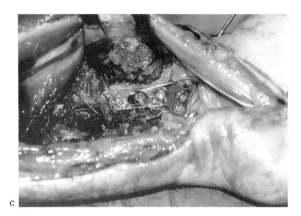
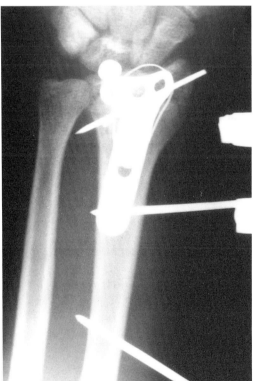

Figure 22.11

A complex intra-articular distal radial fracture in a construction worker who fell 20 feet. a,b) AP and lateral radiographs demonstrate a complex fracture-dislocation. c) The radius was approached anteriorly and the fracture reduced by longitudinal traction and direct manipulation. Internal fixation was accomplished with an anterior buttress plate, interfragmentary screws, and a cerclage wire. d) Radiograph demonstrating the addition of external fixation. e,f) AP and lateral radiographs taken 12 weeks postoperatively.

(Continued)

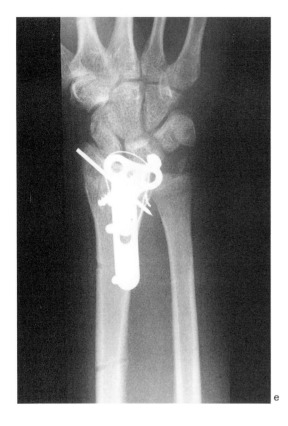
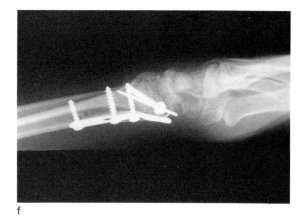

Figure 22.11
(Continued)

reduction and careful maintenance of the reduction will lead to a good functional outcome. If the articular fragments heal within 2 mm of normal alignment, little if any post-traumatic arthrosis will result. By the same token, articular fractures that have healed with a greater degree of residual articular displacement do indeed demonstrate post-traumatic arthrosis which, in most patients, is symptomatic (Knirk and Jupiter 1986).

With those fractures undergoing open reduction and internal fixation, one can anticipate a return of function to within two-thirds to three-quarters of that of the opposite uninjured wrist. Grip strength will return to near normal, although it may require an extended period of time to gain this functional status.

Complications of these fractures can be significant, including loss of strength, post-traumatic arthrosis with associated pain, dysfunction of the distal radio-ulnar joint, and soft tissue sequalae, such as median nerve dysfunction, reflex sympathetic dystrophy, and stiffness of the small joints of the hand.

References

Axelrod TJ, McMurtry RY. Open reduction and internal fixation of comminuted intrarticular fractures of the distal radius. *J Hand Surg* 1990; **15A**: 1–11.

Axelrod T, Paley D, Green J, McMurtry RY. Limited open reduction of the lunate facet in comminuted intraarticular fractures of the distal radius. *J Hand Surg* 1988; **13A**: 372–77.

Bickerstaff DR, Bell MJ. Carpal malalignment in Colles' fractures. *J Hand Surg* 1989; **14B**: 155–60.

Clancey GJ. Percutaneous Kirschner wire fixation of Colles' fractures. *J Bone Joint Surg* 1984; **66A**: 1008–14.

Collert S, Isaacson J. Management of re-dislocated Colles' fractures. *Clin Orthop* 1978; **135**: 183–86.

De Oliveira JC. Barton's fractures. *J Bone Joint Surg* 1973; **55A**: 586–94.

Dowling JJ, Sawyer B Jr. Comminuted Colles' fractures. Evaluation of a method of treatment. *J Bone Joint Surg* 1952; **34A**: 651–62.

Ellis J. Smith's and Barton's fractures — a method of treatment. *J Bone Joint Surg* 1965; **47B**: 724–27.

Frykman G. Fracture of the distal radius including sequelae — shoulder-hand-finger-syndrome, disturbance in the distal radioulnar joint and impairment of nerve function. A clinical and experimental study. *Acta Orthop Scand* 1967; **108(Suppl)**: 1–155.

Gartland JJ Jr, Werley CW. Evaluation of healed Colles' fractures. *J Bone Joint Surg* 1951; **33**: 895–907.

Howard PW, Steward HD, Hind RE, Burke FD. External fixation or plaster for severely displaced comminuted Colles' fractures? *J Bone Joint Surg* 1989; **71B**: 68–73.

Jupiter JB, Lipton H. The operative treatment of intraarticular fractures of the distal radius. *Clin Orthop Rel Res* 1993. **292**: 48–61.

Kapandji A. Les broches intra-focales a "effet de réduction" de type "ARUM" dans l'osteosynthèse des fractures de l'extrémité inférieure du radius. *Ann Chir Memb Super* 1991; **10(2)**: 138–45.

Knirk JL, Jupiter JB. Intraarticular fractures of the distal end of the radius in young adults. *J Bone Joint Surg* 1986; **68A**: 647–59.

Leung KS, Tsang HK, Chiu KH et al. An effective treatment of comminuted fractures of the distal radius. *J Hand Surg* 1990; **15A**: 11–17.

McMurtry RY, Jupiter JB. Fractures of the distal radius. In: Browner B, Jupiter J, Levine A, Trafton P, eds. *Skeletal trauma*. Philadelphia: WB Saunders, 1992.

McQueen M, Caspers J. Colles' fracture: Does the anatomic result affect the final function? *J Bone Joint Surg* 1988; **70B**: 649–51.

Melone CP Jr. Articular fractures of the distal radius. *Orthop Clin North Am* 1984; **15**: 217–36.

Müller ME. The comprehensive classification of fractures of the long bones. In: Müller ME, Allgöwer M, Schneider R, Willenegger M, eds. *Manual of internal fixation*. New York, Heidelberg: Springer-Verlag, 1991.

Pattee GA, Thompson GH. Anterior and posterior marginal fracture-dislocations of the distal radius. *Clin Orthop* 1988; **231**: 183–95.

Rubinovich RM, Rennie WR. Colles' fracture: End results in relation to radiologic parameters. *Can J Surg* 1983; **26**: 361–63.

Seitz WH Jr, Putnam MD, Dick HM. Limited open surgical approach for external fixation of distal radius fractures. *J Hand Surg* 1990; **15A**: 288–93.

Thompson GH, Grant TT. Barton's fractures — reverse Barton's fractures: Confusing eponyms. *Clin Orthop* 1977; **122**: 210–21.

Van der Linden W, Ericson R. Colles' fracture: How should its placement be measured and how should it be immobilized? *J Bone Joint Surg* 1981; **63A**: 1285–91.

23
The role of bone grafting in comminuted distal radial fractures

KS Leung, PC Leung

The treatment of comminuted fractures of the distal radius is challenging. There are multiple options which include casting, bracing, internal fixation, external fixation and various combinations of all of these (Gartland and Werley 1951, Jakob and Fernandez 1982, Knirk and Jupiter 1986). There has been growing interest in the use of external fixators in the treatment of these unstable fractures, along with recognition of the complications that result from the long duration of their application (Cole and Obletz 1986, Frykman 1967).

To overcome these complications a prospective trial was completed using ligamentotaxis, primary bone grafting and functional bracing as a treatment protocol for unstable intra-articular fractures of the distal radius. Several hundred patients were treated according to this protocol, and the first 100 patients were analysed and reported (Leung et al. 1989). Subsequently, 54 patients, after long-term follow-up periods of 2–5 years, were reassessed to review the late results (Leung et al. 1991). Our emphasis of treatment was on accurate reduction which was maintained by distraction across the wrist joint (ligamentotaxis). Bone graft of the fracture site, early mobilization of the fingers, removal of the external fixation, and motion of the wrist was the treatment programme that we established.

The fracture patterns were grouped according to Frykman's classification (1969). The distribution of the different types of fracture were very similar in both series. The radiocarpal joint was involved in 80% of cases, the distal radio-ulnar joint in 67% of cases, and both joints in 65% of cases.

Method of treatment

The operation was performed under general anaesthesia. A Hoffman half-frame (small 'C' series model) external fixator was constructed across the wrist. The half pins were carefully placed to provide a secure anchorage in the metacarpals distally and the radius proximally. Manipulation and closed reduction were performed under fluoroscopic control. Ligamentotaxis was achieved by distraction with the adjustable rod of the 'C' series fixator. Although the Hoffman external fixator was used in this study, there are no contraindications for the use of other models.

Bone grafting was performed through a dorsal approach to the radius in each of our patients. Cancellous bone chips were taken from the iliac crest through a small incision. The grafts were packed tightly through the fracture site and towards the distal joint line. In most cases, a substantial amount of graft, which was very loose was used as a result of the severe degree of comminution.

Postoperatively, the external fixator was maintained in place for the first three weeks; finger and forearm mobilization was begun. At the end of the third week, the external fixator was removed and a short arm brace was applied, which left the hand free and allowed only wrist flexion and forearm rotation. Wrist extension was not allowed, and the brace was kept in place for three more weeks. At the end of the sixth week, mobilization and strengthening exercises of the wrist were started without restriction (Leung et al. 1989).

The patients were assessed clinically and radiologically.

The clinical assessment included distal radio-ulnar joint instability, pain, grip power compared with the normal side, range of movement, and normal daily activities. The results were quantified using the Demerit system (Table 23.1) which was suggested by Gartland and Werley (1951) and subsequently modified by Sarmiento et al (1975).

Radiological assessment included the volar tilt angle, radio-articular angle, degree of arthrosis (Szabo and Weber 1988) (Table 23.2) and condition of the distal radio-ulnar joint.

Results of treatment

The analysis of the first 100 patients revealed very few complications and excellent overall results. There was no pin-tract infection since the distractors were all removed after three weeks. In one case, distractor loosening gave a poor result because the reoperation lengthened the time needed for fracture union and limited the return of joint function. The perfect engagement of the distal pins into the proximal second metacarpal should be emphasized so that this complication can be avoided (Seitz et al. 1990). Other complications included radial sensory irritation, transient median nerve paresis and sympathetic dystrophia, all of which were self-limiting. The results of joint function and the radiological appearances were well illustrated by the long-term follow-up of 54 cases.

Table 23.1 Demerit Point System used to evaluate end results of healed Colles' fractures (after Gartland and Werley 1951, and Sarmiento et al 1975).

	Points
Residual deformity (range: 0–3 points)	1
Prominent ulnar styloid	2
Residual dorsal tilt	2 or 3
Radial deviation of hand	
Subjective evaluation (range: 0–6 points)	
Excellent — no pain, disability, or limitation of movement	0
Good — occasional pain, slight limitation of motion, and no disability	2
Fair — occasional pain, some limitation of motion, feeling of weakness in wrist, no particular disability if careful, and activities slightly restricted	4
Poor — pain, limitation of motion, disability, and activities more or less markedly restricted	6
Objective evaluation* (range: 0–5 points)	
Loss of dorsiflexion	5
Loss of ulnar deviation	3
Loss of supination	2
Loss of palmar flexion	1
Loss of radial deviation	1
Loss of circumduction	1
Pain in distal radio-ulnar joint	1
Grip strength — 60% or less than on opposite side	1
Loss of pronation	2
Complications (range: 0–5 points)	
Arthritic change	
Minimum	1
Minimum with pain	3
Moderate	2
Moderate with pain	4
Severe	3
Severe with pain	5
Nerve complications (median)	1–3
Poor finger function due to cast	1 or 2
Final result (ranges of points)	
Excellent	0–2
Good	3–8
Fair	9–20
Poor	≥21

*The objective evaluation is based on the following ranges of motion as being the minimum for normal function: dorsiflexion, 45°; palmar flexion, 30°; radial deviation, 15°; ulnar deviation, 15°; pronation, 50°; and supination, 50°.

Table 23.2 Arthritis grading (after Szabo and Weber 1988)

Grade	Findings
0	None
1	Slight joint space narrowing
2	Marked joint space narrowing, osteophyte formation
3	Bone-on-bone, osteophyte formation, cyst formation

Joint function at long-term follow-up

Gross appearance. No deformity was detected around the wrist on inspection from all angles.

Pain. Three patients experienced pain in the ulnar styloid when making a strong grip. Four patients had pain when pronating the forearm. One patient had pain on wrist movement.

Grip power. This ranged from 69.2% to 122% (average 92%) of the unaffected side.

Range of movement. Finger movements were normal in all patients. Six (11.1%) patients had less than 20° limitation in total wrist movement (flexion and extension). Ten (18.5%) patients had limitations in forearm rotational movements of less than 20°, while one patient (1.9%) had limitation of over 20°. The remaining patients had a normal range of joint motion.

Normal daily activity. Five (9.3%) patients experienced slight restriction in their daily activities; one (1.9%) patient claimed significant restriction and could not return to his original job. The rest resumed their previous work.

Status of distal radio-ulnar joint (DRUJ). Six (11.1%) patients had evidence of subluxation of the distal radio-ulnar joints and three patients (5.6%) had frank dislocations.

Radiological assessment at long-term follow-up

Bone healing was achieved in all cases. Using the Uhthoff and Rahn system of analysis (1981), the majority of patients showed contact or gap healing (Table 23.3). The radial articular angle and volar tilt angle were within normal ranges. The radial articular angle measured from 19° to 26°, with a mean of 22°. The volar tilt angle measured from 0° to 15°, with a mean of 9°. When compared with the postoperative radiographs taken one year after operation, no observable changes were detected.

Table 23.3 Healing pattern (after Uhthoff and Rahn 1981)

Type	Description	No.	%
Ia	Contact healing	17	31.5
Ib	Gap healing	35	64.8
II	External callus	2	3.7

In radiographic analysis, a normal articular surface and joint space was displayed by 49 patients (Fig. 23.1). Four patients had slight joint narrowing when compared with the uninjured side. One patient had significant narrowing with a bony spur on the dorsal edge of the distal radius (Fig. 23.2), but in spite of this radiological finding in this last patient, clinical symptoms of loss of motion or strength were not present.

In 14 patients, a fracture of the ulnar styloid resulted in non-union. Of these patients, six demonstrated concomitant DRUJ instability, while three others had clinical and radiological evidence of dislocation. Only four of these patients experienced pain, either in the ulnar wrist area or generally in the wrist joint.

The overall results were quantified using the demerit point system. Over 90.7% of patients had excellent and good results while 9.3% showed only fair results. Using this method of assessment, none had poor results. Table 23.4 shows a comparative analysis of the results of this study classified by the demerit system, compared with five other studies using five different systems of assessment in the initial period. Table 23.5

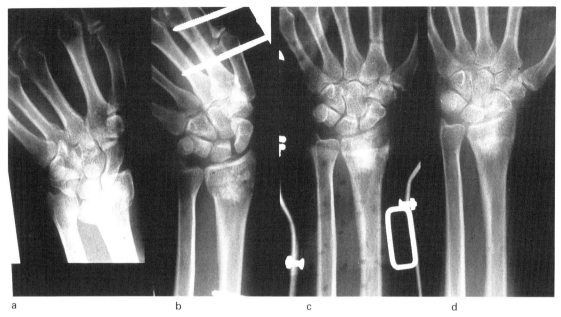

Figure 23.1

Comminuted distal radial fracture in a 38-year-old man treated by distraction and bone grafting. Normal articular surfaces are obvious $2\frac{1}{2}$ years after the treatment. a) Preoperative radiography. b) Fracture fixed with external fixator and bone graft. c) Fracture fixed with brace. d) Wrist $2\frac{1}{2}$ years after fracture.

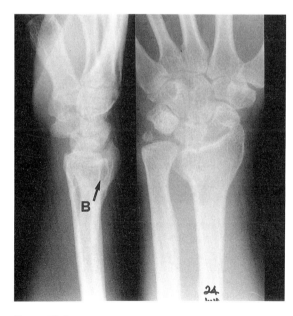

Figure 23.2

Dorsal bone spurs (B) over the distal radius, 3 years after treatment.

illustrates the final results of this study three years later.

The late complication of DRUJ instability, ranging from subluxation to frank dislocation, did not produce marked clinical symptoms but continuous observation and monitoring of these cases is necessary. Likewise, early radiocarpal joint changes should be an area of concern. The only patient with definite evidence of early osteoarthritis received treatment a week after injury and the bone graft procedure aimed at restoration of the distal radial articular integrity proved not to be effective.

Discussion

Treating comminuted fractures of the distal radius by ligamentotaxis alone may give satisfactory results, but the distracting external fixator provides a great degree of mechanical stability for these unstable fractures. Although it has been reported that the external fixator cannot maintain the volar tilt angle satisfactorily (Schuind et al.

1984), bone grafting was not used in those cases. In the study presented here, both the volar tilt and radio-articular angles were maintained within the normal range when bone grafting was combined with external fixation. In a few patients, there was a slight decrease in the radio-articular angle when the external fixator was removed. Nevertheless, this phenomenon did not progress.

The unique feature of this method of treatment is the addition of primary cancellous grafting in all cases. This is an essential component of the treatment modality and we believe that this procedure was responsible for the excellent results.

A metaphyseal fracture, resulting from a high-velocity injury, produces bony comminution and impaction. This leaves a deficiency of bone support and empty spaces after fracture distraction and reduction. If these spaces are not filled with bone to the comminution of the bone cortex, the fracture will remain unstable. The external fixator does provide stability to maintain the reduction, but it takes a long time for the fracture gap to be filled by new bone formation in order that sufficient stability is present to allow for wrist mobilization. Because of this, many studies recommend that the fixator should stay in place for six to ten weeks to allow fracture consolidation (Szabo and Weber 1988, Seitz et al. 1990, Uhthoff and Rahn 1981, Vidal et al. 1983). The complications of external fixators, such as pin-tract infection, wrist stiffness and Sudeck's atrophy are proportional to the duration of application of the external fixator. With cancellous bone intra-fracture grafting, this period of time is shortened significantly and hence the complications are minimized. A laboratory study on cadaveric wrist models demonstrated that bone grafting conferred at least a four-fold increase in stability. Thus, filling the bone gaps that result from a comminuted fracture significantly supports the ligamentotaxis as a means of maintaining fracture reduction. The bone grafts supply an intraosseous distension force which enhances the effect of ligamentotaxis, and at the same time helps to line up the juxta-articular bone fragments to maintain the integrity of the distal radius.

Cancellous bone grafts are biological tissues that facilitate bone healing by their osteogenic properties of osteoconduction and osteoinduction. These effects are demonstrated by the analysis of the healing pattern using the Uhthoff and Rahn (1981) shown in Table 23.3. The majority of fractures showed type I healing which indicated interfragment stability.

By pushing the grafts towards the distal radial articular surface, many of the die-punch fragments, which cannot be reduced by ligamentotaxis alone (Weber and Szabo 1986, Liggs and Cooney 1983), can be adequately lifted, reduced and supported to achieve a congruent joint surface (Fig. 23.3). The restoration of the congruency to the distal radial articular surfaces accounts for the low incidence of arthrosis after 2–5 years. As in all intra-articular fractures, early mobilization is mandatory if a good range of motion is to be restored. By shortening the period of external fixation and the use of functional bracing, controlled motion is started at a very early stage to ensure a good range of motion and return of strength.

Serial radiographs of a typical fracture show minimal changes in the radio-articular angle (Fig. 23.4). This illustrates that reduction stability, healing and structural integrity are not jeopardized by early removal of the external fixator and subsequent controlled movement by functional bracing.

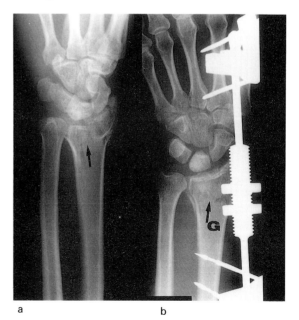

Figure 23.3

a) Comminuted distal radial fracture with die-punch fragments (arrow). b) These fragments are adequately reduced and supported by distraction and bone grafting (G).

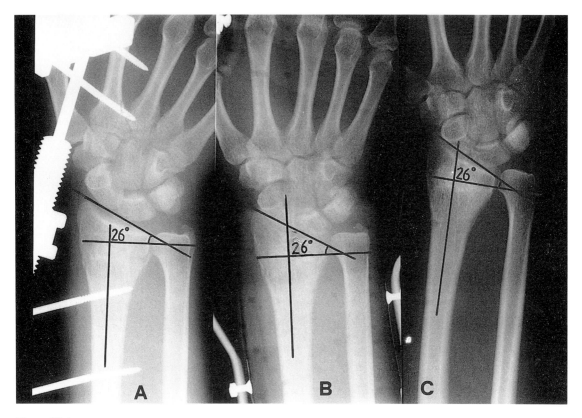

Figure 23.4

Serial radiographs of the same fracture shown in Fig. 23.3, illustrating good maintenance of the radio-articular angle.

Late complications are observed among fractures involving the ulnar wrist complex (types VI and VIII). On reducing these fractures, it was found that pronating the forearm displaced the fracture (Fig. 23.5a) and with full supination of the forearm, the fracture could be satisfactorily reduced (Fig. 23.5b). This indicates that when the forearm is pronated, considerable dorsal stress is put upon the ulnar wrist complex and the fracture remains displaced. With this in mind, the treatment protocol for type VI and VIII fractures was modified. After the radial component of the fracture was reduced and the external fixator inserted across the wrist, the forearm was immobilized in full supination with an ulnar connection rod fixed to two ulnar pins (Fig. 23.6). Pronation was allowed only after removal of the external fixator.

The long-term results achieved using this treatment were better than those of studies using different treatment protocols (see Tables 23.4 and 23.5). As we have already mentioned, the addition of a primary cancellous bone graft significantly shortens the duration of external fixation, thus enabling early mobilization and strengthening exercises. The cancellous graft also helps to restore the congruency of the radial articular surface and prevent post-traumatic arthrosis. Coronal axial tomographic pictures clearly show the multiple spaces in the distal radius resulting from a comminuted fracture and the elimination of these spaces after bone grafting. If such spaces do occur in all comminuted distal radial fractures, it would be good practice to fill them, to prevent further collapse and maintain early healing.

If an external fixator is not available for distraction ligamentotaxis, then intrafracture bone graft followed by cast immobilization could be a reasonable and effective method of management — much better than casting alone. This graft

Table 23.4 Results of present study compared with those of other studies

Results	Gartland and Werley (1951)	Cole and Obletz (1966)	Sarmiento et al. (1966)	Cooney et al. (1979)	Knirk and Jupiter (1985)	Leung et al. (1989)
No. of patients	60	33	44	60	43	54
Mean age (years)	53	18–81	40s	63	27.6	40.9
% Intra-articular	88	NA	100	88	100	96.4
Method	Plaster cast	Pins and plaster	Functional brace	External fixator	Varied	Fixator and brace
Average follow-up (years)	1.5	1.5–5.0	0.5	2.4	6.7	2.65
% Arthritis	22	NA	NA	2	65	9.2
% Finger stiffness	18	0	12	0	0	0
Final result (%)						
Excellent	22 69	51 94	42 81	32 87	26 61	33 90.4
Good	47	43	39	55	35	57.4
Fair	28	6	18	13	33	9.6
Poor	3	0	0	0	6	0

NA = not applicable

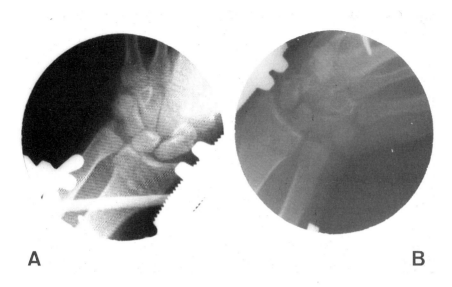

Figure 23.5

Comminuted fracture affecting ulnar wrist complex. A) There is obvious displacement when the forearm is pronated. B) Good reduction is achieved when the forearm is supinated.

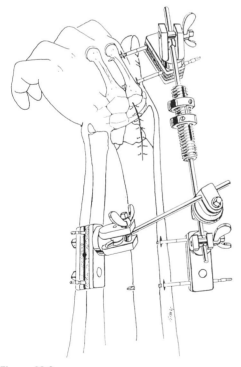

Figure 23.6

Full supination is maintained by applying an extension rod, bridging two additional pins through the ulnar shaft, as well as an external fixator

Table 23.5 Final result according to Demerit Point System (after Gartland and Werley 1951, and Sarmiento et al. 1975)

	Points	No.	%
Excellent	0–2	18	33.3
Good	4–8	31	57.4
Fair	9–20	5	9.3
Poor	>20	0	

should be able to maintain its unique role of supporting the fragments from within the fracture, thus inducing rapid bone union.

Unless expensive investigations like CAT scanning are routinely performed for this type of fracture, the empty spaces are not identifiable. It is therefore logical to include bone grafting as a routine procedure in the treatment of comminuted distal radial fractures among young and active patients. In this current era of bone substitute application, the next step should be the replacement of cancellous graft with a bone substitute to eliminate morbidity of the donor site and thus make this treatment modality even more acceptable.

Conclusions

Treating comminuted fractures of the distal radius with ligamentotaxis, primary cancellous bone graft and functional bracing gives good long-term results both clinically and radiologically. With the addition of the bone graft, the duration of external fixation is significantly shortened and early rehabilitation is facilitated. In spite of the obviously good results, however, the problem of DRUJ dislocation needs further evaluation.

References

Cole JM, Obletz BE. Comminuted fractures of the distal end of the radius treated by skeletal transfixion in plaster case — A result study of thirty-three cases. *J Bone Joint Surg* 1986; **48A**: 931–45.

Cooney WP, Linsheid RL, Dobyns JH. External pin fixation for unstable Colles' fractures. *J Bone J Surg* 1979; **61A**: 840–45.

Frykman G. Fracture of the distal radius including sequelae — Shoulder-hand-finger syndrome, disturbance in the distal radio-ulnar joint and impairment of nerve function. A clinical and experimental study. *Acta Orthop Scand* 1967; **108 (suppl)**: 1–155.

Gartland JJ, Werley CW. Evaluation of healed Colles' fractures. *J Bone Joint Surg* 1951; **33A**: 895–907.

Jakob RP, Fernandez DL. The treatment of wrist fractures with the small AO external fixation device. In Uhthoff HK. *Current Concepts of External Fixation of Fractures.* Berlin: Springer-Verlag, 1982: 307–14.

Knirk JL, Jupiter JB. Intraarticular fractures of the distal end of the radius in young adults. *J Bone Joint Surg* 1986; **68A**: 647–59.

Leung KS, So WS, Chiu VDF, Leung PC. Ligamentotaxis for comminuted distal radial fractures modified by primary cancellous grafting and functional bracing: Long-term results. *J Orthop Trauma* 1991; **5,3**: 265–71.

Leung KS, Kwan M, Wong J, Shen WY, Tsang A. Therapeutic functional bracing in upper limb fracture-dislocations. *J Orthop Trauma* 1989; **2,4**: 308–13.

Leung KS, Shen WY, Kinninmonth AWG, Leung PC, Chang JCW, Chan GPY. Ligamentotaxis and bone grafting for comminuted fractures of the distal radius. *J Bone Joint Surg* 1989; **71B**: 838–42.

Riggs SA, Cooney WP. External fixation of complex hand and wrist fractures. *J Trauma* 1983; **23**: 332–36.

Sarmiento A, Pratt GW, Berry NC, Sinclair WF. Colles' fracture. *J Bone Joint Surg* 1975; **57A**: 311–17.

Schuind F, Donkerwolcke M, Burny F. External fixation of wrist fractures. *Orthopaedics* 1984; **7**: 841–44.

Seitz WH, Froimson AI, Brooks DB, Postak PD, Parker RD, LaPorte JM, Greenwald AS. Biomechanical analysis of pin placement and pin size for external fixation of distal radius fractures. *Clin Orthop Rel Res* 1990; **251**: 207–12.

Szabo RM, Weber SC. Comminuted intraarticular fractures of the distal radius. *Clin Orthop Rel Res* 1988; **230**: 39–48.

Uhthoff HK, Rahn BA. Healing patterns of metaphyseal fractures. *Clin Orthop Rel Res* 1981; **160**: 295–303.

Vidal J, Buscayret C, Paran M, Melka J. Ligamentotaxis. In Mears DC, ed. *External Skeletal Fixation.* Baltimore, London: Williams & Wilkins, 1983: 493–96.

Weber SC, Szabo RM. Severely comminuted distal radial fracture as an unsolved problem: Complications associated with external fixation and pins and plaster techniques. *J Hand Surg* 1986; **11A**: 157–65.

24
Open reduction of intra-articular fractures of the distal radius

Peter C Amadio

Introduction

Intra-articular fractures of the distal radius are notorious for their difficult management and their poor results, especially with closed treatment. Bradway et al. (1989) have emphasized that the adverse effects of residual incongruity after reduction are a major determinant of poor results, a point also made in the reports of Knirk and Jupiter (1986), Seitz et al. (1991), Axelrod and McMurtry (1990), and Fernandez and Geissler (1991). Long-term results have generally shown that post-traumatic arthritis is well correlated both with residual incongruity, especially when the articular 'step-off' is greater than two millimeters (Knirk and Jupiter 1986, Bradway et al. 1989), and when symptoms include persistent pain and weakness (Bradway et al. 1989). This chapter will review the indications and techniques of open reduction and fixation of displaced intra-articular fractures of the distal radius favored by the author.

Indications

Closed reduction should be the first option considered when approaching a patient with a fracture of the distal end of the radius, regardless of the patient's age, handedness, or occupation. In general, closed reduction is best achieved by longitudinal traction, to which manipulation can be added to provide 'fine tuning' of translation and angulation of the distal fragment. An acceptable reduction at this stage would include length to within 3–4 mm of normal, at least neutral palmar flexion angulation, and radial inclination of 15–20°. Any intra-articular displacement should be corrected to within 1 mm of anatomic position. If such a reduction is achieved by closed means, the goal should be to maintain this reduction, whether by cast support, percutaneous pin fixation, or external skeletal fixation, as described elsewhere in this monograph. It is only when a satisfactory reduction cannot be achieved by closed means, or is achieved but then irretrievably lost, that open reduction should be considered.

The lack of a satisfactory closed reduction should not be considered an absolute indication for open reduction. As will be discussed below, the results in patients over the age of 50 may be less uniform, with a higher rate of complication and failure, than those in younger patients. Patients with severe osteoporosis may lack sufficient bone stock for stable internal or external fixation. Thus, although the presence of residual articular incongruity is the basic prerequisite, other criteria of patient vitality and bone sufficiency must be met before deciding on the appropriateness of open reduction in a given case.

Technique

There are three issues which must be addressed in deciding the ideal fixation in any specific case: the choice of internal fixation, the need for supplemental external fixation, and the need for bone graft. In general, the key feature which will drive these decisions is the degree of comminution. For this reason, the AO classification is recommended; this is the only scheme that specifically addresses comminution as a classification factor (Bradway et al. 1989, Fernandez and

Geissler 1991). An additional feature which must be considered nowadays is the question of arthroscopically controlled percutaneous reduction. The availability of arthroscopy can reduce the need for arthrotomy.

In the AO scheme, intra-articular fractures are types B and C (Fig. 24.1). Type B fractures involve a single corner of the radius, such as the styloid, or the volar and dorsal articular surfaces (i.e. Barton's fractures). Some intra-articular Smith's fractures, those classified as type 2 by Thomas (1957), would also fit in this category, a point confirmed by De Oliveira (1973). Type C fractures include all intra-articular fractures with a metaphyseal component. If neither of the two parts are comminuted, the fracture is classified as type C1;

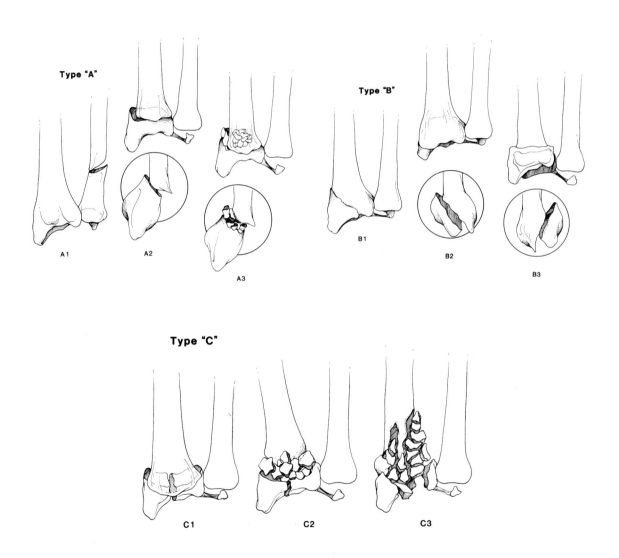

Figure 24.1

The AO Classification. Type B fractures include those of the radial styloid (B1) and the volar (B2) and dorsal (B3) rims. Type C fractures are characterized by comminution of the articular surface. (Copyright Mayo Foundation.)

if only the metaphyseal portion is comminuted, it is considered as type C2; and if both the metaphysis and articular surface are comminuted, it is classified as type C3.

Type B fractures are often unstable, and frequently require internal fixation. In many cases, a buttress plate will be appropriate, as this provides stable fixation, and may reduce the need for external plaster support.

Technique of volar plate fixation (Volar approach)

For volar Barton's fractures and type 2 Smith's fractures, the radius is approached through the interval between the brachioradialis and flexor carpi radialis, as described by Henry (1973). The distal radial metaphysis is exposed by elevating the pronator quadratus and, if necessary, the distal fibers of the flexor pollicis longus can be released from the radius subperiosteally. It is often advisable to extend the incision distally and to release the carpal tunnel through it. This approach not only aids exposure, but also reduces the risk of postoperative carpal tunnel syndrome. With such an exposure, the fracture reduction is usually easy to view directly. This approach may also be used with some type C fractures, but it can be difficult to evaluate the articular surface accurately from the volar approach. Therefore, even if the plate is placed anteriorly for reasons of a lower profile and less interference with tendon gliding and joint movement, a second dorsal incision is often made to inspect the joint surface when fixing a type C fracture from a volar approach.

Once the fracture is adequately exposed, it is reduced under direct vision. The provisional reduction is fixed with Kirschner wires under radiographic control. Once a satisfactory reduction is assured, a T-shaped or angled buttress plate is applied, and fixed to the shaft fragment with two or three 3.5 mm cortical screws (Fig. 24.2). If the distal fragment is large enough, additional screws can be inserted into it through the plate. These screws may be either cortical or cancellous, depending on the quality of the bone. Again, depending on the security of the total fixation construct, the Kirschner wires may or may not be removed at this point. Additional radiographs should be obtained to confirm satisfactory plate and screw position and fracture reduction. Postoperatively, a well-padded dressing with a plaster splint is usually applied to support the wrist, and the wound is inspected a few days later. If the wound is healing satisfactorily, a below-elbow fiberglass cast is applied. The fracture is X-rayed again after one month, by which time healing is usually sufficient to begin motion exercises for the wrist, with a plastic molded wrist support used for support between motion exercises. In the occasional trustworthy, well-motivated patient with good bone stock and solid fixation, motion exercises can begin as soon as the wrist is comfortable, usually within seven to ten days postoperatively.

Technique of dorsal plate fixation

When open reduction is necessary and the fracture fragments are displaced dorsally, as is the usual case with dorsal Barton's and Colles-type fractures, it is often easiest to achieve reduction through a dorsal approach. In some cases, comminution and the small size of the articular fractures will preclude plate fixation, but in the major plate fixation this will be possible. In such cases, the distal radius is exposed by opening the extensor retinaculum between the third and fourth compartments, and the entire sheath of the finger extensors as a flap with the dorsal periosteum is elevated, which causes minimal interference with tendon gliding. Deep to this flap, the terminal portion of the posterior interosseous nerve can be seen. A segment of this nerve is usually excised, as this helps to reduce postoperative pain. A proximally based T-shape flap is used to open the wrist capsule, and the articular surface is inspected. As in the volar approach, a provisional reduction is obtained with Kirschner wires and confirmed radiographically. The plate application principles are also similar to those for the volar approach. It is often necessary to osteotomize Lister's tubercle to achieve optimal plate apposition. It is usually necessary to split the extensor retinaculum to provide an interval between the plate and the external tendons.

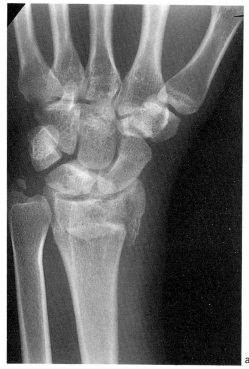
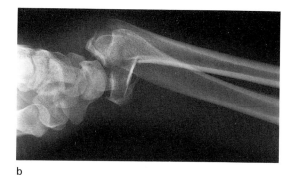
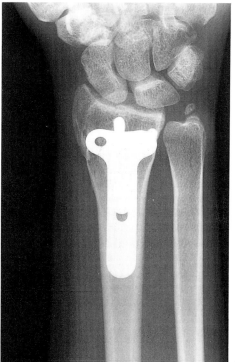
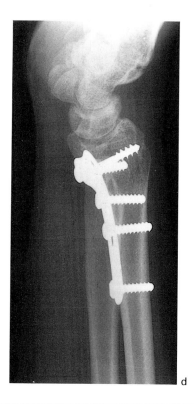

Figure 24.2

Fixation with plate through a volar approach. a) Preoperative view (anteroposterior). b) Preoperative view (lateral). c) Postoperative view (anteroposterior). d) Postoperative view (lateral).

Arthroscopically controlled fracture reduction

The advent of arthroscopy of the wrist has permitted some intra-articular fractures to benefit from arthroscopically directed percutaneus pin fixation. In general, this technique is limited to type B fractures, especially of the radial styloid, and perhaps some type C1 fractures which require only elevation of a depressed styloid or lunate facet fragment. Fractures with intra-articular comminution are not suitable for this technique because the fragments are too difficult to control percutaneously and because the arthroscopic lavage fluid can extravasate beyond the wrist capsule, aggravating the risk of postoperative neurovascular compromise.

Arthroscopic reduction of intra-articular fractures of the distal radius is performed like any other wrist arthroscopy, except that there is a need for intraoperative radiographic control. The joint must be irrigated thoroughly to remove all clotted blood. For this reason, this technique is best reserved for fresh fractures, which can be treated within a few days of injury. A shaver or suction punch can be quite helpful in clearing away the clotted blood. Once the fracture line is clearly seen, the fracture fragment can be manipulated back into position. A 1.5 mm Kirschner wire is drilled into the fragment, and then used as a joystick to guide the fragment back into anatomic position. A second 1.5 mm wire is then drilled across the fracture site, securing the reduction. The first wire can then also be advanced to provide additional fixation. The arthroscope is used to inspect the wrist to ensure that no inadvertent penetration of the joint has occurred. Final radiographs should also be obtained to confirm pin position. Postoperatively, the wrist is protected in a below-elbow cast for six weeks.

Bone grafting — indications, source and technique

Comminution, which cannot be reduced by closed means or which leaves a significant bone defect, is frequently present in distal radial fractures. In such cases, a cancellous bone graft can supply both structural and osteogenic support. Often, when a comminuted fracture is finally reduced, there is a large gap in the metaphysis, representing the region crushed at the moment of impact. This gap, if maintained, will result in a prolonged healing time (Cooney et al. 1979). The gap also poses a risk of collapse, with loss of reduction. Filling the gap with bone graft addresses both of these problems.

Of the many sources of bone graft that are theoretically available, autogenous cancellous bone, preferably from the iliac crest, is recommended. It should be autogenous, to eliminate the risk of viral disease transmission — in 1988, a case of AIDS was reported by the Center for Disease Control, in which the disease was transmitted by a bone allograft; cancellous, because this tissue is more osteogenic, and incorporates faster than cortical bone (Friedlaender 1987); and from the iliac crest, because this source of bone remains of high quality even in the elderly, when sources such as the olecranon may be deficient. When the degree of comminution is modest, the requisite iliac bone can be harvested by trephine, perhaps avoiding the need for a general anesthetic. Larger amounts (and usually the need is significant) will require a formal surgical exposure of the crest. The bone should be packed firmly into the recipient site, from distal to proximal, as this will provide some structural support for the articular 'pavement'.

Combined internal and external fixation with bone graft

Usually, when distal radial fractures are not amenable to closed or percutaneous treatment, the reason relates to comminution of the metaphysis, the joint surface, or both. Such fractures (AO types C2 and C3) are not typically suitable for plate fixation. There is simply not enough distal bone stock to support the plate. In such cases, an external fixator can provide the neutralization of joint compressive force needed to achieve and maintain reduction. Fine tuning of the articular surface can then be obtained with fine Kirschner wires, 0.8 mm, or even 0.6 mm in diameter. Fine wires can be used because the forces on them are low — only that needed to maintain a smooth joint surface. Such pins are ideally suited to the subchondral bone, which may be all that remains for purchase distally. These pins are further reinforced in their action by cancellous bone graft packed in the metaphyseal defect beneath them.

The first coherent English language description of this method of treatment for difficult distal radial fractures was provided by Palmer in 1988. Melone (1986), summarized by Palmer (1988) and also described in German by Sennwald (1987). This method, with some variations, is now generally accepted as a useful approach for these fractures (Bradway et al. 1989, Seitz et al. 1991, Axelrod and McMurtry 1990, Fernandez and Geissler 1991).

The method begins with application of an external fixator of choice. Traction may be applied during fixator placement to facilitate the provisional reduction, or the reduction can be performed after the fixator is applied. In the latter circumstance, it is important to place the fixator pins so that the fixator can be applied after reduction, and not necessarily with the fracture in its unreduced position. This is especially important when using fixators with some constraint on pin position, such as the Agee and Clyburn frames. If this point is not addressed at the beginning of the procedure, and a frame of this type is used, adequate correction might not be permissible within the constraints of the frame, and the pins will need to be repositioned; otherwise, a less than adequate reduction will have to be accepted (Berger et al. 1991).

Two other points are important when selecting a frame configuration. First, uniplanar constructs will be more useful than biplanar ones, because the dorsal plane of the biplanar construct will interfere with surgical exposure of the fracture. Secondly, ease of intraoperative adjustability is an advantage, as occasionally the fracture will require temporary intraoperative overdistraction during final reduction. A frame which permits change in length without loss of stability, such as the Agee or Hoffman C-series frames, are particularly useful in these circumstances.

Once the frame is applied and provisional reduction confirmed, then frame application and alteration are employed in a standard fashion, as described elsewhere in this monograph. After the frame has been applied, the fracture can be exposed, as described in the section on dorsal plate fixation. The exposure must be ample enough to clearly view the joint surface and to expose the metaphysis for bone grafting. It need not be as extensive an exposure as for plate fixation (Fernandez and Geissler 1991). The joint surface is carefully reconstructed using a small Freer elevator or dental probe to guide the fragments into place. Major fragments are fixed to each other with fine Kirschner wires; smaller pieces can usually be adequately wedged into the interstices without metal fixation. If fibrin glue is available, it can be quite helpful in holding these smaller fragments.

Once the joint surface is reconstructed and proper length has been restored, any metaphyseal defects that remain should be packed with cancellous bone graft (Fig. 24.3). As mentioned earlier, this not only supports the articular construct, but also speeds bony healing. Postoperatively, additional ulnar wrist support is provided in the form of a molded plastic orthosis. The pins and fixator can usually be removed in six to eight weeks, with the final determination depending, of course, on the radiographic appearance.

Results

A number of reports are now available which discuss the results of open treatment of comminuted distal radial fractures (Bradway et al. 1989, Seitz et al. 1991, Axelrod and McMurtry 1990, Fernandez and Geissler 1991), but unfortunately some series have not separated the clinical results of patients with open treatment from those treated percutaneously (Seitz et al. 1991, Fernandez and Geissler 1991). Others have used grading such as 'satisfactory/unsatisfactory', which does not allow easy comparison with other series (Axelrod and McMurtry 1990).

At the Mayo Clinic, open reduction has been employed for comminuted distal radial fractures since 1977 (Bradway et al. 1989). Our initial experience with 16 AO type C2 and C3 fractures, followed for a minimum of two years, was reported in 1989. Since that time an additional 48 patients have been treated by this method. Combining the two groups, this series includes 29 patients treated with a combination of internal and external fixation, 16 treated with Kirschner

OPEN REDUCTION OF INTRA-ARTICULAR FRACTURES OF THE DISTAL RADIUS 199

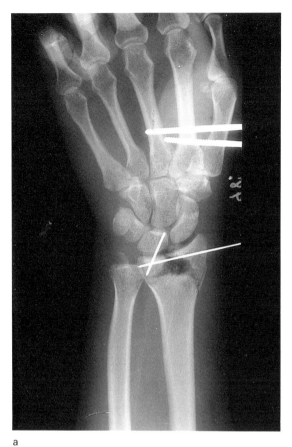
a

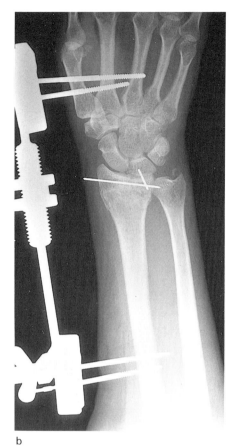
b

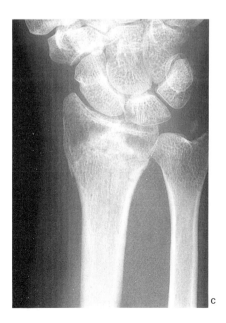
c

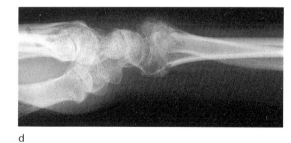
d

Figure 24.3

Combined internal and external fixation with bone graft. a) Intra-operative radiograph showing external fixator and Kirschner wires in place. Note the excellent restoration of overall anatomy, with a large metaphyseal defect. b) Intraoperative radiograph after bone graft is inserted. Note the obliteration of metaphyseal defect. c) Final result (anteroposterior view). d) Final result (lateral view).

wires alone, and 19 treated with plate fixation. Out of the total of 64 patients, 40 required bone grafting. Ages ranged from 17 to 86 years, with 36 of the 64 patients being under the age of 50.

Follow-up on the most recent group is not yet sufficient to draw independent conclusions, but a preliminary review suggests that the results have tended to improve as experience with the techniques has increased. In general, however, the conclusions of the initial report still appear valid. The quality of the final result appears to be strongly linked to the quality of the intra-articular reduction (Fig. 24.4), whereas the degree of initial displacement did not correlate well either with the quality of the final reduction, or with the incidence of post-traumatic arthritis. Post-traumatic arthritis did correlate well in several studies with clinical score of wrist function (Fig. 24.5).

In this regard, it is important to make a plea for more stringent clinical scoring of the wrist. All too often, as mentioned above, results are listed as satisfactory or unsatisfactory with either no definition, a broad definition, or some loose tie to either 'normal', which is not further defined, or to the opposite side, which again is not well defined, or it may even be adjusted for handedness.

Another common option is the use of the Gartland and Werley score (1951). Although this has the advantage of being commonly used, permitting comparison between series, it makes assumptions regarding the gradation of wrist and hand function that seem outdated at best. For example, an excellent result can be achieved with 45° extension, 30° flexion, 50° each of pronation and supination, carpal tunnel syndrome, and a grip strength less than half the opposite side, provided only that the patient has no pain, no gross deformity, and no radiographic evidence of arthritis. The addition of a gross deformity moves the patient down only as far as the good category. Disabling pain and arthritis are necessary for a fair or poor result.

A modification of the Green and O'Brien system (Green and O'Brien 1978, Bradway et al. 1989) is recommended instead. This modified score can be used for evaluation of any condition or treatment of the wrist. It provides independent scores for motion, strength, pain, and activity level which can be objectively graded (Table 24.1). More importantly, to achieve an excellent result, truly excellent motion, strength, function, and comfort must be present. The features of an excellent result under the Gartland and Werley system listed above, would rate only fair under the modified Green–O'Brien score, which is probably a truer assessment of the situation.

One clinical aspect in our series correlated well with both clinical and radiographic outcome. An age of over 50 years was associated with a

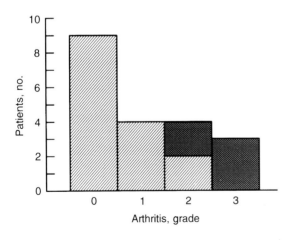

Figure 24.4

Reduction grade versus arthritis. Ligher shade: less than 2 mm of joint surface incongruity; darker shade: 2 mm or more of incongruity. Arthritis is graded from 0 (arthritis) to 3 (severe arthritis).

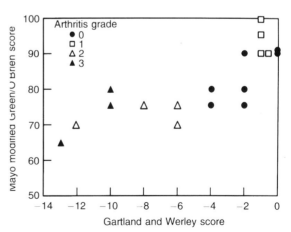

Figure 24.5

Arthritis grade versus clinical score. Mayo modified score: 100 points is normal. Gartland–Werley score: 0 points is normal. Arthritis is graded from 0 (no arthritis) to 3 (severe arthritis).

Table 24.1 The modified Green–O'Brien score (after Green and O'Brien 1978)

Category	Score	Findings
Pain	25	None
	20	Mild
	15	Moderate (requires medication)
	0	Severe (requires narcotic)
Function	25	Same job
	20	Different job
	15	Able; no job
	0	Unable
Motion	25	100%
	15	75–99%
	10	50–74%
	5	25–49%
	0	0–24%
Strength	25	100%
	15	75–99%
	10	50–74%
	5	25–49%
	0	0–24%

Motion and strength as percent of opposite side

SCORING:
- Excellent 90–100%
- Good 80–89%
- Fair 65–79%
- Poor <65%

significantly lower rate of success than that seen overall. Two-thirds of the patients under the age of 50 had a good or excellent result; this was true for only one-third of the older patients. Although no one specific cause for this difference could be established, several features seem salient. Older patients are more likely to suffer from osteoporosis, and this may limit the holding power of the fixation used, or make it more likely to loosen. Older patients may also predispose to arthrofibrosis (joint stiffness), limiting ultimate motion and strength. Whatever the reason or reasons, one clearly must take extra precautions both in selecting older patients for open reduction, and in managing them postoperatively.

Conclusions

Open reduction is indicated for intra-articular fractures of the distal radius which cannot be reduced anatomically by closed means. Often, such fractures show extreme comminution, and a combination of internal and external fixation and bone grafting is necessary to achieve and maintain reduction. The results achieved with this technique are related more to reduction quality than to initial displacement, especially when strict scoring criteria are used. Special case should be taken in selecting patients over the age of 50 for open reduction, as they may be at increased risk of a poor result.

References

Axelrod TS, McMurtry RY. Open reduction and internal fixation of comminuted intraarticular fractures of the distal radius. *J Hand Surg* 1990; **15A**: 1–11.

Berger RA, Beckenbaugh RD, Amadio PC, Cooney WP. Preliminary experience with the Agee Wrist Jack external fixator. Presented at the 46th Annual Meeting of the American Society for Surgery of the Hand, Orlando, Florida, 1991.

Bradway JK, Amadio PC, Cooney WP. Open reduction and internal fixation of displaced, comminuted intra-articular fractures of the distal end of the radius. *J Bone Joint Surg* 1989; **71A**: 839–47.

Center for Disease Control. Transmission of HIV through bone transplantation: case report and public health recommendations. *Morbidity and Mortality Weekly Report*. 1988; **37**: 597–99.

Cooney WP, Linscheid RL, Dobyns JH. External pin fixation for unstable Colles' fractures. *J Bone Joint Surg* 1979; **61A**: 840–45.

De Oliveira JC. Barton's fractures. *J Bone Joint Surg* 1973; **55A**: 586–94.

Fernandez DL, Geissler WB. Treatment of displaced articular fractures of the radius. *J Hand Surg* 1991; **16A**: 375–84.

Friedlaender GE. Bone grafts. The basic science rationale for clinical application. *J Bone Joint Surg* 1987; **69A**: 786–90.

Gartland JJ, Werley CW. Evaluation of healed Colles' fractures. *J Bone Joint Surg* 1951; **33A**: 895–907.

Green DP, O'Brien ET. Open reduction of carpal dislocations. *J Hand Surg* 1978; **3**: 250–65.

Henry AK. *Extensile Exposure*. London: Churchill Livingstone, 1973; 102–4.

Knirk JL, Jupiter JB. Intraarticular fractures of the distal end of the radius in young adults. *J Bone Joint Surg* 1986; **68A**: 647–59.

Melone CP. Open treatment for displaced articular fractures of the distal radius. *Clin Orthop* 1986; **202**: 103–11.

Palmar AK. Fractures of the distal radius. In Green DP, ed. *Operative Hand Surgery*. New York: Churchill Livingstone, 1988: 1010–12.

Sennwald G. *L'entite radius-carpe*. Heidelberg: Springer Verlag, 1987: 230–34.

Seitz WH, Froimson AI, Leb R, Shapiro JD. Augmented external fixation of unstable distal radius fractures. *J Hand Surg* 1991; **16A**: 1010–16.

Thomas FB. Reduction of Smith's fractures. *J Bone Joint Surg* 1957; **39B**: 463–70.

25
Treatment of distal radial fractures by external fixation: techniques and indications

Frédéric Schuind, Monique Donkerwolcke, Franz Burny

Introduction

It is well known that in comminuted fractures of the distal radius, reduction may be obtained by transarticular distraction, as the capsular and ligamentous structures are usually preserved. This principle, termed 'ligamentotaxis' by Vidal et al. (1977 and 1980), also applies to other fractures, for example the unstable fractures of the dorsal and lumbar spine, which are treated with the Harrington distraction system (Willen et al. 1984, Yosipovitch et al. 1977), and the fractures of the base of the thumb metacarpal, which are treated by external fixation and distraction (Schuind et al. 1988).

At the wrist, like at other locations, it is usually not very difficult to obtain a satisfactory reduction of most comminuted or unstable distal radial fractures by traction. The problem is to maintain this reduction, as immobilization by a plaster cast is frequently insufficient. Prolonged transarticular traction maintained by an external fixator between the distal radius and the second metacarpal was first described by Vidal et al. in 1977 and then by Rasquin et al. in 1979. This chapter is based on the clinical experience of over 400 cases with this technique. The first 225 cases have been reported in previous papers (Schuind et al. 1984, 1985, and 1989).

Biomechanics

External fixation is based on the principle of 'load transfer' (Burny and Bourgois 1972, Chao 1987). A portion of the forces, or the totality of the forces normally transmitted from the metacarpals to the radius are bypassed through the fixator frame and the bone-pin interfaces. Such load transfer characteristics depend on the stiffness of the external fixator.

The frame stability may be quantified using the concept of fracture stiffness. Fracture stiffness is defined as the ratio of the applied load on the bone ends versus the displacement, measured at the fracture site (Briggs and Chao 1982, Chao 1987). Frykman et al. (1989) have compared the fracture stiffness of several common external fixators. The C-Hoffman device appears to have an intermediate stiffness, similar to the small AO fixator and higher than the Roger Anderson or the Jaquet minifixator devices. It should be noted, of course, that the optimal fracture stiffness is not known (Chao et al. 1979, Schuind and Burny 1990). In the authors' clinical practice, the C-Hoffman model appears to provide sufficient stability to maintain length and reduction.

Little is known about the biomechanics of ligamentous distraction. Research should be undertaken to assess which ligaments are in tension and the mechanical consequences of prolonged traction on these structures. Atmospheric pressure might play a role: a substantial decrease in intra-articular pressure has been measured during wrist distraction. This negative pressure could produce a suction effect, which in turn could play a significant role in the reduction of intra-articular fragments (Schuind et al. 1994).

Surgical technique

The standard Hoffman external fixator was used. This apparatus is simple to apply, and the versatility of the device allows various configurations, multiple attempts at reduction, and release of distraction at the third week.

The surgical technique has been described in detail in several papers (Rasquin et al. 1979, Schuind et al. 1984, 1985, and 1989, Schuind and Burny 1990). It must be applied following the general biomechanical requirements of osteosynthesis:

- secure anchorage of the components to strong bone, that is, the radius and the second metacarpal; and
- an adapted frame configuration to the bone lesion.

Anaesthetics

The surgery is performed under general or regional anaesthesia (usually under axillary nerve block or with intravenous regional anaesthetics), not only to avoid pain but also to relieve muscle spasm. The patient is positioned on the operating table with the upper limb on a lateral radiolucent table. A pneumatic tourniquet may be used. The entire upper limb is sterilized and draped.

Insertion of the pins

Continuous 3 mm Hoffman threaded half pins (C38-80-20 or S30) are used. Because of anatomical considerations (the superficial branch of the radial nerve), the proximal pins are inserted 5–10 cm above the joint, in the postero-lateral aspect of the middle third of the radius. The distal pins are inserted in the postero-lateral aspect of the second metacarpal shaft, which is subcutaneous. Two pins are inserted in each bone, in a parallel direction (Fig. 25.1). In patients with marked osteoporosis, the use of three pins is recommended. The pins are manually tested to ensure that they are solidly anchored. Fluoroscopy is also used, to confirm that the pins are actually inserted in both cortices of the bones, without excessive (more than 2 mm) protrusion within the soft tissues of the hand or forearm.

Reduction of the fracture

For most cases, a single half-frame configuration is recommended. After insertion of the pins, the fracture is reduced using longitudinal traction and closed manipulation under fluoroscopic control. After reduction, the traction is maintained by locking the fixator, without use of a distraction rod. It is frequently necessary, during the first three weeks, to fix the wrist with some palmar flexion and ulnar deviation (Figs 25.1 and 25.2).

In the case of persistent impaction of a 'die-punch' fragment, complementary adjunctive internal fixation may be advisable (Gainor and Groh 1990).

Open fractures

In open fractures with bone defects, immediate bone grafting is dangerous. The defect may be

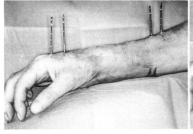
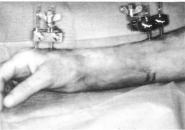
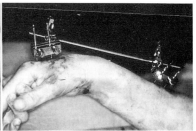

a b c

Figure 25.1

Surgical technique. a) Insertion of the pins. Note the proximal position of the pins inserted in the radius. b) After tightening of the clamps. c) After reduction of the fracture. Note the immobilization of the wrist in palmar flexion.

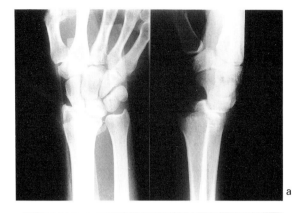
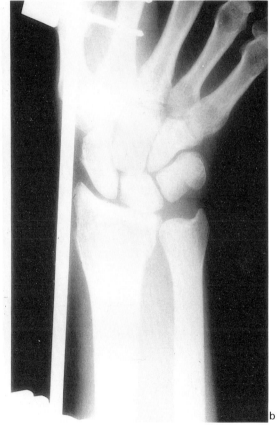

Figure 25.2
Radio-metacarpal half-frame external fixator for unstable fracture of the distal radius. a) Preoperative radiographs. b) After implantation of the external fixator.

temporarily filled with gentamycin PMMA minichains (Asche et al. 1979, Schuind and Burny 1990). In addition to their antibiotic activity, the minichains serve as a space holder. The minichains should be removed after three to six weeks to be replaced by cancellous bone graft.

Other configurations

Other configurations are possible using external fixation frames. The triangular frame, with transfixing pins implanted in the second and third metacarpals is not recommended. A few cases have been treated by radial-radial or radial-metacarpal external minifixators. The pins should be implanted in the distal radius only after a preliminary dissection of the soft tissues to avoid an iatrogenic injury to the superficial branch of the radial nerve or to the tendons of the first dorsal compartments.

Postoperative treatment

A light dressing is placed around the external fixator to avoid local compression. Elevation of the hand is recommended for the first few postoperative days. Early motion of the fingers, elbow and shoulder is encouraged as early as possible, with the assistance of physiotherapists. During the short postoperative hospitalization, the patient learns how to clean the skin at the pin exit sites, so that this cleaning can continue after discharge.

The patient is followed-up by the surgeon at the External Fixation Clinic. With the aim of minimizing reflex sympathetic dystrophy, distraction is discontinued after three weeks. External fixation is removed when the fracture is healed. The decision is made on the basis of control radiographs (usually after six weeks). The pins are removed without anaesthesia.

Active and passive wrist exercises are then initiated and physiotheraphy is continued until maximal functional recovery is obtained (Vanderhaegen 1980).

Indications

Traditional methods of closed reduction and cast application are still used for stable wrist fractures.

The authors' indications of external fixation for distal radial fractures are as follows:

1. unstable or open fractures;
2. fractures occurring in patients with multiple injuries;
3. loss of reduction following closed orthopaedic treatment;
4. bilateral fractures.

The aim is to obtain a perfect reduction of the fracture. It is very important to perfectly restore the joint surfaces (Riggs and Cooney 1983).

Results

The results have been presented in detail in previous publications (Schuind et al. 1984, 1985, and 1989).

An uneventful postoperative course of recovery is usual (78%), but 7% of patients complain of moderate pain during the early postoperative period. Moderate oedema and digital stiffness can be seen in 16% and 7% of the cases. Bone and skin reactions to pins can be minor problems. The quality of pin anchorage is satisfactory in most cases (Burny 1984) (Table 25.1).

In this series, the average length of retention of the fixator was 49 days. The mean duration of the subsequent physiotherapy was 74 days.

Clinical results

The clinical results are usually good. However, 20% of the patients complain from time to time of pain. Occasional oedema and slight digital stiffness occurred in 2% and 7% respectively. Reflex sympathetic dystrophy (Mackinnon and Holder 1984) is observed in less than 1% of the patients. However, persistent wrist stiffness and decrease of grip strength of the hand are usual (Table 25.2).

Roentgenographic results

The restoration of the anatomy of the distal end of the radius is evaluated according to the Lidström–Frykman anatomic gradation system (Frykman 1967, Lidström 1959). The reduction is perfect in 68% (grade I), good in 19% (grade II) and fair in 3%. No patients were classified as the 'poor' category (grade IV).

Persistent osteoporosis was present in 17% of patients.

Table 25.1 Bone and skin reactions to pins and anchorage of pins (manual evaluation)

	Radius N = 125	Metacarpal bone N = 100
Skin reactions		
No reaction	87%	90%
Inflammatory reaction	5%	7%
Infection (drainage)	4%	0%
Tissue proliferation	4%	2%
Other	0%	1%
Radiological reactions		
No reaction	89%	90%
Osteolysis in the 'in' cortex	5%	7%
Osteolysis in the 'out' cortex	2%	0%
Osteolysis in both cortices	4%	3%
Brodie abcess	0%	0%
Clinical anchorage (manual evaluation)		
Perfect anchorage	91%	83%
Slight motion	4%	4%
Important motion	2%	11%
Manual extraction	2%	1%
Spontaneous pull-out	1%	1%

Table 25.2 Functional results (after a mean follow-up duration of 6 months) (N=225 cases)

Mobility (% of normal side)	
Palmar flexion	67%
Dorsal flexion	64%
Radial flexion	61%
Ulnar flexion	79%
Pronation	93%
Supination	81%
Strength of the hand	52%

Complications of wrist fractures

Post-traumatic carpal tunnel syndrome occurred in 3%. No cases of tendon rupture, osteomyelitis or non-union at the site of the fracture have been observed.

Complications of external fixation

Fractures at the site of a pin, either of the radius or of the metacarpal shaft, occurred in 1% of patients. Secondary displacements, which required a repetition of reduction, occurred in 1% of the cases.

A major complication was neuroma of the superficial sensory branch of the radial nerve. This complication is always related to an inadequate insertion of the external fixator pins, with the proximal pins too close to the wrist joint. This complication was present in 2% of the cases in this series.

Discussion

Skeletal traction maintained by a half-frame external fixator between the radius and the second metacarpal appears to provide appropriate stabilization of the fragments (Cooney et al. 1979, Cooney 1983, D'Anca et al. 1984, Grana and Kopta 1979, Jenkins and Jones 1986, Nakata et al. 1985, Rasquin et al. 1979, Riggs and Cooney 1983, Schuind et al. 1984, 1985, and 1989, Schuind and Burny 1990, Vidal et al. 1977 and 1980, Weber and Szabo 1986, Wild et al. 1982). Skeletal traction maintained by pins in plaster (Boehler 1944, Cartier et al. 1975, Green 1975, Ledoux et al. 1973) may also achieve this aim but is technically more demanding than external fixation, and does not avoid constrictive cast complications (Schuind, Louvard et al. 1990).

The external fixator provides easy accessibility for wound care, and can be combined with either pedicle or free-flap coverage. Fracture management is also simplified, by allowing the patient elbow and hand freedom for daily activities.

As with any other method of treatment of wrist fractures, osteoporosis is a frequent postoperative complication, usually without any clinical sign of reflex sympathetic dystrophy. Osteoporosis, which is likely to be related to the immobilization of the wrist, can also be caused by prolonged skeletal traction. In an attempt to minimize this complication, distraction is always released at the third week.

We believe that it is the quality of reduction that determines the final clinical outcome (Castaing et al. 1964, De Wulf and Razemon 1968). Thus, the aim of external fixation with distraction is to obtain an anatomic reduction of the fracture. However, in spite of a satisfactory reduction in most cases, persistent wrist stiffness (except in pronation-supination) and decrease of grip strength of the hand are frequent. This limitation of the joint motion is probably well tolerated by patients, as the majority of common hand tasks can be accomplished with 70% of the maximal range of wrist flexion-extension and lateral deviations (Ryu et al. 1991). The treatment of extra-articular fractures of the distal radius by radio-radial external minifixation, sparing the wrist joint (Cooney 1983, Nakata et al. 1985, Riggs and Cooney 1983), or the use of articulated radio-metacarpal external fixators (Asche 1989) could provide better functional results, although the potential benefits of these methods have not yet been clearly demonstrated.

The complications of wrist external fixation are infrequent. Carpal tunnel syndrome occurs significantly less frequently ($p < 0.05$) than after plaster immobilization (Schuind et al. 1989), probably because of better reduction of the fracture, less wrist flexion, and avoidance of supplementary local constriction (Schuind et al. 1990, Schuind and Burny 1990). No tendinitis or tendon rupture, which are frequent complications after percutaneous pinning (Epinette et al. 1982, Kapandji 1976), were observed. Fractures at the site of a pin were rare when 3 mm pins were used (Gainor and Groh 1990). Radial sensory neuromas result from a technical fault that can be avoided by optimal implantation of the radial pins.

In conclusion, external fixation with distraction between the radius and second metacarpal is a simple and efficient technique for the treatment of distal fractures of the distal radius. The technique is so satisfactory that the indications have now been extended to comminuted fractures of the base of the first metacarpal bone (Schuind et al. 1988), fractures of the carpal bones (Schuind et al. 1985) and total or partial wrist arthrodeses (Schuind et al. 1986, Schuind and Burny 1988 and 1990).

References

Asche G, Haas HG, Klemm K. Lokalantiobiotische Behandlung mit Gentamycin-PMMA-Miniketten in der septischen Chirurgie der Hand. *Handchir* 1979; **11**: 37–38.

Asche G. The moving fixator in the treatment of wrist-fractures. Proceedings, 13th International Conference on Hoffmann External Fixation, Rochester, 1989: 143.

Boehler L. *Technique du traitement des fractures*. Paris: Ed Med de France, 1944.

Briggs BT, Chao EYS. The mechanical performance of the standard Hoffmann-Vidal external fixation apparatus. *J Bone Joint Surg* 1982; **64A**: 566–73.

Burny F, Bourgois R. Etude biomécanique du fixateur externe d'Hoffmann. *Acta Orthop Belg* 1972; **38**: 265–301.

Burny F. The pin as a percutaneous implant: general and related studies. *Orthopedics* 1984; **7**: 610–15.

Cartier P, Tiesse J, Père C. Traitement des fractures comminutives du poignet par la méthode de traction bipolaire. *Rev Chir Orthop* 1975; **61**: 517–31.

Castaing J, le Club des Dix. Les fractures récentes de l'extrémité inférieure du radius chez l'adulte. Rapport de la XXXIXème Réunion Annuelle de la SOFCOT. *Rev Chir Orthop* 1964; **50**: 581–666.

Chao EYS, Briggs BT, McCoy MT. Theoretical and experimental analyses of Hoffmann-Vidal external fixation system. In Brooker AF, Edwards CC. *External fixation — The current state of the art*. Baltimore: Williams & Wilkins, 1979: 345–70.

Chao EYS. Biomechanics of external fixation. In Lane J. *Fracture Healing*. New York: Churchill-Livingstone, 1987: 105–22.

Cooney WP, Linscheid RL, Dobyns JH. External pin fixation for unstable Colles' fractures. *J Bone Joint Surg* 1979; **61A**: 840–45.

Cooney WP. External fixation of distal radial fractures. *Clin Orthop* 1983; **180**: 44–49.

D'Anca AF, Sternlieb SB, Byron TW, Feinstein PA. External fixation management of unstable Colles' fractures. An alternative method. *Orthopedics* 1984; **7**: 853–59.

De Wulf A, Razemon JP. Les séquelles des fractures du poignet. *Acta Orthop Belg* 1968; **34**: 14–201.

Epinette JA, Lehut JM, Cavenaille M, Bouretz JC, Decoulx J. Fracture de Pouteau–Colles: double embrochage intrafocal en berceau salon Kapandji. *Ann Chir Main* 1982; **1**: 71–83.

Frykman G. Fractures of the distal end of the radius, including sequelae — shoulder, hand, finger syndrome, disturbance in the distal radio-ulnar joint and impairment of nerve function. *Acta Orthop Scand* 1967; **108 (Suppl)**: 27.

Frykman GK, Tooma GS, Boyko K, Henderson R. Comparison of eleven external fixators for treatment of unstable wrist fractures. *J Hand Surg* 1989; **14A**: 247–54.

Gainor BJ, Groh GI. Early clinical experience with Orthofix external fixation of complex distal radial fractures. *Orthopedics* 1990; **13**: 329–33.

Grana WA, Kopta JA. The Roger Anderson device in the treatment of fractures of the distal end of the radius. *J Bone Joint Surg* 1979; **61A**: 1234–38.

Green DB. Pins and plaster treatment of comminuted fractures of the distal end of the radius. *J Bone Joint Surg* 1975; **57A**: 304.

Jenkins NH, Jones DG. Simultaneous Colles' and scaphoid fractures: treatment by combined internal and external fixation. *Am J Emerg Med* 1986; **4**: 229–30.

Kapandji A. L'ostéosynthèse par double embrochage intrafocal. Traitement fonctionnel des fractures non articulaires de l'extrémité inférieure du radius. *Ann Chir* 1976; **30**: 903–8.

Ledoux A, Rauis A, Van Der Ghinst M. L'embrochage des fractures inférieures du radius. *Rev Chir Orthop* 1973; **59**: 427–38.

Lidström A. Fractures of the distal end of the radius. A clinical and statistical study of end-results. *Acta Orthop Scand* 1959; **41 (suppl)**: 1–95.

Mackinnon SE, Holder LE. The use of three-phase radionuclide bone scanning in the diagnosis of reflex sympathetic dystrophy. *J Hand Surg* 1984; **9A**: 556–63.

Nakata RY, Chand Y, Matiko JD, Frykman GK, Wood JE. External fixators for wrist fractures: a biomechanical and clinical study. *J Hand Surg* 1985; **10A**: 845–51.

Rasquin C, Burny F, Andrianne Y, Quintin J. Traitement des fractures du poignet par fixateur externe. *Acta Orthop Belg* 1979; **45**: 678–83.

Riggs SA, Cooney WP. External fixation of complex hand and wrist fractures. *J Trauma* 1983; **23**: 332–36.

Ryu J, Cooney WP, Askew LJ, An KN, Chao EYS. Functional ranges of motion of the wrist joint. *J Hand Surg* 1991; **16A**: 409–19.

Schuind F, Donkerwolcke M, Burny F. External fixation of wrist fractures. *Orthopedics* 1984; **7**: 841–44.

Schuind F, Donkerwolcke M, Burny F. External fixation of wrist fractures — a study of 182 cases. In Scheiberer L, Eitel F, eds. *Emergency surgery — trends, techniques, results*. Munich: W. Zuckschwerdt Verlag, 1985: 236–39.

Schuind F, Burny F, Donkerwolcke M, Hinsenkamp M. Applications particulières de la fixation externe au poignet. Société Française de Chirurgie de la Main (GEM), Paris, 1986.

Schuind F, Noorbergen M, Andrianne Y, Burny F. New technique. Comminuted fractures of the base of the first metacarpal treated by distraction-external fixation. *J Orthop Trauma* 1988; **2**: 314–21.

Schuind F, Burny F. Ostéonécroses du semi-lunaire: nouvelle approche thérapeutique. *Acta Orthop Belg* 1988; **54**: 127–32.

Schuind F, Donkerwolcke M, Rasquin C, Burny F. External fixation of fractures of the distal radius: a study of 225 cases. *J Hand Surg* 1989; **14A(2)**: 404–7.

Schuind F, Louvard A, Schoutens A, Itzkowitch D. The use of three-phase radionuclide bone scan after limb surgery. In Arlet J, Mazières B. *Bone circulation and bone necrosis*. Berlin: Springer-Verlag 1990: 219–21.

Schuind F, Burny F. New techniques of osteosynthesis of the hand. Principles, clinical applications and biomechanics with special reference to external minifixation. Basel: Karger, 1990: 1–156.

Schuind F, Fabeck L, Burny F. Etude des pressions articulaires lors de la réduction des fractures de l'extrémité distale du radius. Belgian Hand Group, Ottignies, 1994.

Vanderhaegen Y. Kinésithérapie après fracture du poignet: revue de 434 cas. Mémoire, licence en kinésithérapie. Université Libre de Bruxelles, 1980: 1–127.

Vidal J, Buscayret C, Fischbach C, Brakin B, Paran M, Escare P. Une méthode originale dans le traitement des fractures comminutives de l'extrémité inférieure du radius: le taxis ligamentaire. *Acta Orthop Belg* 1977; **43**: 781–89.

Vidal J, Paran M. Ligamentotaxis. 7èmes *Journées Internationales sur la Fixation Externe d'Hoffmann — Montpellier 1979*, Diffinco, Genève, 1980: 180–86.

Weber SC, Szabo RM. Severely comminuted distal radial fracture as an unsolved problem: complications associated with external fixation and pins and plaster techniques. *J Hand Surg* 1986; **11A**: 157–65.

Wild JJ, Hanson GW, Bennett JB, Tullos HS. External fixation use in the management of massive upper extremity trauma. *Clin Orthop* 1982; **164**: 172–76.

Willen J, Lindahl S, Irstam L, Nordwall A. A study by CT and conventional roentgenology of the reduction effect of Harrington instrumentation. *Spine* 1984; **9**: 214–19.

Yosipovitch Z, Robin GC, Makin M. Open reduction of unstable thoracolumbar spinal injuries and fixation with Harrington rods. *J Bone Joint Surg* 1977; **59A**: 1003–14.

26
Treatment of articular fractures of the distal radius with external fixation and pinning

Diego L Fernandez

Among the wide spectrum of wrist injuries, traumatic disruption of the articular surface of the distal radius represents a therapeutic challenge. These fractures are generally caused by a high-energy impact, resulting in articular and metaphyseal comminution, and are therefore less amenable to the traditional methods of closed manipulation and casting. Excessive fragmentation is responsible for skeletal instability. These fractures have an inherent tendency for shortening and articular collapse due to impaction of the cancellous metaphyseal bone of the distal radius. If treated conservatively, intra-articular and extra-articular malunion with secondary shortening and incongruity of the distal radioulnar joint are the rule (Bacorn and Kurtzke 1953, Cassebaum 1950, Cooney et al. 1980, Fernandez 1982, Gartland and Werley 1951, McQueen and Caspers 1988, Scheck 1962, Villar et al. 1987). Although extra-articular post-traumatic deformity can be corrected at a later date, intra-articular incongruity leads to rapid joint deterioration that can only be solved with salvage procedures such as arthroplasty or arthrodesis. It is for this reason that displaced fractures involving the articular surface deserve an aggressive initial treatment in an effort to reduce the incidence of post-traumatic osteoarthritis, at least in the young, manually active individual (Bradway et al. 1989, Knirk and Jupiter 1985 and 1986, Martini 1986).

Although restoration of the joint surface can be obtained by a variety of treatment modalities (closed reduction, skeletal traction, percutaneous manipulation, open reduction), prevention of secondary displacment of the initial anatomic reduction of the articular surface, together with maintenance of radial length and metaphyseal alignment in the first four weeks, constitutes the key to a successful result. This can be achieved with minimal internal fixation using Kirschner wires or plates in simple fracture types when the fragments are of reasonable size and there is no metaphyseal comminution (Axelrod and McMurtry 1990, Axelrod et al. 1988, Bradway et al. 1989, Fernandez and Geissler 1991, Fernandez and Maeder 1977). Otherwise, an external fixation that will neutralize axial loading of the carpus on the comminuted surface of the radius, in combination with autologous bone grafting of the metaphyseal defect for a period of five weeks, becomes mandatory (Anderson and O'Neil 1944, Cooney 1988, Cooney et al. 1979, Grana and Kopta 1979, Howard et al. 1989, Jakob and Fernandez 1982, Leung et al. 1990, Sanders et al. 1991, Vidal et al. 1979, Wagner and Jakob 1985, Weber and Szabo 1986). This chapter will cover the indications, surgical technique, and complications of combined internal and external fixation, used to manage articular fractures of the distal end of the radius.

Classification of fractures of the distal radius

Modern classification systems of fractures of the distal radius have become a valuable aid in helping to decide the best possible treatment for each specific injury. Current classifications are based on the analysis of the mechanism of injury (Castaing 1964, Frykman 1967), stability (Cooney et al. 1979), number of fragments (McMurtry and Jupiter 1991, Melone 1986), displacement pattern

(Melone 1984, 1986 and 1988), and degree of joint and metaphyseal involvement (Fernandez 1987, Müller et al. 1987). Some include a prognostic parameter by separating simple and complex articular fractures, which readily orients the surgeon for the election of the appropriate method for each fracture. The author prefers a classification based on the mechanism of injury, because manual reduction and realignment of the fracture is usually achieved by applying a force opposite to that which produced the injury. Moreover, associated ligamentous lesions, subluxation, and fractures of the neighbouring carpal bones, as well as concomitant soft tissue damage, are in direct relationship to the quality and degree of violence sustained. Since the basic mechanical features of each fracture are strictly dependent on the mechanism of injury, fractures of the distal radius may be classified as shown in Table 26.1 (Fernandez, 1993).

These five basic main groups are easily recognized with plain AP and lateral radiographs of the wrist. However, special imaging such as traction views following reduction, tomograms or CT scans provide a more accurate diagnosis of the displacement pattern, number of fragments and degree of joint involvement both at the radiocarpal and radio-ulnar level. Careful assessment of the carpus in the initial radiographs, or in those taken after reduction of the radial fracture, is imperative to rule out associated carpal ligament injuries or fractures of the neighbouring carpal bones. Ideally, these lesions should be treated along with the radial fracture in the acute stage, in an effort to restore carpal integrity with primary ligament repair. Both late ligamentoplasties and limited carpal fusions are of questionable long-term efficacy, and result in abnormal carpal kinematics and limited overall function of the wrist (Cooney et al. 1991). Critical assessment of concomitant soft tissue lesions (median nerve compression, compartment syndrome, soft tissue defects, tendon injuries), and ipsilateral fractures of the upper extremity will also influence the treatment selected.

From a biomechanical standpoint, this simple classification points out the ideal method of fixation for each basic type.

Type I: Bending fractures are best treated by a counterforce that will exert tension forces on the side of the concavity of the angulation. This is achieved in cases with adequate bone quality and absence of metaphyseal comminution with a well-moulded three-point contact cast.

Type II: Shearing fractures usually occur in hard cancellous bone, are extremely unstable due to the obliquity of the fracture line and are therefore suitable for internal fixation with buttress plates (DeOliveira 1973; Ellis 1968, Fernandez 1980).

Type III: Compression fractures. Restoration of the joint surface can be achieved in most cases by applying tension to the joint capsule with finger traps, external fixators, or pins and plaster techniques. In a number of cases, however, disimpaction of cartilage-bearing fragments may require limited or extensile open reduction and replacement of the cancellous defect with a bone graft.

Type IV: Avulsion fractures are a constant component of radiocarpal dislocations, occurring after a wrist sprain in which rotational forces are part of the mechanism of injury. Tension wiring or screw fixation is the method of choice if such fractures remain displaced.

Type V: Combined fracture (High-velocity injury). A combined method of fixation will be selected for treatment.

It must be pointed out that this classification also provides prognostic information, since the complexity of the bony lesions and the probability of occurrence of associated soft tissue disruption increases consistently from type I through to type V fractures.

Indications and contraindications of operative treatment

Open reduction of articular fractures of the distal radius is indicated when intra-articular congruity

Table 26.1 Classification of fractures of the distal radius based on mechanism of injury

Fracture types (adults) based on the mechanism of injury	Children fracture equivalent	Stability/ instability: high risk of secondary displacement after initial adequate reduction	Displacement pattern	Number of fragments	Associated lesions (ligaments, carpus, median ulnar nerve, tendons, ipsilateral fractures upper extremity, compartment syndrome)	Treatment
TYPE I Bending fracture of the metaphysis	Distal forearm fracture Salter II	Stable Unstable	Non-displaced Dorsally (Colles–Pouteau) Volarly (Smith) Proximal Combined	Always 2 main fragments Metaphyseal comminution (varying degree = instability)	Uncommon	Conservative (stable fractures) Percutaneous pins Percutaneous pins External fixation (exceptionally Bone graft)
TYPE II Shearing fracture of the joint surface	Salter IV	Unstable	Dorsal Radial Volar Proximal Combined	Two-part Three-part Comminuted	Common	Open reduction Screw/plate fixation
TYPE III Compression fracture of the joint surface	Salter III, IV, V	Stable Unstable	Non-displaced Dorsal Radial Volar Proximal Combined	Two-part Three-part Four-part Comminuted	Frequent	Conservative Closed, limited, or extensile open reduction Percutaneous pins combined ext. and int. fixation bone graft
TYPE IV Avulsion fractures, radiocarpal fracture-dislocation	Very rare	Unstable	Dorsal Radial Volar Proximal Combined	Two-part (radial styloid, ulnar styloid) Three-part (volar, dorsal margin) Comminuted	Very frequent	Closed or open reduction Pin or screw fixation Tension wiring
TYPE V Combined fractures (I–II–III–IV) high-velocity injury	Very rare	Unstable	Dorsal Radial Volar Proximal Combined	Comminuted (frequently intra-articular, open, bone loss, seldom extra-articular)	Always present	Combined method

of the fracture cannot be achieved by closed manipulation, joint distraction, or percutaneous reduction manoeuvres in manually active patients with good bone quality and absence of pre-existing wrist pathology. Open reduction and internal fixation is also indicated in open fractures and in fractures with associated carpal disruption, tendon or nerve injuries, since immediate skeletal stability is a prerequisite for undisturbed soft tissue healing. Delayed open reduction may be indicated for secondary intra-articular displacement in a fracture that undergoes loss of reduction after a conservative trial with closed reduction and plaster fixation.

Articular fractures in elderly inactive patients and those with massive osteoporosis are a formal contraindication to open reduction due to the high risk of complications, such as inadequate purchase of internal fixation material, iatrogenic non-union, and reflex sympathetic dystrophy, in this age group (Bradway et al. 1989, Fernandez et al. 1983, Wagner and Jakob 1985). Other contraindications, not related to the fracture itself, include the general condition of the patient, associated diseases, and the presence of degenerative changes of the wrist joint prior to injury (non-union of the scaphoid, Kienböck's disease, rheumatoid arthritis). Operative treatment is also contraindicated in unreliable, unmotivated, non-cooperative patients.

In our experience, the limitation of surgical restoration of an articular fracture of the distal radius is given by the number of fragments, their size, the amount cancellous bone impaction and the presence of associated primary lesions of the articular cartilage. Exact anatomic restoration should not be pursued if articular comminution exceeds five to six good-sized fragments; over that limit, the chances of obtaining a perfect anatomic reduction of the joint surface are low. However, this does not preclude the necessity of improving extra- and intra-articular alignment in these cases. Restoration of radial length can be achieved with external fixators, in an effort to improve the anatomic relationship of the radius and ulna and to ensure the normal alignment of the hand and carpus with the long axis of the forearm.

Healing of the fracture without extra-articular malunion and normal radial length greatly facilitates secondary wrist procedures such as partial or total wrist fusion, or resection arthroplasty, which may be necessary to treat painful radio-carpal and radio-ulnar arthritis.

Surgical technique

The technique of limited and extensile open reduction of type III, IV, and V fractures, stabilized with combined internal and external fixation will be described in this section.

If a type III compression fracture has a simple intra-articular component (not more than two fragments) and no metaphyseal comminution, it usually responds well to closed or percutaneous reduction and seldom needs formal open reduction (Fernandez and Geissler 1991).

A percutaneous reduction implies the manipulation of cartilage-bearing fragments with an awl or a periosteal elevator through a small skin incision, with a minimum of soft tissue dissection under fluoroscopic and/or arthroscopic guidance (Axelrod et al. 1988, Fernandez and Geissler 1991). The great majority of these cases may be stabilized with percutaneous pinning. If the fracture has a simple intra-articular component and extensive metaphyseal comminution, external fixation is the method of choice to control radial shortening and metaphyseal angulation. If the articular congruity is not adequately restored with ligamentotaxis following application of the external fixator, then a percutaneous or limited open reduction in combination with bone grafting is advocated (Fig. 26.1).

If the fracture has more than two articular fragments and an increasing degree of metaphyseal or even diaphyseal comminution, open reduction and bone grafting become more suitable, because joint distraction with external fixators does not always allow for disimpaction of small cartilage-bearing fragments. This technique will not produce reduction of severely rotated volar ulnar lip fragments in the so-called four-part fractures (Melone 1986). These injuries are the result of high-velocity trauma, with a higher incidence of associated fractures of the distal ulna, a fact that increases the instability of the distal forearm and may therefore require additional specific treatment.

A displaced intra-articular fracture should be treated in the operating room under adequate anaesthesia, with the iliac crest draped and sterile.

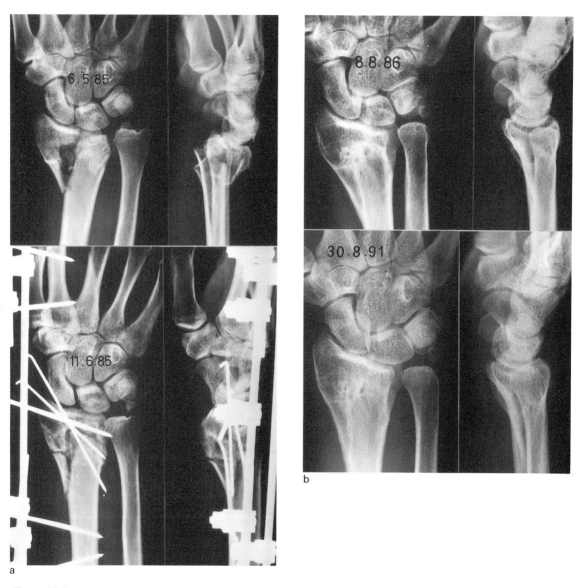

Figure 26.1

a) Top: Type III 4-part articular fracture with metaphyseal comminution. Bottom: 5 weeks after open reduction, bone grafting and combined internal and external fixation. The fixator is shortly to be removed.
b) Radiographs taken 15 months (top) and 6 years (bottom) after injury. Note the complete bone remodelling and absence of late degenerative changes.

A tourniquet should be applied if limited or formal open reduction becomes necessary. With the image intensifier properly draped, a classical closed manipulation with traction, palmar flexion, and ulnar deviation is performed. The quality of reduction is assessed under fluoroscopy, while traction is maintained by the surgeon and countertraction by the assistant. Alternatively, horizontal longitudinal traction can be applied using sterile finger traps with 2.5–5 kg weights, and countertraction across the upper arm. This frees both the surgeon's hands for manipulation and pinning.

Restoration of radial length, volar tilt, and articular congruity is assessed at this point. If there is no metaphyseal comminution and reduction of the joint fragments is acceptable, a conventional percutaneous pinning of the fracture is carried out. If reduction of the 'medial complex fragments' (Melone 1988) is anatomic with no articular step-off, additional pinning from the radial styloid towards the sigmoid notch is performed using 1.2 mm Kirschner wires, and being careful not to enter the radio-ulnar joint. If a satisfactory reduction of the dorso-medial fragment cannot be achieved by radial deviation and palmar flexion (Mortier et al. 1986), then a 2 cm long skin incision is placed between the fourth and fifth dorsal compartments and, with a minimum of soft tissue dissection, an awl or periosteal elevator is introduced. Under fluoroscopy, the displaced fragment is reduced against the lunate and pinned transversely as described above.

When the medial fragments are split into dorsal and volar components (four-part fracture) and the volar fragment is severely displaced, then limited open reduction through a volar approach is mandatory. This volar ulnar fragment cannot be reduced anatomically by closed manipulation or traction due to its tendency to rotate dorsally when tension is applied to the volar capsule. An extended incision for carpal tunnel release is used in this situation. The skin incision follows the thenar crease, is reflected towards the ulna and over the volar wrist skin crease and is continued in the forearm with a slight curve radially. The carpal tunnel is opened and the interval between the ulnar artery and the ulnar nerve and the flexor tendons is developed. Then the distal border of the pronator quadratus is partially incised and separated from the displaced volar ulnar fragment. Flexion of the wrist releases tension in the flexor tendons, allowing easy separation towards the radial aspect of the forearm. Reduction is performed without additional soft tissue dissection, taking care not to disturb the important attachments of this fragment to the triangular fibrocartilage. If the fragment is small, fixation is carried out with a single Kirschner wire, which is introduced obliquely from the volar surface of the fragment, across the metaphysis, and is retrieved through the dorsal skin of the forearm (Fig. 26.2). For bigger fragments a small L- or T-plate may be applied to buttress the fragment, as in the classical technique for reversed Barton's fractures (Ellis 1968).

When the articular fracture shows a considerable degree of metaphyseal and even diaphyseal comminution, external fixation is the most reliable method of stabilization to prevent radial shortening. However, if radiocarpal and radio-ulnar congruity cannot be achieved with external fixation alone, a percutaneous or formal open reduction of the joint surface should be used, in combination with the external fixator. Before applying the external fixator, the gross displacement of the fracture is reduced with a conventional closed manipulation, and the quality of reduction is assessed with the image intensifier.

If satisfactory reduction is obtained with adequate correction of the radial inclination and radial length, as well as the volar tilt, a temporary percutaneous fixation of the radial styloid is performed. Then two 2.5 mm half-threaded pins are inserted into the base and the shaft of the second metacarpal, as shown in Fig. 26.3. The pins are inserted through small stab wounds, spreading the underlying soft tissues with a haemostat and using a protection guide. If the bone is osteoporotic, the pins may be inserted directly, otherwise predrilling with a 2 mm drill-bit is advisable. In the second metacarpal the pins are inserted in a converging manner, at 40–50° to each other, to increase their holding power in the bone. A second pair of pins is then inserted into the distal third of the radius, just proximal to the bellies of the abductor pollicis longus and extensor pollicis brevis muscles. Again, the use of small skin incisions, blunt dissection of the soft tissues and the protection guide will minimize iatrogenic lesions of the superficial radial nerve branch at this level.

If a longer distance has to be bridged with the external fixator due to diaphyseal comminution, stability of the frame should be increased by using either three pins in the proximal fragment, or 4 mm half-threaded pins in the proximal radius. If the fracture is stable with the wrist in neutral position, a straight frame with two long connecting rods is used. If wrist flexion and deviation is needed to restore the volar tilt, two short rods are connected to the two pairs of half-pins with a universal clamp. However, unnatural wrist positioning is undesirable because of the high risk of delayed finger motion and median nerve compression neuropathy.

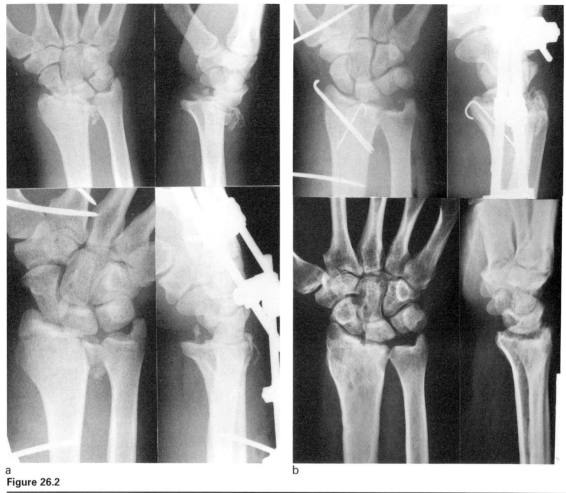

Figure 26.2

a) Top: Type IV radiocarpal fracture-dislocation with significant comminution of the joint surface. Bottom: Attempted closed reduction and external fixation shows persistent dorsal subluxation of the carpus and articular fragment displacement.
b) Top: Restoration of joint congruity with open reduction and palmar capsular repair. Notice antero-posterior pin fixation of the volar ulnar joint fragment. Bottom: Radiographs at one year after surgery showing adequate joint congruity and normal carpal alignment.

After tightening the fixator clamps, the quality of joint reduction is again assessed under fluoroscopy. If articular congruity is unacceptable (more than 1–2 mm step-off), a percutaneous or formal open reduction, as described previously, is performed with the fixator in place. The choice of surgical approach depends on the localization of the fragment needing additional reduction. Most commonly, the approach between the third and fourth extensor compartments is used. The proximal part of the extensor retinaculum is divided up to the level of the radiocarpal joint and the extensor pollicis longus tendon is freed at the level of Lister's tubercule. The wrist joint capsule is opened transversely and the fragments are manually elevated and reduced against the scaphoid and lunate.

The remaining bone defect after reduction of the fragment should be grafted with autologous iliac bone graft in every case. Bone grafting not only provides additional mechanical support for the articular fragments, but also accelerates bone healing. Even in cases where adequate joint congruity has been obtained with ligamentotaxis

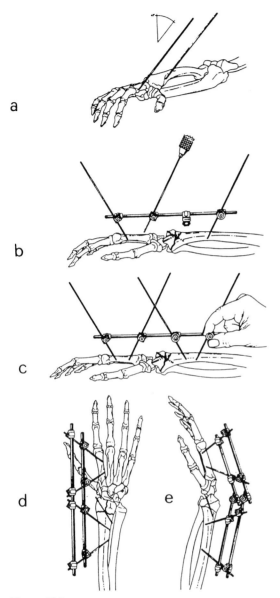

Figure 26.3

Technique of application of a wrist fixator. a) First, two pins are inserted into the second metacarpal and distal third of the radius. b) A single bar is connected with the first pair of pins. The third and fourth pins are inserted through the free clamps. c) The screws are tightened proximally and ligamentotaxis is achieved with longitudinal traction applied to the thumb, index and middle fingers. d) The stability of the frame is increased by adding a second bar. Note the converging pin positioning, which increases the pin purchase distance in the bone. e) If wrist flexion and ulnar deviation are desired, the two pairs of short bars are connected to each other with universal clamps, which permit free wrist positioning.

alone, primary bone grafting is strongly recommended if massive metaphyseal defects persist after the application of the wrist fixator, since grafting enhances fracture healing and permits early removal of the fixator, allowing early wrist rehabilitation. The use of transverse Kirschner wire fixation from the radial styloid towards the distal radio-ulnar joint depends on the size of the fragments.

Associated distal radioulnar joint lesions

Fractures of the distal radius are often accompanied by traumatic disruption of the distal radioulnar joint (DRUJ). In order to guarantee a satisfactory outcome, these lesions should be recognized and treated at the time of injury. In fact the most common cause of disability after distal radius fractures is the DRUJ, often referred to by Cooney as the 'forgotten joint'. Since final adverse results depend basically on residual DRUJ instability and/or post-traumatic arthritic changes, DRUJ lesions associated with radius fractures may be classified into stable, unstable and potentially unstable lesions, depending on the residual stability of the DRUJ after the fracture of the distal radius has been adequately reduced and stabilized (Table 26.2). This implies that the anatomic relationship of the sigmoid notch to the ulnar head has been re-established through restoration of radial length, rotation, and sagittal and frontal tilt of the distal fragment.

Type I are stable DRUJ lesions, meaning that the joint is clinically stable and the radiograph shows articular congruity. These lesions include avulsion of the tip of the ulnar styloid, and stable fractures of the neck of the ulna. In both the primary stabilizers of the joint (TFCC and capsular ligament) are intact. These injuries carry a good prognosis and are best treated by early motion postoperatively.

Type II are unstable DRUJ lesions with clinical and radiographic evidence of subluxation and/or dislocation of the ulnar head due to a massive

Table 26.2 Fracture of the distal radius: associated distal radioulnar joint (DRUJ) lesions

	PATHO-ANATOMY OF THE LESION	DEGREE OF JOINT SURFACE INVOLVEMENT	PROGNOSIS	RECOMMENDED TREATMENT	
TYPE I STABLE (following reduction of the radius the DRUJ is congruous and stable) A AVULSION FRACTURE TIP ULNAR STYLOID / B STABLE FRACTURE ULNAR NECK		NONE	GOOD	A+B	FUNCTIONAL AFTERTREATMENT
					ENCOURAGE EARLY PRONATION-SUPINATION EXERCISES
				NOTE:	EXTRAARTICULAR UNSTABLE FRACTURES OF THE ULNA AT THE METAPHYSEAL LEVEL OR DISTAL SHAFT REQUIRE STABLE PLATE FIXATION
TYPE II UNSTABLE (subluxation or dislocation of the ulnar head present) A SUBSTANCE TEAR OF TFCC AND/OR PALMAR AND DORSAL CAPSULAR LIGAMENTS / B AVULSION FRACTURE BASE OF THE ULNAR STYLOID		NONE	– CHRONIC INSTABILITY – PAINFUL LIMITATION OF SUPINATION IF LEFT UNREDUCED – POSSIBLE LATE ARTHRITIC CHANGES	A	CLOSED TREATMENT REDUCE SUBLUXATION, SUGAR TONG SPLINT IN 45° OF SUPINATION FOUR TO SIX WEEKS
				A+B	OPERATIVE TREATMENT REPAIR TFCC OR FIX ULNAR STYLOID WITH TENSION BAND WIRING IMMOBILIZE WRIST AND ELBOW IN SUPINATION (CAST) OR TRANSFIX ULNA/RADIUS WITH K-WIRE AND FOREARM CAST
TYPE III POTENTIALLY UNSTABLE (subluxation possible) A INTRAARTICULAR FRACTURE OF THE SIGMOID NOTCH / B INTRAARTICULAR FRACTURE OF THE ULNAR HEAD		PRESENT	– DORSAL SUBLUXATION POSSIBLE TOGETHER WITH DORSALLY DISPLACED DIE PUNCH OR DORSOULNAR FRAGMENT	A	ANATOMIC REDUCTION OF PALMAR AND DORSAL SIGMOID NOTCH FRAGMENTS. IF RESIDUAL SUBLUXATION TENDENCY PRESENT IMMOBILIZE AS IN TYPE II INJURY
			– RISK OF EARLY DEGENERATIVE CHANGES AND SEVERE LIMITATION OF FOREARM ROTATION IF LEFT UNREDUCED	B	FUNCTIONAL AFTERTREATMENT TO ENHANCE REMODELLING OF ULNAR HEAD.
					IF DRUJ REMAINS PAINFUL: PARTIAL ULNAR RESECTION, DARRACH OR SAUVÉ-KAPANDJI PROCEDURE AT A LATER DATE

substance tear of the TFCC or an avulsion fracture of the base of the ulnar styloid. If the ulnar head is left unreduced, chronic instability with painful limitation of supination and possible late arthritic changes are the rule. Soft tissue injuries with involvement of the TFCC or the capsular ligaments can be treated closed with reduction of the DRUJ and immobilization in 45° of supination for four to six weeks. Fractures of the base of the ulnar styloid require internal fixation using two parallel Kirschner wires with a tension band wire passed in a figure of eight through the ulnocarpal ligaments and a drill hole at the neck of the ulna.

Type III injuries are potentially unstable lesions due to skeletal disruption of the joint surface at either the sigmoid notch (four-part fracture of the distal radius) or the ulnar head. The fracture of the radius involving a dorso-ulnar fragment can allow dorsal subluxation of the distal ulna. Anatomic reduction of the radial fracture should stabilize this injury and minimize the chance of late arthritic changes. Intra-articular fractures of the ulnar head are best treated by early motion to enhance remodelling of the ulnar head. Early resection of the distal ulna is not recommended. If the distal radioulnar joint remains painful, partial ulnar resection, a Darrach procedure, or a Sauvé-Kapandji procedure can be performed at a later date.

Treatment of concomitant injuries

The incidence of associated injuries increases progressively in types III, IV, and V fractures (Table 26.3). These include a wide spectrum of soft tissue lesions, ligamentous carpal disruption, carpal fractures, and ipsilateral fractures of the upper extremity, as well as fractures of the distal ulna (Fig. 26.4). Neurovascular compromise or the presence of massive soft tissue swelling and forearm compartment syndrome in patients with multiple injuries should be carefully ruled out.

Adequate evaluation of the soft tissue condition is required to determine the ideal timing of surgery. Although surgical restoration of the articular surface is best carried out immediately after the accident, significant soft tissue swelling may jeopardize primary skin closure. In such situations the operation must be delayed for five to six days, provided that the initial displacement of the wrist is reduced and held in a plaster splint. The upper extremity should be elevated until surgery can be performed.

Immediate surgery, on the other hand, is an absolute indication if the fracture is open, if there is a forearm compartment syndrome, or if there is primary compression of the median or ulnar nerves. In open fractures, coverage of primary soft tissue is not attempted after fracture reduction. Usually, the wound is left open and a mesh graft applied once the swelling has subsided and there is no evidence of infection. If there is median or ulnar nerve neuropathy with loss of sensitivity immediately after injury, and the radiograph demonstrates a severely displaced fracture on the volar side of the wrist, surgical decompression and neurolysis during open reduction of the fracture is recommended in every case.

Associated skeletal or ligament injuries of the carpus are seldom recognized on the initial radiograph due to the gross displacement of the fracture. Although complete scapholunate dissociation is clearly visible, non-dissociative scapholunate tears can be easily overlooked. This lesion is a relatively frequent component of fractures disrupting the scaphoid and the lunate fossa of the radius with significant initial displacement. If the fracture is initially reduced with ligamentotaxis, attention must be paid to the distal displacement of the scaphoid, together with the distal carpal row, which can produce a definite step-off at the scapholunate junction if there is ligament disruption. This 'axial scaphoid shift sign' disrupts the smooth arc of the proximal contour of the first carpal row (Fig. 26.5). The axial scaphoid shift sign is diagnostic for complete scapholunate disruption whenever traction is applied to the carpus.

Treatment of acute ligament disruption includes the repair of the scapholunate membrane with non-absorbable intraosseuos sutures, as suggested by Laverna, Cohen and Taleisnik (1992). Since carpal alignment is usually maintained by the external fixator, the need for additional pin fixation of the scapholunate junction depends on the stability provided by the primary intraosseous suture. If there is a tendency for the scaphoid to rotate, pin fixation across the scapholunate and scaphocapitate joints is recommended for eight

Table 26.3 Treatment modalities of 115 articular fractures of the distal radius

Fracture pattern	No.	Reduction			Fixation							Additional procedures for concomitant injuries	
		Closed	Percutaneous	Open	Kirschner wires	Plates	Ex. Fixator	Ext. Fixator Int. Fixation	Bone Graft	Primary RSL Fusion			
TYPE II shearing fractures	43	3	–	40	2	38	–	1	–	–		carpal tunnel release ulnar styloid fixation TFFC repair	2 2 1
Type III compression fractures	60	14	21	25	18	–	5	36	38	1		median nerve decompression scapholunate ligament repair scaphoid screw fixation plate fixation ulna ulnar styloid fixation TFFC repair	9 6 3 3 3 1
Type IV avulsion fractures (radiocarpal fracture-dislocations)	7	–	–	7	3	–	–	3	–	1		carpal tunnel release palmar ligament repair ulnar styloid fixation lunate fracture scaphoid fracture triquetrum fracture fasciotomy tendon injury FPL/PQ	6 5 4 2 1 1 1 1
Type V combined fractures, high-velocity injuries	5	–	–	5	–	–	1	4	4	1		median nerve decompression faciotomy ulnar styloid fixation FPL/FS II ipsilateral forearm fracture plating elbow dislocation elbow fracture-dislocation, brachial artery laceration	4 3 1 1 1 1 1
TOTAL	115	17	21	77	23	38	6	44	42	3			63
Averages (%)		14.7	18.2	70	20	33	5	38	36	2.6			54

RSL radioscapholunate; TFCC triangular fibrocartilaginous complex; FPL flexor pollicis longus; PQ pronator quadratus; FS flexor sublimes

weeks. Since healing of the ligaments may take several months, secondary repair should be aided by screw fixation, as proposed by Herbert (1990) (Fig. 11.6).

Additional carpal bone injuries, most commonly a fractured scaphoid, are treated with primary internal fixation before application of the external fixator for the fractured radius. This allows free manipulation of the scaphoid fragments and easy reduction. If the fixator is applied before scaphoid fixation, the frame will separate the scaphoid fragments when traction is applied across the wrist joint.

Technical pitfalls

The most common pitfall in treatment of articular fractures of the distal radius is the discovery of a

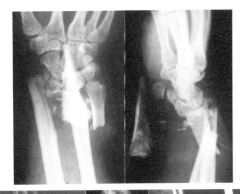
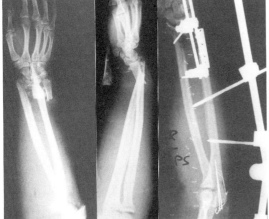
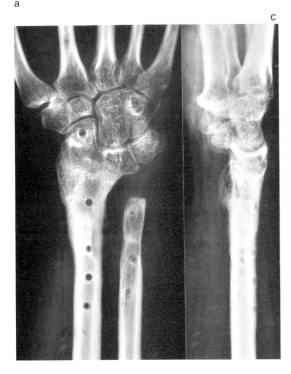

a

c

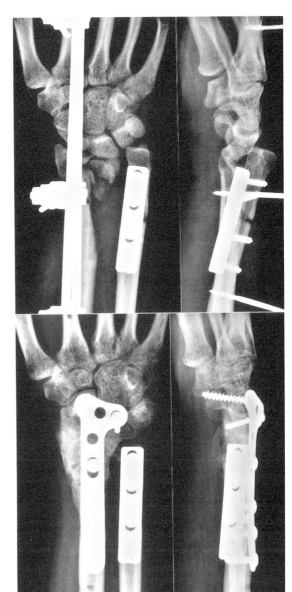

b

Figure 26.4

a) A type V high-velocity injury. Note the massive joint comminution, significant displacement of a joint fragment in the volar soft tissue, fracture of the distal ulna and ipsilateral fracture-dislocation of the elbow. Initial treatment included repair of an associated brachial artery laceration, extensive fasciotomy, internal fixation of the ulna (olecranon and distal shaft) and temporary external fixation of the elbow and wrist (bottom right). b) Due to massive bone loss and distal radio-ulnar dissociation, the wrist was salvaged with a radio-scapholunate fusion and distal ulnar resection 5 weeks after the accident. c) Follow-up roentgenograms 16 months after the injury reveal a solid fusion with a well preserved midcarpal joint space.

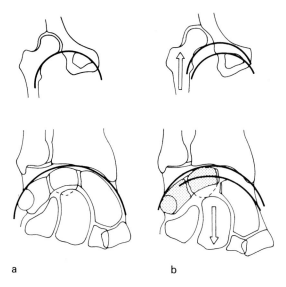

Figure 26.5

The axial scaphoid shift sign. a) The proximal carpal row contour shows a uniform radiographic arc. This is a sign of stability as is the non-disrupted Shenton–Menard arc for a stable hip. b) Whenever traction is applied to the wrist with a scapholunate ligament tear, the scaphoid shifts distally, disrupting the 'carpal Shenton's arc'. c) An intra-articular radial fracture treated with combined internal and external fixation and bone grafting. The axial scaphoid shift is evident. This patient developed an asymptomatic scapholunate dissociation.

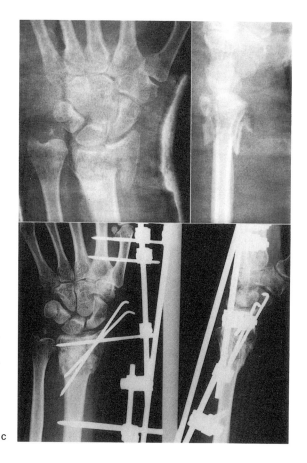

considerably greater amount of articular comminution on opening the joint than that which was expected from the study of the initial radiographs. In these situations, the surgeon must be prepared to obtain the best possible joint congruity with minimal soft tissue disruption, to graft subchondral bone defects and to apply an external fixation device that will provide neutralization of compression forces acting across the wrist until the time of healing. This is especially useful when, because of the size of the fragments, the holding power of screw or pin fixation is greatly diminished. Neutralization of the axial loading of the carpus prevents secondary impaction of small cartilage-bearing fragments. It is important to remain flexible when choosing internal fixation material, and to be able to change the preoperative decision on a particular implant depending on the quality of bone, the amount of comminution, and the quality of fixation obtained during the operation.

Inability to obtain an acceptable reduction of the joint surface depends on technical errors, such as insufficient exposure due to wrong election of surgical approach, and incorrect preoperative evaluation of the size and number of articular fragments, as well as lack of familiarity with internal and external fixation techniques. Most of the problems associated with the reduction of the fracture can be avoided if the procedure is performed on the basis of a careful preoperative plan. This includes a drawing of the separate fracture fragments with the final result and the possible implants to be used, but most importantly, it should include the tactical steps to follow during the procedure. Good preoperative planning orients the surgeon towards systematic reduction of a given fracture situation, and trains the young surgeon to analyse graphically a three-dimensional reconstruction. It also provides adequate choice of implants and reduces operative time, a factor that greatly diminishes tourniquet time and

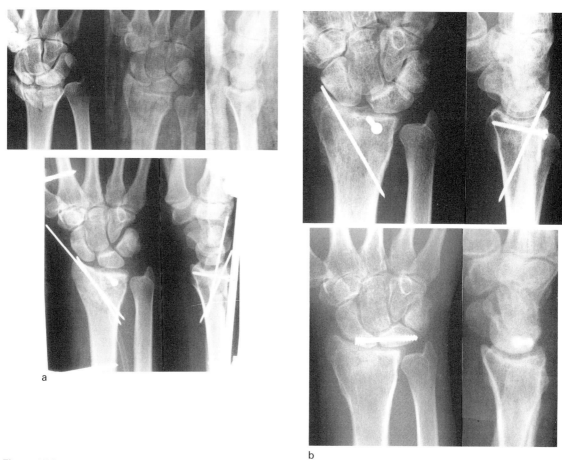

Figure 26.6

a) Top: Type III compression fracture in a patient with multiple injuries. Bottom: Adequate restoration of the joint surface is obtained with limited open reduction, bone grafting, and combined internal and external fixation. Note the mild axial scaphoid shift. b) Top: After removal of the frame at 6 weeks, the fracture is healed, but scapholunate dissociation and rotatory subluxation of the scaphoid are evident. Bottom: Radiographs taken 9 months after scapholunate ligament repair protected with Herbert screw fixation.

wound contamination. Intraoperative fluoroscopy and/or arthroscopy is strongly recommended to control joint reduction. In many cases, this removes the need to disrupt important capsular and ligamentous attachments of the wrist for extensive arthrotomies. Furthermore, the biconcave anatomy of the distal radius does not permit a direct and clear visualization of the whole joint surface.

Loss of reduction, although relatively frequent in conservative treatment with plaster fixation, is practically non-existent in fractures treated with external fixation. It may occur occasionally in osteoporotic patients, whose fractures are treated with percutaneous pinning alone. Loss of reduction is a potential complication if the surgeon has underestimated the degree of metaphyseal comminution and treats the fracture with pin or plate fixation, does not bone graft the metaphyseal area, and does not apply an external fixator to neutralize the axial load on the carpus.

Great care is required during the application of the external fixator. During insertion of the pins, iatrogenic damage to the tendons, nerves, and vascular structures should be avoided. The superficial branch of the radial nerve is at high risk during insertion of the pins for a dorso-radial frame in the distal forearm, or for percutaneous fixation of the radial styloid, and even at the base of the second metacarpal. The use of small stab incisions, or limited exposures as proposed by Seitz (1990), blunt separation of cutaneous nerves and underlying tendons, and the use of a drill guide diminishes this problem.

Prophylaxis to prevent pin-tract infection is achieved by preventing primary skin necrosis, making sure that the skin surrounding the pins is not under excessive tension, and by instructing the patient on daily pin care. Recent reports have shown that the incidence of pin-tract infection has been substantially reduced with refinement of pin insertion techniques, the use of threaded pins, and the pre-drilling of cortical bone to avoid heat necrosis (Cooney 1988, Howard et al. 1989, Wagner and Jakob 1985). However, pin loosening may occur in the early stages of treatment in cases with osteoporotic bone without associated pin-tract infection. This is invariably associated with loss of reduction. If this complication occurs in the first three weeks, pin removal and reapplication of a frame to prevent malunion is the treatment of choice.

Late pin loosening is practically always associated with pin-tract infection. In such situations removal of the frame, debridement of the pin tract and curettage of ring sequestra is imperative. Reapplication of a new external fixator or immobilization of the wrist in a plaster depends on the likelihood of shortening of the radius, as judged by radiographic evaluation of fracture healing at the time of onset of the pin-tract infection.

Since the current management protocol recommends that all fractures are grafted to permit early removal of the fixator (Leung et al. 1990), the potential complications of pin loosening and pin-tract infection have practically disappeared.

Postoperative management

Postoperative management varies, depending on whether or not the fracture of the distal radius is associated with concomitant soft tissue (ligamentous) or other skeletal (carpus, ipsilateral fractures of the upper extremity) injuries.

For simple articular fractures treated with percutaneous pinning or simple internal fixation with Kirschner wires or small plates, a sugar-tong splint is applied for a period of two weeks at the time that the sutures are removed. A short forearm cast with a window to allow for pin care is maintained for a further three weeks. For intra-articular fractures treated with open reduction, bone grafting, internal and external fixation, the frame is maintained for a period of five weeks. If the wrist was initially fixed in flexion and ulnar deviation at three weeks, it is brought to a neutral position to facilitate finger rehabilitation.

If the fracture of the distal radius is associated with primary repair of the triangular fibrocartilage or ulnar styloid fixation, forearm rotation is prevented by a sugar-tong splint applied for a period of three weeks in all cases (with or without external fixators). The arm is positioned at 45° supination to allow initial fibrous healing of the distal radio-ulnar joint capsule. If the fracture is associated with a primary scapholunate repair, forearm cast fixation after removal of the external fixator frame is continued for a total of eight weeks postoperatively.

For fractures of the distal radius with associated carpal bone injuries that have been treated with screw fixation, functional wrist postoperative treatment is begun after removal of the wrist fixator at five weeks. Active physiotherapy for the finger joints and elbow are started the day after surgery. After removal of the fixator a removable protection splint may be used for two more weeks between physiotherapy sessions. Dynamic splints may be necessary if joint contractures or tendon tightness are present. This is more common in open fractures with associated soft tissue lesions and forearm compartment syndrome. There are two indications to maintain a wrist fixator for over five weeks. The first is a complex injury with massive soft tissue defects that need secondary plastic coverage, and the second is a fracture complicated with acute infection.

Conclusions

Despite the fact that restoration of articular congruity to prevent secondary osteoarthritis after articular fractures is a well recognized concept in fracture treatment, fractures of the distal radius did not profit from this management principle for many years. Subsequently, long-term follow-up studies have demonstrated a strict correlation between wrist disability and post-traumatic deformity (Cassebaum 1950, Cooney et al. 1980, Frykman 1967, Gartland and Werley 1951, Knirk and Jupiter 1985, Martini 1986, McQueen and Caspers 1988, Scheck 1962, Smaill 1965, Younger and DeFiore 1977), so that current treatment has become more aggressive in an effort to optimize the functional outcome. The results have been consistently improved with percutaneous pinning (Castaing 1964, Clancey 1984, De Palma 1952, Epinette et al. 1982, Mortier et al. 1983, Mortier et al. 1986, Roth et al. 1977, Ruiz 1981, Stein and Katz 1975) with the use of external fixators (Anderson 1944, Cooney 1988, Cooney et al. 1979, Grana and Kopta 1979, Green 1975, Howard et al. 1989, Jakob and Fernandez 1982, Leung et al. 1990, Vaughn et al. 1985, Vidal et al. 1979, Wagner and Jakob 1985, Weber and Szabo 1986), and with percutaneous or open reduction techniques (Axelrod and McMurtry 1990, Axelrod et al. 1988, Bradway et al. 1989, DeOliveira 1973, Fernandez 1980, Fernandez and Geissler 1991, Fuller 1973, Melone 1984). The initial results of surgical restoration of the articular surface of the distal radius and its correlation with the functional results have been recently documented by various authors (Axelrod and McMurtry 1990, Bradway et al. 1989, Leung et al. 1990, Melone 1988, Sanders et al. 1991).

Our own results (Fernandez and Geissler 1991) have shown a satisfactory extra-articular alignment in 85% of the cases treated, and in 92.5% of the patients there was a residual articular incongruity of 1 mm or less at late follow-up. Although the average follow-up in this series was four years, radiographic evidence of radiocarpal arthritis was present in only 5% of the cases at late follow-up. The clinical results correlated with the radiographic findings in the great majority of patients. The incidence of post-traumatic arthritis seems to depend on the ability to restore the best possible articular congruity. However, the overall functional result depends not only on restoration of the joint surface, but also on early rehabilitation of the wrist and hand, and the initial adequate treatment of concomitant injuries.

Upon reviewing 115 articular fractures of the distal radius (Fernandez, 1993), an additional procedure for concomitant skeletal or soft tissue injuries was performed in 54% of the cases. In this group, Type III compression fractures of the articular surface accounted for 52% of the patient population, type II shearing fractures for 37%, radiocarpal dislocations (avulsion fractures) for 6% and combined fractures (high-velocity injuries — type V) for 4% of the cases.

Out of a total of 115 fractures, restoration of the joint surface was obtained by open reduction in 70% of the cases, by percutaneous manipulation in 18.2%, and by closed reduction in 14.7%. The great majority of the shearing fractures of the joint surface were stabilized with plate fixation. In the type III compression fractures, two-thirds of the patients were treated with external fixation, the majority with combined internal fixation and bone graft, while the remaining one-third represented the simple articular fractures that could be stabilized with percutaneous Kirschner wires alone.

The fact that over two-thirds of the patient population needed open reduction of the joint surface reinforces the author's opinion that it is worth aiming for anatomic reduction or improved articular congruity to a lower limit of a 1 mm step-off at the joint surface. Primary fusion of the joint surface was performed in only 2.6% of the cases treated. Bone grafting is used systematically now to replace cancellous bone loss in compression fractures, to provide mechanical support of small cartilage-bearing fragments, and to accelerate bone healing, allowing early removal of wrist fixators.

References

Anderson R, O'Neil G. Comminuted fractures of the distal end of the radius. *Surg Gynecol Obstet* 1944; **78**: 434–40.

Axelrod TJ, McMurtry RY. Open reduction and internal fixation of comminuted intra-articular fractures of the distal radius. *J Hand Surg* 1990; **15A**: 1–11.

Axelrod, T, Paley D, Green J, McMurtry RY. Limited open reduction of the lunate facet in comminuted intra-articular fractures of the distal radius. *J Hand Surg* 1988; **13A**: 372–77.

Bacorn RW, Kurtzke JF. Colles' fracture: A study of two thousand cases from the New York State Women's Compensation Board. *J Bone Joint Surg* 1953; **35A**: 643–58.

Bradway JK, Amadio PC, Cooney WP. Open reduction and internal fixation of displaced comminuted intra-articular fractures of the distal end of the radius. *J Bone Joint Surg* 1989; **71A**: 839–47.

Bowers WH. Distal radioulnar joint arthroplasty: The hemiresection-interposition technique. *J Hand Surg* 1985; **10A**: 169–78.

Cassebaum WH. Colles' fracture: A study of end results. *JAMA* 1950; **143**: 963–65.

Castaing J. Les fractures recentes de l'extrémité inférieure du radius chez l'adulte. *Rev Chir Orthop* 1964; **50**: 581–696.

Clancey GJ. Percutaneous Kirschner wire fixation of Colles' fractures. A prospective study of thirty-five cases. *J Bone Joint Surg* 1984; **66A**: 1008–14.

Cooney WP. Distal radius fractures: external fixation. In: Barton NJ, ed. *Fractures of the Hand and Wrist*, vol 4. Edinburgh: Churchill Livingstone, 1988: 290–301.

Cooney WP, Dobyns JH, Linscheid RL. Complications of Colles' fractures. *J Bone Joint Surg* 1980; **62A**: 613–19.

Cooney WP, Linscheid RL, Dobyns JH. External pin fixation for unstable Colles' fractures. *J Bone Joint Surg* 1979; **61A**: 840–45.

Cooney WP, Linscheid RL, Dobyns JH. Fractures and dislocations of the wrist (Chapter 8). In: Rockwood CA, Green DP, eds. *Fractures in Adults*, 3rd edn. Philadelphia: JB Lippincott Company, 1991: 563–678.

DeOliveira JC. Barton's fractures. *J Bone Joint Surg* 1973; **55A**: 586–94.

De Palma AF. Comminuted fractures of the distal end of the radius treated by ulnar pinning. *J Bone Joint Surg* 1952; **34A**: 651–62.

Ellis J. Smith's and Barton's fractures — a method of treatment. *J Bone Joint Surg* 1968; **47B**: 724–27.

Epinette JA, Lehut JM, Cavenaile M, Bouretz JC, Decoulx J. Fracture de Pouteau-Colles: Double embrochage intrafocal en berceau selon Kapandji. *Ann Chir Main* 1982; **1**: 71–83.

Fernandez DL. Smith Frakturen. *Hefte zur Unfallheilk* 1980; **148**: 91–95.

Fernandez DL. Irreducible radiocarpal fracture-dislocation and radioulnar dissociation with entrapment of the ulnar nerve, artery and flexor profundus II–V – Case Report. *J Hand Surg* 1981; **6**: 456–61.

Fernandez DL. Correction of post-traumatic wrist deformity in adults by osteotomy, bone grafting and internal fixation. *J Bone Joint Surg* 1982; **64A**: 1164–78.

Fernandez DL. Avant-bras segment distal. In: Mueller ME, Nazarian S, Koch P, eds. *Classification AO des fractures. Les os longs*. Berlin, Heidelberg, New York: Springer-Verlag, 1987: 106–15.

Fernandez DL. Radial osteotomy and Bower's arthroplasty for malunited fractures of the distal end of the radius. *J Bone Joint Surg* 1988; **70A**: 1538–51.

Fernandez DL. Fractures of the distal radius: operative treatment. In: Heckman JD, ed. *Instructional Course Lectures*, American Academy of Orthopaedic Surgeons, volume 42, 1993: 73–88.

Fernandez DL, Geissler WB. Treatment of displaced articular fractures of the radius. *J Hand Surg* 1991; **16A**: 375–84.

Fernandez DL, Maeder G. Die Behandlung der Smith-Frakturen. *Arch Orthop Unfallchir* 1977; **88**: 153–61.

Fernandez DL, Jakob RP, Büchler U. External fixation of the wrist. Current indications and technique. *Ann Chir Gyn* 1983; **72**: 298–302.

Fuller DJ. The Ellis plate operation for Smith's fracture. *J Bone Joint Surg* 1973; **55B**: 173.

Frykman G. Fractures of the distal end of the radius, including sequelae — shoulder, hand, finger syndrome, disturbance in the distal radio-ulnar joint and impairment of nerve function. *Acta Orthop Scand (Suppl)* 1967; **108**: 1–155.

Gartland JJ, Werley CW. Evaluation of healed Colles' fractures. *J Bone Joint Surg* 1951; **33A**: 895–907.

Grana WA, Kopta JA. The Roger Anderson device in the treatment of fractures of the distal end of the radius. *J Bone Joint Surg* 1979; **61A**: 1234.

Green DP. Pins and plaster treatment of comminuted fractures of the distal end of the radius. *J Bone Joint Surg* 1975; **57A**: 304–10.

Herbert TJ. In: *The fractured scaphoid*. St Louis: Quality Medical Publishing, 1990: 184–89.

Howard PW, Stewart HD, Hind RE, Burke FD. External fixation or plaster for severely displaced comminuted Colles' fractures? *J Bone Joint Surg* 1989; **71B**: 68–73.

Jakob RP, Fernandez DL. The treatment of wrist fractures with the small AO external fixation device. In: Uhthoff HK, ed. *Current concepts of external fixation of fractures*. Berlin, Heidelberg: Springer Verlag, 1982: 307–14.

Knirk JL, Jupiter JB. Late results of intra-articular distal radius fractures in young adults. *Orthop Trans* 1985; **9**: 456.

Knirk, JL, Jupiter JB. Intra-articular fractures of the distal end of the radius in young adults. *J Bone Joint Surg* 1986; **68A**: 647–59.

Laverna CJ, Cohen MS, Taleisnik J. Treatment of scapholunate dissociation by ligamentons reqair and scaphilodesis. *J Hand Surg* 1992; **17A**: 354–9.

Leung KS, Tsang HK, Chiu KH et al. An effective treatment of comminuted fractures of the distal radius. *J Hand Surg* 1990; **15A**: 11–17.

Martini AK. Die sekundäre Arthrose des Handgelenkes bei der in Fehlstellung verheilten und nicht korrigierten distalen Radiusfraktur. *Akt Traumatol* 1986; **16**: 143.

McMurtry RY, Jupiter JB. Fractures of the distal radius. In: Browner B, Jupiter J, Levine A, Trafton P, eds. *Skeletal Trauma*. Philadelphia: WB Saunders, 1991: **2**: 1063–94.

McQueen M, Caspers J. Colles fracture: Does the anatomic result affect the final function? *J Bone Joint Surg* 1988; **70B**: 649–51.

Melone CP. Articular fractures of the distal radius. *Orthop Clin North Am* 1984; **15**: 217–36.

Melone CP. Open treatment for displaced articular fractures of the distal radius. *Clin Orthop* 1986; **202**: 103–11.

Melone CP. Unstable fractures of the distal radius (Chapter 11). In: Lichtmann D, ed. *The wrist and its disorders*. Philadelphia: WB Saunders, 1988: 160–77.

Moberg E. Shoulder-hand-finger syndrome, reflex dystrophy, causalgia (Abstract). *Acta Chir Scand* 1963; **125**: 523.

Mortier JP, Kuhlmann JN, Richet C, Baux S. Brochage horizontal cubito-radial dans les fractures de l'extrémité inférieure du radius comportent un fragment postéro-interne. *Rev Chir Orthop* 1986; **72**: 567–71.

Mortier JP, Baux S, Uhl JF, Mimoun M, Mole B. Importance du fragment postéro-interne et son brochage spécifique dans les fractures de l'extrémité inférieure du radius. *Ann Chir Main* 1983; **2**: 219–29.

Müller ME, Nazarian S, Koch P, eds. *AO classification des fractures*. Berlin, Heidelberg, New York: Springer-Verlag, 1987: 106–15.

Roth, B, Müller J, Lusser G, Barone C, Bachmann B. Erfahrungen mit der perkutanen Spickdrahtosteosynthese bei distalen Radiusfrakturen. *Helv Chir Acta* 1977; **44**: 815–20.

Ruiz GR. Percutaneous pinning of comminuted Colles' fractures. *Clin Orthop* 1981; **195**: 290.

Sanders RA, Keppel FL, Waldrop JI. External fixation of distal radial fractures: results and complications. *J Hand Surg* 1991; **16A**: 385–91.

Scheck M. Long-term follow-up treatment of comminuted fractures of the distal end of the radius by transfixation with Kirschner wires and cast. *J Bone Joint Surg* 1962; **44A**: 337.

Seitz WH, Putnam MD, Dick HM. Limited open surgical approach for external fixation of distal radius fractures. *J Hand Surg* **15A**; 1990: 288–93.

Smaill GB. Long-term follow-up of Colles' fracture. *J Bone Joint Surg* 1965; **47B**: 80–85.

Stein AH, Katz SF. Stabilization of comminuted fractures of the distal inch of the radius: percutaneus pinning. *Clin Orthop* 1975; **108**: 174–81.

Stewart HD, Innes AR, Burke FD. Hand complication in Colles's fracture. *J Hand Surg* 1985; **10B(1)**: 103–6.

Vaughn PA, Lui SM, Harrington IJ, Maistrelli GL. Treatment of unstable fractures of the distal radius by external fixation. *J Bone Joint Surg* 1985; **67B**: 385–89.

Vidal J, Buscayret C, Connes H. Treatment of articular fractures by 'ligamentotaxis' with external fixation. In: Brooker A, Edwards CC, eds. *External Fixation. The Current State of the Art*. Baltimore: Williams and Wilkins, 1979: 75–81.

Villar RN, Marsh D, Rushton N, Greatorex RA. Three years after Colles' fracture. *J Bone Joint Surg* 1987; **69B**: 635–38.

Wagner HE, Jakob RP. Operative Behandlung der distalen Radiusfraktur mit Fixateur externe. *Unfallchirurg* 1985; **88**: 473–80.

Weber SC, Szabo RM. Severely comminuted distal radial fracture as an unsolved problem: complications associated with external fixation and pins and plaster techniques. *J Hand Surg* 1986; **11A**: 157–65.

Younger CP, DeFiore JC. Rupture of flexor tendons to the fingers after a Colles' fracture. A cast report. *J Bone Joint Surg* 1977; **59A**: 828.

27
Fixation of distal radial fractures: intramedullary pinning versus external fixation

JL Haas, JY de la Caffinière

Indications for conservative treatment of distal radial fractures, although applied with great care, were restricted after January 1985 in the authors' hospital, due to a significant rate of secondary displacement. The burden of treatment for loss of reduction was difficult to bear both for the patients and the surgical team, and it was decided to extend surgical treatment to all displaced fractures, whatever the patient's age.

Two methods were chosen:

1. fixation by distal to proximal intramedullary pinning (IMP), following the technique described by Py (1987), was used mostly for extra-articular fractures;
2. radiometacarpal external fixation, as described by Thomine and Demesy (1979) was used for communited metaphyseal distal radial fractures. This method was extended to all intra-articular fractures, comminuted or not, if pins were not able to provide a stable fixation.

The cases were reviewed after five years to determine the best indications for these two methods.

Patients

Over a period of four-and-a-half years, 142 distal radial fractures were treated by operation in 136 patients, six of whom had bilateral fractures. Most of the patients were between 40 and 70 years of age; 84 were female and 52 male.

The mechanism of fracture was always a combination of compression and extension: 75 of the fractures were extra-articular and 67 intra-articular. They were classified into 11 types according to the Kapandji system (1976) (Table 27.1).

After reduction, IMP was used in 96 cases and external fixation in 46, the type of fracture and the bone density guiding this choice.

Table 27.1 Anatomical types (Kapandji classification) 142 fractures (9 records lost to follow-up)

KAPANDJI types	PROXIMAL INTRA MEDULLARY pinning	EXTERNAL FIXATION
Type 1	30	0
Type 2	39	6
Type 3	18	18
Type 4	5	2
Type 3+4	4	7
Type 5	0	2
Type 6	0	1
Type 9	0	10

Methods

Intramedullary pinning

The principle of this technique is determined by the elastic characteristics of the two long, intramedullary transepiphyseal pins (Fig. 27.1):

- the first pin, inserted through the apex of the radial styloid prevents loss of the radial angulation;

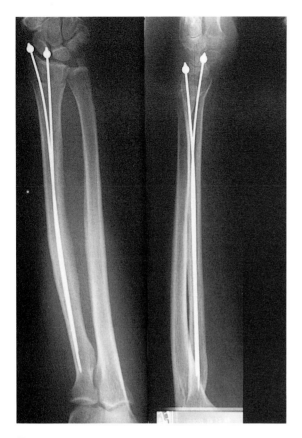

Figure 27.1

Intramedullary pinning: one pin is inserted laterally and the other posteriorly.

- the second pin, inserted posteriorly near Lister's tubercle, prevents dorsal tilt.

In this study the pins were positioned after dorsal reduction, unlike Py's technique. Great care should be taken to avoid injury to the tendons, vessels and nerves and two small approaches are necessary. Fluoroscopy will aid in directing the pins. The pins are based on those used by Ilizarov (1971); these have been modified by the addition of an 'olive' to the end of the pin (de la Caffinière and Vignes 1989). This provides optimal support for the bone, prevents distal migration, is a protection for tendinous structures and makes proximal migration more difficult. This method is not indicated in young people with a good bone density when the medullary canal is narrow and difficult to penetrate. In these cases, double radiostyloid pin fixation is still used.

Postoperative immobilization is achieved using a removable splint which is worn constantly for three weeks, and then progressively weaned from the patient over a further three weeks.

Radiometacarpal external fixation

This procedure is intended to prevent recurrence of dorsal tilt. The fixator is mainly posterior and composed of two groups of two pins, linked by a posterior rod. The pins for the radius penetrate through a short dorsal approach at the distal quarter of the postero-lateral surface of the radius. Great care should be taken to avoid injuries of the nervous and tendinous structures. The metacarpal pins are inserted under fluoroscopic control at the postero-lateral border of the proximal epiphysis of the second metacarpal, preserving the index extensor tendons. The rod is fixed without applying longitudinal distraction (Fig. 27.2).

Early rehabilitation is performed particularly on forearm prono-supination and finger motion.

Results of intramedullary pinning

Global anatomical results

Anatomy was assessed on antero-posterior (AP) and lateral radiographic views, using the standard four criteria (Fig. 27.3):

- radial angulation;
- dorsal angulation;
- line passing through the radial and ulnar styloid (the bistyloid line);
- ulnar variance.

These radiographic measurements (Table 27.2) allow classification of the anatomical results into four groups:

a) anatomical reduction;
b) under-reduced;
c) grossly under-reduced;
d) failures (non-reduced or over-reduced).

The initial anatomical reduction was quoted as 'good' anatomical result or under-reduced in 61

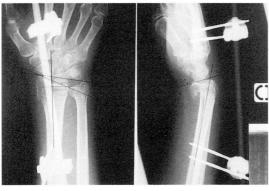
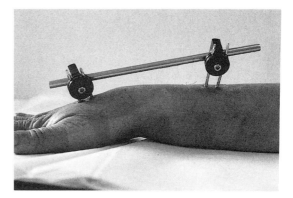
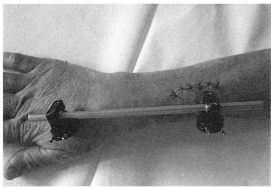

Figure 27.2

Radiometacarpal external fixation. The pins are inserted postero-laterally and linked by a posterior rod. The short dorsal control approach is distant from the pins' points of entry.

out of 87 fractures (70%) with a complete radiological record: of the remainder, 21 were categorized as inadequate and 5 as failures.

The final anatomical result, measured after 45 days, was not so good. Only 34 out of 77 fractures (44%) were judged to be 'good' (note that 10 patients were lost for follow-up). Of the remainder, 17 were categorized as inadequate and 26 as failures. Secondary displacement occurred in 46 out of 77 patients.

Secondary displacement

Two different types of secondary displacement were observed:

- Secondary displacements, usual in these types of fractures, reproducing the initial displacement in a more or less complete way, with dorsal tilt or loss of radial angulation of the epiphysis (Fig. 27.4). This pattern was seen in 12 cases, 8 with dorsal tilt, 2 with loss of radial angulation, and 2 with dorsal tilt and loss of radial angulation. All of the cases with a dorsal tilt were observed when the posterior pin had been inserted in too lateral a position (Fig. 27.5).
- Over-reduction with a progressive verticalization of the radial angulation on the AP view, without noted modification on the lateral view (Fig. 27.6). This is not found with classical pinning, and occurs more frequently: 34 cases were found in this series.

Increase in dorsal angulation of extra-articular fractures is explained in two out of three cases by inadequate fixation, when the two pins are inserted laterally and their combined elastic action pushes on the distal fragment (Fig. 27.7). Posterior comminution concentrated on the medial part of the radius exacerbates the increase in

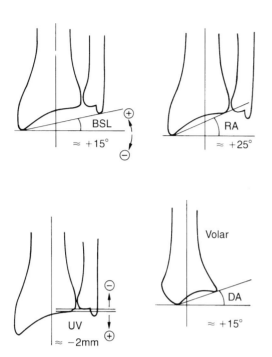

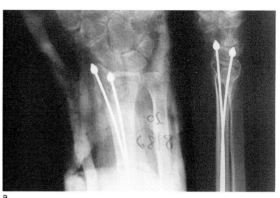

Figure 27.3

Radiographic measurements: bistyloid line (BSL), radial angulation (RA), AP view, dorsal angulation (DA), lateral view, and ulnar variance (UV).

Figure 27.4

Secondary dorsal tilt complicating intramedullary pinning. Two examples of bad fixation: a) the lateral pin is too anteriorly inserted (anterior border of the styloid); b) the posterior pin is too lateral (posterior border of the styloid).

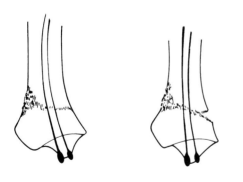

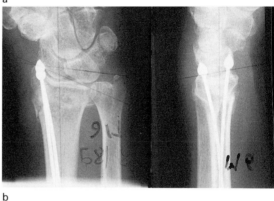

Figure 27.5

IMP: pathomechanism of the secondary dorsal tilt. The posterior pin is too lateral and cannot prevent the dorsal displacement. The lateral pin is too anterior and pushes the epiphysis backwards.

dorsal angulation. In some cases, verticalization occurred although the fixation was adequate: these cases were extra-articular fractures associated with an ulnar neck or head fracture where there is nothing to oppose the elastic action of the pin (Fig. 27.8). Therefore, ulnar fractures are a contraindication to this method.

Other extra-articular fractures had the same displacement with an adequate fixation. This included the very distal fractures in elderly people with a comminuted postero-medial fragment and porotic bone (Figs 27.9 and 27.10).

Increase in dorsal angulation of intra-articular fractures is an almost constant feature and is related to the inadequacy of internal fixation. More than two-thirds of fractures with a frontal

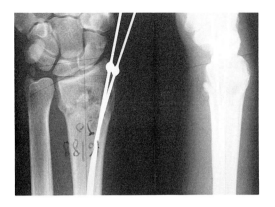

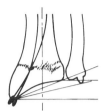 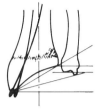

Figure 27.7

IMP: pathomechanism of secondary verticalization. The two pins are inserted laterally and their elastic action in the frontal plane causes verticalization of the epiphysis.

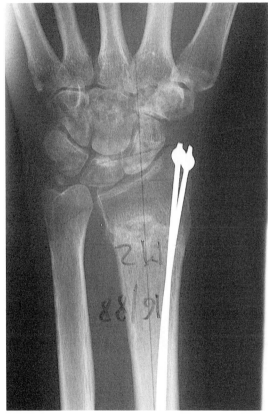

Figure 27.6

Secondary verticalization. Imperfect fixation: the two pins are lateral. Loss of pin curvature and positive ulnar variance are indicative of secondary displacement.

T-line or with a postero-medial fragment and all four fragment fractures have resulted in dorsal angulation of the distal radius (Figs 27.11 and 27.12). Anterior tilt is very rare (two cases in this series).

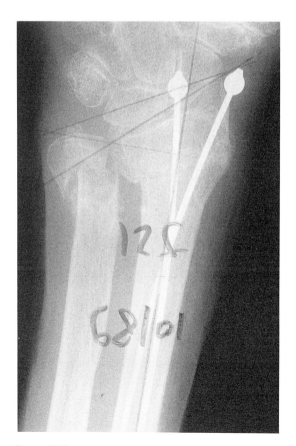

Figure 27.8

IMP: extra-articular fracture of the distal radius associated with an ulnar head fracture. There is secondary verticalization with ulnar shift due to loss of medial support.

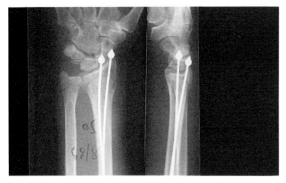
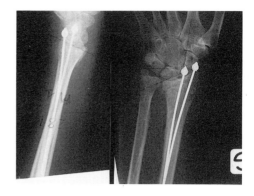

Figure 27.9

IMP: verticalization of a correctly fixed distal radial fracture in an elderly patient.

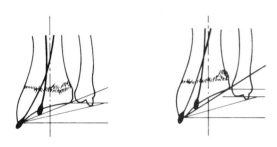

Figure 27.10

Pathomechanism of verticalization with a correct fixation. There is impaction at the site of medial comminution.

Thus, there are two contraindications to intramedullary pinning: intra-articular fractures and distal radius fractures associated with an ulnar neck fracture.

Complications

Few complications were noted. There was only one superficial infection. One case of sympathic dystrophy and one case of paresthesia in the radial nerve area were noted. Extensor pollicis longus (EPL) tendon rupture, or pin rupture or migration, were not noted.

Results of external fixation

This method was used to treat 46 cases: 6 extra-articular fractures and 40 intra-articular fractures, half of which were three-fragment and half four-fragments fractures. The mean age was lower than for the entire series.

Anatomical results

These were assessed using the measurements shown in Table 27.2. Four records were not complete, so out of 42 cases, the initial anatomical result was considered 'good' (perfect reduction or under-reduced) in 23 (55%), inadequate in 11 and a failure in 8 cases. After three months, the number categorized as 'good' had dropped to 18 (43%), the number judged inadequate had risen to 13 and the number deemed a failure had increased to 11. There were only six secondary displacements: less than with intramedullary pinning.

Secondary displacement

Two different types of displacement were observed:

- secondary displacement of apparently healed distal fracture component with total posterior displacement, and with a displaced radial joint orientation (Fig. 27.13). This was seen in six cases;
- secondary displacement of one fragment, usually involving a medial or postero-medial fragment, proximally and dorsally displaced (Fig. 27.14). This was seen in five cases. In one

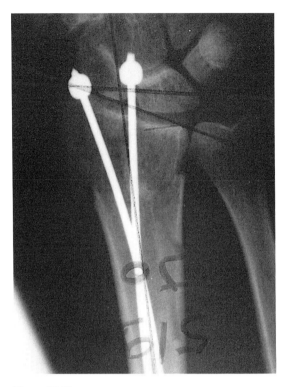 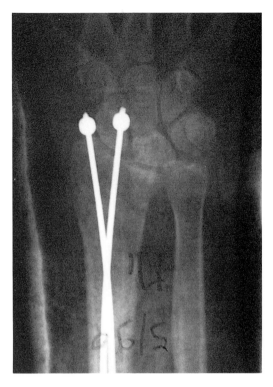

Figure 27.11

IMP: verticalization of a correctly fixed intra-articular T frontal fracture.

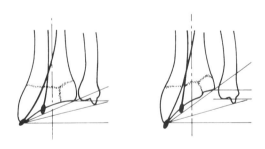

Figure 27.12

Pathomechanism of the verticalization of a T frontal fracture. The proximal migration of the medial fragment allows the verticalization of the epiphysis.

case, it involved a small radial styloid fragment. These fragment displacements do not alter the global radiograph measurements.

These two types of displacement do not take place at the same stage of therapy, except for one case (Fig. 27.15) where the global displacement occurred early, explained by an antero-lateral instead of a postero-lateral external fixation. The global displacement is seen if the external fixator is removed before two months, whereas the fragment displacement takes place earlier, when the external fixator is still in place.

It can be concluded, therefore, that an extra-articular fracture needs two months to heal and the posterior empty space left after reduction needs much longer. The external fixator does not stabilize an articular postero-medial or radial styloid fragment. In these cases, additional pin fixation is necessary (Fig. 27.16).

Complications

Again, few complications were noted. There was just one case of sympathetic dystrophy and three cases of pin infection.

Table 27.2 Analysis of radiological results

	BSL	RA	UV	DA
Perfect reduction	10–20°	20–30°	−2–0 mm	10–20°
Under-reduced	5–10°	10–20°	0–2 mm	0–10°
Grossly under-reduced	0–5°	0–10°	−2–4 mm	−10–0°
Failure	>20° <0°	>30° <0°	>4 mm	<−10°

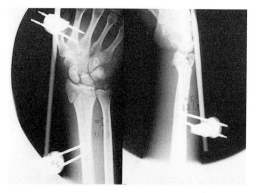
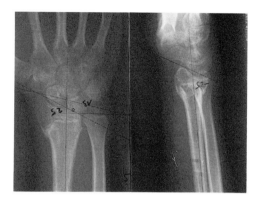

Figure 27.13
Secondary displacement after external fixation. Dorsal tilt has occurred after early removal of an external fixator that was correctly inserted.

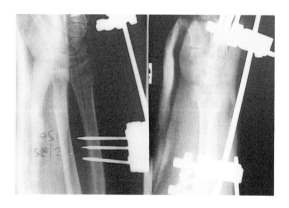
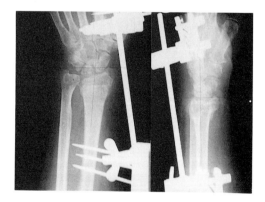

Figure 27.14
Secondary displacement after external fixation. The postero-medial fragment was not fixed and has displaced proximally and dorsally. There is positive ulnar variance.

Functional results

The follow-up time for this series was short: 33 out of 96 fractures treated by intramedullary fixation (IMF) had a mean five-and-a-half months follow-up while 20 out of 46 fractures treated by external fixation had a mean five months follow-up.

The final result can be assessed only after one year, but some remarks can be made. The two methods have similar results but each has its own indications (Table 27.3). Motion in

Table 27.3 Results of mobility in flexion-extension

Method of treatment		30°	30–50°	50–70°
External fixation (20 cases)	Flexion	1	17	2
	Extension	11	7	2
Intramedullary fixation (33 cases)	Flexion	4	24	5
	Extension	11	18	4

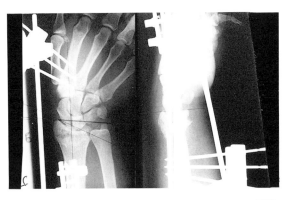
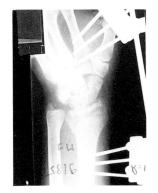
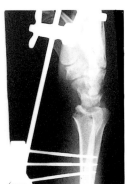
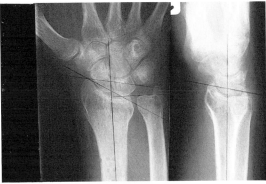

Figure 27.15

External antero-lateral fixation. Early dorsal tilt (M1), leading to a dorsal orientation of the radial articular surface.

prono-supination (mainly supination) was limited in half of the patients treated by IMF and in two-thirds of the patients treated by external fixation, although the elbow had never been immobilized (Table 27.4). This loss of pronation and supination was not related to the ulnar variance but it could possibly be related to a rotary malunion: the reduction maneuver promoted by Castaing in flexion and pronation can lead to an over-reduction and healing in pronation of the distal fragment, thus reducing motion in supination.

Discussion

Extra-articular fractures

A simple, secure and rapid method of treatment should be applied to the very frequent Colles' fracture. Direct pin fixation combined with a cast was utilized by Castaing in 1964. The disadvantage of this treatment was a high recurrence of redisplacement due to poor bone density and the inability to prevent dorsal tilt. In 1976, Kapandji

Table 27.4 Results of mobility in prono-supination

Method of treatment	Normal	Pronation	Supination	Prono-supination
External fixation (20 cases)	7	0	10	3
Intramedullary fixation (33 cases)	17	1	10	5

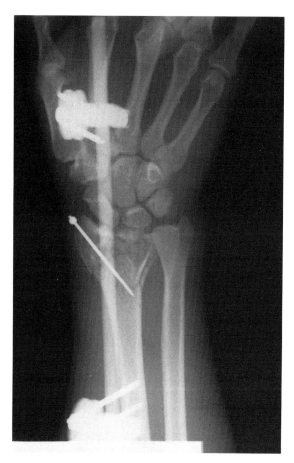

Figure 27.16
External fixator combined with pin fixation of an unstable radial styloid fragment.

proposed an intrafocal pinning with modified pins to prevent the dorsal tilt.

IMF uses transepiphyseal pins inserted into the medullary canal, with an elastic support on the proximal cortical bone, which is of better density. The use of special pins (Desmanet 1989) avoids tendon injuries and migration problems (de la Caffinière and Vignes 1989). Rehabilitation is possible when this method is applied to Colles' fractures, but not to intra-articular fractures or radial styloid fractures. Great care should be taken in positioning the pins with the aid of fluoroscopy.

Intra-articular fractures

Treatment of intra-articular fractures has two aims: to restore the anatomy of the intra-articular fractures, and to maintain the epiphysis (distal radius fracture components) in this good position during healing.

Fractures with a postero-medial fragment are a contraindication to the methods described here. This fragment can be treated by direct ulnar-radial pinning (Mortier and Baux 1983), intrafocal pinning (Kapandji 1991) or direct pinning (Desmanet 1989). Direct ulnar-radial pinning involves the insertion of a pin, under fluoroscopy, 3–4 cm proximal to the radial styloid and then directed distally and obliquely to the PMF to fix it.

Complex fractures cannot be fixed by pins alone. After reduction, loss of dorsal bone will result in secondary displacement. This can be treated either by a direct surgical approach, with operative reduction, K-wire fixation, and filling of the defect with bone graft or other material, or by external fixation, relying on the spontaneous ossification of the defect while the normal radio-carpal length is restored. One or several pins can be added to the external fixator, which should be left in place for two months.

Conclusions

IMF is appropriate for extra-articular Colles' fractures. External fixation is appropriate for complex or comminuted intra-articular fractures.

Application of the external fixator must follow several rules:

- gentle, but not permanent, distractions;
- no skin tension or interference with tendons by the pins;
- additional pins for unstable fragments;
- external fixation removal after two months.

Early rehabilitation of forearm prono-supination and finger flexion gives good functional results for complex fractures. External fixation has been extended to some extra-articular fractures. In six cases with osteoporotic bones it has produced good results without secondary displacement or complications. In these cases, the external fixator can be removed before the end of the second month.

The current treatment recommendations for extra-articular fractures are:

- undisplaced or with little displacement: conservative treatment;
- displaced: IMF;
- displaced in a young patient, or with associated ulnar fractures: direct intraosseous pins penetrating the radial styloid;
- distal fracture in an old osteoporotic patient: external fixation.

The current treatment recommendations for intra-articular fractures are:

- with a postero-medial fragment or with three fragments (T shape): two direct intraosseous pins plus one oblique pin for the PMF;
- complex intra-articular fractures: external fixation plus direct pinning of unstable fragments.

References

Boudot O. Les fractures complexes de l'extrémité inférieure du radius traitées par fixateur externe métacarpo-radial. Résultats. (A propos d'une série de 68 cas.) Service du Pr. Thomine. Thèse 1981. Rouen.

Castaing J, le Club des Dix. Les fractures récentes de l'extrémité inférieure du radius chez l'adulte. Rapport de la XXXIX Réunion Annuelle de la SOFCOT. Rev Chir Orthop 1964; **50**: 581–696.

Cooney WP, Linscheid RL, Dobyns JH. External pin fixation for unstable Colles' fractures. J Bone Joint Surg 1979; **61A**: 840–45.

de la Caffinière JY, Vignes B. Saint Denis. La broche boutonnée: un moyen simple d'éviter la migration dans les ostéosynthèses légères. Rev Chir Orthop 1989; **75**: 573–74.

Desmanet E. L'ostéosynthèse par double embrochage du radius. Traitement fonctionnel des fractures de l'extrémité inférieure du radius. A propos d'une série de 130 cas. Ann Chir Main 1989; **8,3**: 193–206.

Ilizarov GA. Basic principle of transosseous compression and distraction osteosynthesis. Rev Orthop Traumatol Protes 1971; **11**: 7–15.

Kapandji A. L'ostéosynthèse par double embrochage intra-focal. Traîtement fonctionnel des fractures non articulaires de l'extrémité inférieure du radius. Ann Chir 1976; **30(11–12)**: 903–8.

Kapandji A. L'embrochage intra-focal des fracture de l'extrémité inférieure du radius dix ans après. Ann Chir Main 1987; **6,1**: 57–63.

Kapandji A. Les broches intra-focales à "effet de réduction" de type "ARUM" dans l'ostéosynthèse des fractures de l'extrémité inférieure du radius. Ann Chir Main 1991; **10,2**: 138–45.

Mortier JP, Baux S. Importance du fragment postéro-interne, et son brochage spécifique dans les fractures de l'extrémité inférieure du radius. Ann Chir Main 1983; **2**: 219–29.

Py C. Embrochage des fractures de l'extrémité inférieure du radius, technique Py. Communication aux journées militaires de Chirurgie Orthopédique et Traumatologique de l'Hôpital Begin. 1987.

Rossillon D, Boute B, Hubert M. Etude sur le fixateur externe dans le traitement des fractures de l'extrémité inférieure des deux os de l'avant-bras de l'adulte. A propos de 55 cas. Ann Chir Main 1987; **6,1**: 25–30.

Thomine JM, Demesy M. Le fixateur externe dans le traitement des fractures graves de l'extrémité inférieure du radius. Ann Chir 1979; **33**: 731–34.

28
Indications for open treatment of intra-articular fractures of the distal radius

Ch Mathoulin, E de Thomasson, Th Judet, Ph Saffar

Introduction

The therapeutic difficulties encountered with articular fractures are far from simple. Reduction should be performed as early as possible to avoid development of edema which can impede a successful outcome. In addition to controlling swelling, a precise radiological analysis can be made following reduction with traction in the operating room. Open surgical reduction is needed quite frequently in these cases to obtain adequate fracture stabilization. When possible local anaesthesia should be used during the procedure.

The indications for treatment in this chapter are based on the classification system described in Chapter 16. The study of a series of 137 articular fractures in the young adult (Mathoulin 1990) showed the following:

1. Whatever the type of fracture, orthopaedic treatment was not shown to be completely effective for articular fractures.
2. Certain fractures were underestimated or overestimated by the classification when considering the degree of displacement; this resulted in therapeutic errors.

For this reason, we chose to treat the patients in this study according to the stages of our classification only after post reduction radiological assessment. Stable fixation was easier to obtain in type 1 than in type 4 fractures.

Choice of therapy according to fracture type

Type 1

These are fractures with one articular fracture line in the frontal plane. The use of an anterior (volar) plate is well accepted and has been shown to be effective (Augerau 1983). The approach should be palmar and systematically associated with an opening of the flexor retinaculum of the forearm and wrist (transverse carpal ligament).

V or Kerboul-type plates can be used with proximal screws. The anterior curvature of the moulded plate effectively maintains the anterior marginal fragment in a reduced position. In certain cases, distal screws can be used. The posterior (dorsal) cortex must not be transfixed to avoid the risk of tendinous lesions. Articular dorsal and palmar marginal fractures are not included in type 1 of this classification system and the use of a simple plate to treat these cases is usually a failure.

For posterior (dorsal) marginal fractures, closed reduction treatment can be used in cases in which there is no significant displacement. However, the technique described by Judet (1958) is preferable; this utilizes palmar flexion and ulnar deviation for three weeks. In fact, this technique should avoid secondary dorsal displacement. Palmar flexion is released after the third week and replaced by a straight plaster cast for a further three weeks. Because a short cast is used, this technique avoids stiffness of the elbow. It is without risk so long as the rules mentioned above are strictly applied.

In dorsal marginal fractures with marked displacement, a dorsal approach with posterior-anterior screws is recommended to hold the fracture reduction. It is important not to injure tendons or nerves during this procedure.

Type 2

Type 2 fractures have one fracture line in the sagittal plane, which extends into one of the articular facets of the distal radius (scaphoid, lunar or distal radio-ulnar joints).

Pins in two different axes

This technique should be used in fractures into the scaphoid and lunate fossae (type 2 fractures). In these cases the styloid pin described by DePalma (1952) is used. A skin incision is made so that muscles and nerves which might be involved in the procedure can be identified or protected. Two cross pins are inserted. One pin passes into the radial styloid between the radial wrist extensor tendons and the short extensor and long abductor tendons of the thumb, while the second pin passes ulnar to Lister's turbercle. These pins are inserted across the opposite cortex to secure rigid fixation. This technique usually requires plaster cast immobilization in addition to the pinning.

In cases of incomplete reduction of the fracture fragments, the surgical approach can be enlarged radially. A screw can also be used, which provides quite stable fixation.

Evidence of scapholunate instability is an absolute indication for surgery. A dorsal approach is used so that reduction of the radial styloid fragment can be verified and the scapholunate ligament repaired. Two pins should be inserted across the scapholunate joint for six weeks (Fig. 28.1).

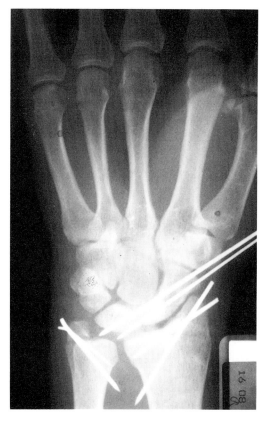

Figure 28.1

Distal radial fracture type II. This fracture has been treated by double crossed pinning of the lateral fragment, double scapholunate pinning after ligament repair and ulnar styloid pinning.

Type 3

Type 3 fractures are T-fractures with a horizontal extra-articular line and a vertical articular line.

Closed reduction and cast immobilization

This technique should be limited to the rare cases of fractures without or with only minimal displacement. It requires regular radiographic supervision. When used for type 2 radio-ulnar fractures treated by reduction with palmar flexion-pronation and ulnar deviation, close radiographic supervisions and follow-up are also indicated.

Triple intrafocal pinning

Triple intrafocal pinning is performed according to the technique described by Kapandji (1976). This procedure, which is the authors' technique of choice, seems to be the simplest and most effective for these cases (Fig. 28.2) but it requires adherence to several strict rules:

- always place the pins after the reduction;
- insert the pins through cortical bone using a

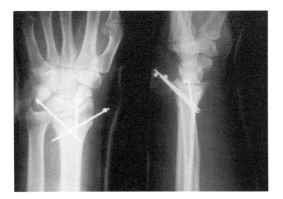

Figure 28.2

Triple intrafocal pinning for distal radial fracture type III.

power drill at low speed. Back and forth movement should be avoided to limit pin loosening;
- two pins must be placed dorsally, with at least one to hold the postero-medial fragment in the correct position;
- the pins are left sticking out of the skin and protected by strict and regular dressing changes.

Utilizing this technique, we have not had any tendon ruptures or pin infections, and the pins can be removed easily in the consultation room without local anaesthesia. A resting splint should be used for three weeks to avoid pain during the first few days and to give any existing intra-carpal ligament lesions the time to heal.

In some cases, operative treatment may be necessary to reduce the medial fragments. In this case a dorsal approach is used for pin insertion and in some cases a radio-ulnar pin, as described by Mortier (1986), can be used. In cases with significant displacement where stability is uncertain, the anterior (palmar) approach makes it possible to perform accurate reduction followed by application of an anterior T-plate for immobilization.

Type 4

Type 4 fractures have four fragments, an extra-articular horizontal fracture line, and two articular lines in the frontal and sagittal planes.

In these cases an operative approach is generally recommended, especially for young patients (Bassett 1987, Knirk and Jupiter 1986, Melone 1986). The fractures have a high potential for displacement, and are generally treated with triple pins (Kapandji technique) supported by an anterior plate, which provides the correct curvature for the distal end of the radius (Fig. 28.3). In certain type 4 fractures with minimal displacement, a triple pin associated with an anterior splint may be sufficient. In these cases, the fracture must be closely supervised and surgery performed at the first sign of displacement.

The anterior plate is applied by a palmar approach after initial reduction and K-wire fixation. Distal screws cannot be used with multifragment fractures. Thus, reduction fixation is

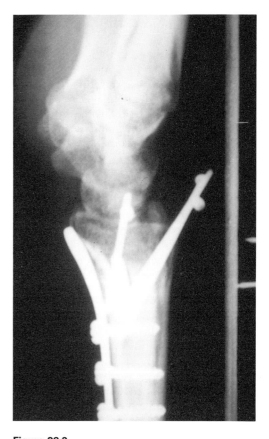

Figure 28.3

Distal radial fracture type IV. This fracture has been treated by triple intrafocal pinning (dorsal and lateral) and an anterior plate.

achieved first, using either a classic intrafocal pin as described by Kapandji, or by fragment-to-fragment fixation to assure proper stability. A double approach, both palmar and dorsal, may be necessary either to reduce a postero-medial fragment (which cannot be achieved by simple traction), or to pull down a central fragment.

Surgical treatment of type 4 fractures by bone fixation and wrist distraction

An external fixator can be used to treat the type 4 complex fracture. However, the use of external fixation does not solve all the eventual problems and ligamentotaxis, as shown by Bartosh and Saldana (1990), cannot reduce all of the displacement, especially dorsal angulation and fracture displacement. Axelrod (1990) has also shown that the use of an external fixator alone cannot reduce all medial and central fragments, especially if there is depression of the articular surface.

Simple internal bone fixation, with or without a bone graft, can result in malunion, secondary to loss of reduction and displacement (about 50% of our cases). Rigid internal bone fixation should be considered in these cases, combining K-wire plate fixation and external fixation. This technique, combining internal and external fixation, avoids secondary collapse which may occur in 10–50% of cases (Chamay et al. 1983) without internal bone fixation after removal of a simple fixator. The use of an external fixator, however, can be associated with a significant number of complications (10–61% of patients) (Chamay 1987 and 1983, Clyburne 1984, Cooney 1983, Jenkins et al. 1987) and therefore must be carefully applied and the patient closely followed.

Although infections from the pins usually heal easily, this is not true for neurosympathetic dystrophy and articular stiffness, which may delay normal activity for 6–18 months. Careful K-wire insertion and application of external fixation is necessary to avoid the subcutaneous peripheral nerves.

With external fixation, early physiotherapy is impossible. However, reports associating internal bone fixation and external articulated fixation (wrist distraction) with early motion and immediate physiotherapy appear promising.

Function of the wrist distractor

The wrist distractor has been created in the Orthopedic Traumatology Unit of the Hôpital Tenon. It is an external device temporarily implanted with rods in the radial and second metacarpal diaphyses. The anatomical reduction is obtained with internal fixation.

The goals of this treatment include restoration of the articular profile of the proximal part of the joint while an axial loading force must be avoided as far as possible in order to prevent secondary displacement; there is early active and passive mobilization. The wrist distractor has two orthogonal axes allowing physiological motion. It supports two hinges whose rotation axes make a right angle. This 'Cardan' system allows all motion in flexion extension, radio-ulnar deviation and combined movements, while shielding the reduction from longitudinal stress. In addition, a longitudinal distraction can be adapted.

The wrist distractor is used in order to protect the internal fixation during the first 6 weeks, and the wrist is mobilized early in the post-operative period.

Presentation of the series

Surgery was performed in 19 patients with a type 4 fracture with central depression over a period of almost three years. This technique was used exclusively in the Orthopaedic Trauma Unit of the Tenon Hospital. In our series, there were 12 men and 7 women. The dominant wrist was involved in 14 cases. The average age at the time of the accident was 54.5 years with an age range of 29 to 87 years. The average follow-up was 13.5 months (minimum: 4 months; maximum: 28 months). There was significant posterior comminution in 13 cases.

The distractor was applied in neutralization in all cases, and released for immediate physiotherapy in 16 cases. In three cases, the distractor was released on the 15th day. Internal bone fixation consisted of:

- Kapandji pins alone (three cases);
- isolated anterior plate (nine cases);
- plate plus Kapandji pins (six cases);
- in one case no bone fixation was performed.

Complications

Complications were relatively frequent but generally not severe:

- one fracture of the second metacarpal;
- three pin infections: two healed with a local treatment; one required early pin removal and appropriate antibiotic therapy.
- Two patients presented with a neurogenic osteoporosis.

Results

Clinical result

At the last follow-up, 16 patients had no pain at rest but some during activity. Complications occurred in three patients:

- one patient is being treated for neurogenic osteoporosis
- one patient presented with pseudarthrosis;
- one patient presented with painful intra-articular malunion.

The patients returned to work, or their former activities, an average of 3.5 months after the accident (16 patients) with a minimum of 2.5 months and a maximum of 5.5 months.

Wrist motion

Wrist motion was generally good. Only one patient, markedly limited by pseudarthrosis, had a poor range of motion. The results of the series were as follows: average pronation of 84% (minimum 30°; maximum 90°); average supination of 78° (minimum 20°; maximum 80°); average palmar flexion of 57° (minimum 20°; maximum 70°); average dorsal flexion of 46° (minimum 20°; maximum 70°); and average ulnar deviation of 18.5° (minimum 10°; maximum 40°).

Radiological result

The relatively short follow-up period of this study does not allow an analysis of the complications or sequelae of this method of reduction. However, radiographic analysis provided information about the quality of the initial reduction and the stability during consolidation. The patients were followed up with AP and lateral radiographs at 8, 15, 21, 45 and 90 days after treatment, and then every three months. The criteria established by Castaing (1964) were used to analyse the results.

Articular surface: Initially, the articular surface in 13 patients were considered anatomical; one joint was congruent but enlarged; and five patients presented with a defect in the articular reduction of at least 1 mm. In one case, this was due to a poor reduction and because external fixation alone was used. At the latest follow-up, no changes in articular surface contour were noted.

Radio-ulnar index or dorsal-volar angulation. At follow-up, there were no changes in either the radio-ulnar index or the dorsal-volar angulation. A few cases had limitation of motion.

This technique appears to be effective in providing stability for the fracture during the healing period. There were only two secondary displacements due to an obvious mistake in K-wire placement.

Distraction during the procedure facilitated reduction. The use of a hinge-distractor allows immediate physiotherapy, and early rehabilitation. Out of 19 patients, 16 returned to work an average of 3.5 months after surgery. The low rate of reflex sympathetic dystrophy (2 cases out of 19 in this study) is encouraging, but does not eliminate the importance of releasing the carpal tunnel which was performed in 11 cases.

Conclusion

Intra-articular fractures pose more complex problems than are generally attributed to classical wrist fractures.

A precise radiological analysis can only be based on post-reduction images following traction and reduction in the operating room. Once the potential instability of the fracture has been assessed, treatment should achieve anatomical reduction with stable fixation. This stability is only rarely achieved by cast immobilization; most cases require surgical treatment. Analysis of radiological criteria allows evaluation of the quality of reduction. Careful follow-up and supervision of the fracture reduction in the four first weeks will help prevent loss of reduction and other complications. Treatment should be as precise and complete as possible to maximize the outcome and avoid the secondary problems associated with intra-articular fractures of the distal radius, which can be difficult to treat.

References

Augerau B, Lance D, Kerboul M.: L'ostéosynthèse par plaque des fractures instables du poignet à déplacement antérieur. *Int Orthop (SICOT)* 1983; **7**: 55–59.

Axelrod TS, McMurtry RY. Open reduction and internal fixation of comminuted, intra-articular fractures of the distal radius. *J Hand Surg* 1990; **15A**: 1–11.

Bartosh RA, Saldana MJ. Intra-articular fractures of the distal radius: a cadaver study to determine if ligamentotaxis restores radio-palmar tilt. *J Hand Surg* 1990; **15A**: 18–22.

Bassett R. Displaced intra-articular fractures of the distal radius. *Clin Orthop* 1987; **214**: 148–52.

Castaing J, le Club des Dix. Les fractures récentes de l'extrémité inférieure du radius chez l'adulté. *Rev Chir Orthop* 1964; **50**: 581–96.

Chamay A. Considérations sur les limites de tolérance du traitement conservateur des fractures du poignet. *Ann Chir* 1987; **3**: 340–42.

Chamay A, Meythias AM, Della Santa D. Le traitement des fractures instables du poignet par fixateur externe de Hoffman. Etude d'une série de 40 cas. *Rev Chir Orthop* 1983; **69**: 637–43.

Clyburne TA. Dynamic external fixation for comminuted intra-articular fractures of the distal end of radius. *J Bone Joint Surg* 1984; **66A7**: 1008–14.

Cooney WP, Linscheid RL, Dobyns JH. External pin fixation for unstable Colles' fractures. *J Bone Joint Surg* 1979; **61A**: 840–45.

DePalma AF. Comminuted fracture of the distal end of the radius treated by ulnar pinning. *J Bone Joint Surg* 1952; **34A**: 651.

Jenkins NH, Jones DG, Johnson SR. External fixation of Colles' fractures. An anatomical study. *J Bone Joint Surg* 1987; **69B**: 207–11.

Judet J, Judet R, Carcosta S. Le traitement des fractures de l'extrémité inférieure du radius. *Mém Acad Chir* 1958; **84**: 1035.

Kapandji A. L'ostéosynthèse par double brochage intrafocal: traitement fonctionnel des fractures articulaires de l'extrémité inférieure du radius. *Ann Chir* 1976; **30**: 903–6.

Knirk JL, Jupiter JB. Intra-articular fractures of the distal end of the radius in young adults. *J Bone Joint Surg* 1986; **68A**: 647–59.

Mathoulin Ch. *Fractures articulaires du radius chez l'adulte*. Expansion Scientifique Fr., cahier d'enseignement de la Société Française de Chirurgie de la Main, Tome 2, 1990.

Melone Jr CP. Open treatment for displaced articular fractures of the distal radius. *Clin Orthop Rel Res* 1986; **202**: 103–11.

Mortier JP, Kuhlmann JN, Richet C, Baux S. Brochage horizontal cubito-radial dans les fractures de l'extrémité inférieure du radius comportant un fragment postéro-interne. *Rev Chir Orthop* 1986; **72**: 467–571.

29
Treatment of complex comminuted fractures of the distal radius utilizing the internal distraction plate

Edward F Burke

Introduction

Comminuted intra-articular fractures of the distal radius are fraught with many problems including post-traumatic arthritis, joint stiffness, finger stiffness, malunion, non-union, compression neuropathies, and reflex sympathetic dystrophy. Achieving an anatomic closed reduction and maintaining the reduction can be almost impossible. The goals of care are to anatomically reduce the fracture and to prevent collapse of the fracture site once reduction has been achieved. To realize these goals, many procedures have been attempted, such as closed reduction with casting, percutaneous pinning, pins and plaster, and the use of external fixators. However, complications with these methods, including pin-tract infection, pin loosening, finger and elbow stiffness, and fracture collapse have been encountered. Incongruity of the joint surface is the main cause of post-traumatic arthritis (Knirk and Jupiter 1986). If the articular surface is not reduced anatomically, treatment of the fracture by closed means has yielded poor results (Knirk and Jupiter 1986, Scheck 1962). Anatomic reduction should be achieved, and fixation should be performed to hold the reduction. The external fixator, as well as pins and plaster, have been used to hold the reduction; however, there are significant complications associated with this protocol.

In an attempt to eliminate these problems, a novel approach was developed for treatment of this fracture. The fracture is opened and anatomically fixed; however, in addition to this, the fracture is rigidly held with an internal distraction plate.

Patients and methods

Ten consecutive patients with severely comminuted intra-articular fractures of the distal radius were treated with open reduction and the insertion of an internal distraction plate (Fig. 29.1) The Frykman fracture classification was used — seven patients were classified as Frykman type VIII, and three as Frykman type VII. The age of the patients ranged from 29 to 65 years, with an average age of 40.9 years. There were 7 male and 3 female patients.

Each patient underwent surgical intervention consisting of open reduction and internal fixation through a longitudinal dorsal incision. After anatomical reduction was achieved, application

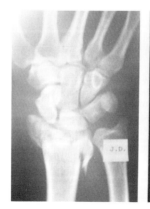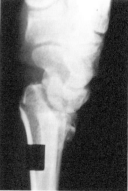

Figure 29.1

AP and lateral radiographs demonstrating a marked comminuted Frykman type VII fracture of the right radius in a 30-year-old man who fell from a ladder.

of the plate was approached between the third and fourth compartments. A dynamic compression plate was used as a neutralization plate and was applied extending from the shaft of the radius, over the top of the fracture and the joint, to the third metacarpal (Fig. 29.2). Two screws were used for fixation of the plate to the radius, proximal to the fracture site, and two screws were used distally for fixation to the third metacarpal. Slight distraction was used to ensure that there would be no compression of the joint surface. If indicated, a bone graft was harvested from the shaft of the radius and was packed behind the comminuted articular fracture surface.

When radiographic healing occurred — approximately eight weeks postoperatively, the plate was removed through two small incisions made proximally and distally over the original incision (Fig. 29.3). To facilitate early resumption of motion, tendolyses were carried out at the time of plate removal. Regional anesthesia was used for both procedures.

During serial follow-up, no patient exhibited postoperative complications of wound infection or fracture collapse. All patients regained functional wrist motion in all planes without pain (Table 29.1) All patients returned to work and normal daily activities in a timely fashion. After three years, no patient had shown evidence of developing arthritis.

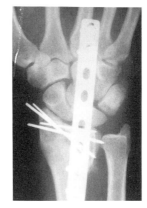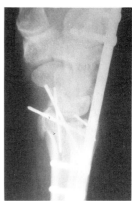

Figure 29.2

AP and lateral radiographs following open reduction and internal fixation and application of an internal distraction plate.

Discussion

Comminuted intra-articular fractures of the distal radius are difficult, particularly in the young adult. Anatomic reduction must be achieved otherwise the incidence of complications, particularly arthritis, is quite significant. The method of maintaining reduction is of equal importance because once reduction has been achieved, there is no inherent stability due to the amount of comminution, and therefore these fractures are extremely prone to collapse.

Table 29.1 During the 3 year follow-up, all patients had regained a functional range of motion.

Patient	Frykman classification	Age	Sex	Range of motion	
				Extension/Flexion	Supination/Pronation
1	VII	30	M	60°/60°	full
2	VIII	65	F	56°/56°	full
3	VIII	65	M	50°/80°	full
4	VIII	41	F	65°/70°	full
5	VIII	45	M	67°/50°	full
6	VIII	23	M	63°/70°	full
7	VIII	30	M	35°/56°	full
8	VIII	22	M	65°/68°	full
9	VII	59	F	46°/52°	full
10	VII	29	M	50°/55°	full

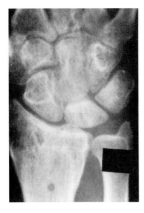
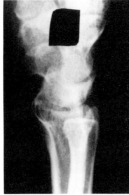

Figure 29.3

AP and lateral radiographs of the right wrist joint following removal of the plate and pins.

The use of the internal distraction plate is a unique way of stabilizing the fracture as it is allowed to heal without collapse. This approach restores and maintains the length of the radius and the angles of the distal radius and, in so doing, achieves and maintains the anatomical position of the articular surface. Patient compliance with this method is excellent and, in the author's opinion, far exceeds the compliance and acceptance with an external fixator. Since there are no pins protruding through the skin, there is no need for pin-tract care.

The internal distraction plate technique appears to be an acceptable method when used in combination with open reduction and K-wire fixation in the treatment of comminuted intra-articular fractures of the distal radius.

References

Knirk JL, Jupiter JB. Intra-articular fractures of the distal end of the radius in adults. *J Bone Joint Surg* 1986; **68A(5)**: 647–59.

Scheck M. Long term follow-up of treatment of comminuted fractures of the distal end of the radius by transfixation with Kirschner wires and cast. *J Bone Joint Surg* 1962; **44A(2)**: 337–51.

30
Treatment of distal radial intra-articular malunions

Ph Saffar

The consequences of distal radial intra-articular malunions have been widely discussed in the literature. Some authors have advocated that these types of malunions can be easily tolerated. More recently, Cooney et al. (1980) found 177 complications after 565 distal radial fractures. Of these complications, 37 were osteoarthritis (OA), 27 were malunions of the distal radio-ulnar joint (DRUJ), and 10 were malunions of the radiocarpal joint: the treatments for these malunions were three dorsal osteotomies, two proximal row carpectomies, two wrist arthrodeses and two prostheses.

In 43 intra-articular fractures in young adults, Knirk and Jupiter (1986) found that, after a mean follow-up of six to seven years, 28 patients (65%) showed evidence of OA, 26 of them (93%) being symptomatic: three showed DRUJ malunion, 14 radiocarpal malunion and 11 had malunion of both joints. If the intra-articular step-off was greater than 2 mm, OA was constant and was found in 91% of the cases with any amount of articular step-off. When congruity was restored after intra-articular fracture, however much the extent of the initial disruption, only 15% of cases were complicated by OA.

Altissimi et al. (1986) found that 18% of cases showed OA after Frykman type VII and VIII fractures. Bradway et al. (1989) confirmed that a step-off of 2 mm always results in OA (with a follow-up of 4.8 years).

These differences in the long-term results depend on the patient's age and occupation, the nature of the original fracture, and any associated injuries, among other features. Distal radial intra-articular malunions may decrease wrist strength and range of motion, but are not always painful, and radiocarpal OA often has a slow evolution. Young manual workers, however, may require more aggressive treatment of intra-articular malunions of distal radial fractures than other patients do.

The intra-articular malunion is often associated with shortening (loss of radial length), loss of radial inclination and dorsal tilt of the distal epiphysis radius usually secondary to excessive dorsal comminution (Fig. 30.1). Intra-articular malunions can also be the consequence of either

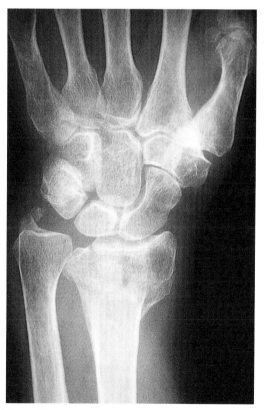

Figure 30.1

Distal radial intra-articular malunion with intra-articular step-off.

an anterior rim, or a postero-medial fragment, with healing in a displaced position and leading to a radiocarpal subluxation.

Malunion can occur at the radioscaphoid, radiolunate or radio-ulnar articulations alone, or it can involve all three joint articulations. This chapter will not describe the problems of the radioulnar compartment.

As for extra-articular malunions, a deformity of the distal radius can result in subluxation of the carpus dorsally or palmarly, with adaptation of the carpus at the level of the midcarpal joint reacting to this malalignment.

There have been several publications dealing with these extra-articular malunions, but very few papers have appeared in the literature dealing with the treatment of intra-articular distal radial malunion. In a series of 20 cases of malunions, Fernandez (1982) treated three cases of intra-articular malunion by extra-articular osteotomy. One case was reported by Light (1987) but the technique used is not indicated.

Patients and methods

Various techniques are available for treatment of these malunions, and the indications vary with the location, the degree of OA, and the functional needs of the patient. The oldest technique is total wrist arthrodesis, but if one tries to preserve a certain amount of motion, other methods are possible, for example extra- or intra-articular osteotomy, bone resections (styloidectomy, anterior or posterior rim resection), radiolunate or radioscapholunate limited arthrodeses, wrist denervation, proximal row carpectomy and finally, wrist prosthesis.

The aims of treatment are to decrease pain, to increase strength, to stop the progression of OA and, when possible, to preserve or increase the range of motion.

In this series, 38 cases of intra-articular malunions were operated on over a ten-year period (Table 30.1). Many techniques were used, apart from radioscapholunate limited arthrodeses and total wrist prosthesis. The age, sex, professional and recreational needs of the patients were recorded, as well as the intensity of pain, range of motion and strength compared with the opposite side.

Table 30.1 Techniques used

Wrist arthrodesis	5
PRC	1
Bone resection	6
Radiolunate arthrodesis	12
Extra-articular osteotomy	4
Intra-articular osteotomy	10
	38 cases

Plain radiographs were taken in AP, lateral and oblique views and in motion series. A CT scan with 3D reconstruction, when available, can help (Fig. 30.2). Evaluation of the site and extent of the normal cartilage preserved can be obtained by arthrography (Fig. 30.3), MRI or arthroscopy. However, as this is a retrospective study, these examinations were, in most cases, not available, apart from preoperative arthroscopy which was performed in three of the cases. With these examinations, it is possible to assess the existence of associated carpal injuries and the status of the DRUJ.

There were 32 male and 6 female patients. The mean age was 39.5 years, ranging from 19 to 63 years (the only proximal row carpectomy performed). Patient occupation was mainly manual: 28 were manual workers and 16 were workers' compensation cases. The mean time elapsed since injury was 17.5 months. The mean preoperative motion (measured in 26 cases) was 37.2° in flexion, 30.6° in extension, 14.7° in radial deviation and 25.3° in ulnar deviation (Table 30.2). The mean preoperative pain was 3 (2.96) in a fourth-grade scale (Table 30.3). The mean grip strength (measured in 25 cases) was 40.8% of the opposite normal side (Table 30.4).

Operative technique and results

Total wrist arthrodesis

This operation was performed in five cases using the usual technique of a posterior graft inserted into a trough hollowed at the dorsal aspect of the carpus and extending up to the metacarpals. Fixation was performed with screws. These cases were treated at the beginning of the series.

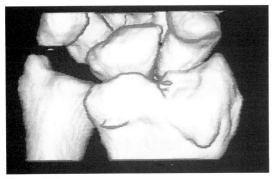 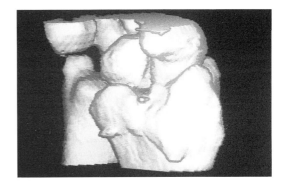

Figure 30.2

CT scan with 3D reconstruction.

Table 30.2 Range of motion

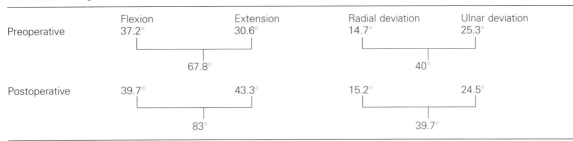

Table 30.3 Quotation of pain

No pain	0
Climatic pain or intermittent pain	1
Pain at strenuous work	2
Pain at light work	3
Permanent pain	4

Extra-articular osteotomy

This was performed in four cases. The site of osteotomy was usually situated 2.5 cm proximal to the articular surface. A triangular or trapezoid corticocancellous graft was inserted to correct the associated deformities of the distal radius. Comparison of postoperative pain, motion and grip strength between this group and the general series did not show significant differences.

Proximal row carpectomy

This treatment was used in only one case, for the oldest patient of the series (63 years of age). Pain

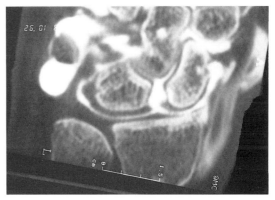

Figure 30.3

Post-arthrography CT scan. Cartilage is present (black line), except at the external part of the scaphoid facet of the radius, where it progressively disappears. It is thinner over the scaphoid proximal pole than on the lunate. Note the scapholunate ligament tear.

decreased from four to zero, flexion-extension from 85° to 75° and deviation increased from 20° to 30°. Grip strength went from 18% to 30% of the opposite side.

Table 30.4 Pain and grip strength

	Pain	Grip strength/Opposite side
Preoperative	2.96	40.8%
Postoperative	0.37	85.8%

New techniques

Three techniques were of special interest: localized bone resections, intra-articular osteotomy and radiolunate arthrodesis.

Bone resection

This was performed (in six cases) by the most direct approach, to remove a radial styloid process in four cases (Fig. 30.4a), a styloid and posterior rim fragment in one case (Fig. 30.4b) and a malunion at the level of the scapholunate crest where a localized step-off was present in the last case. In cases of radial styloid resection, care was taken to preserve the volar ligament insertions. The time elapsed since accident was a mean 15.1 months (range 9–24 months). All of the patients in this group were male manual workers. The mean age of the patients was 50. The results were decrease of pain from 3 to 1, a slight increase in the range of motion and significant increase in grip strength (almost doubled). One case was associated with wrist denervation.

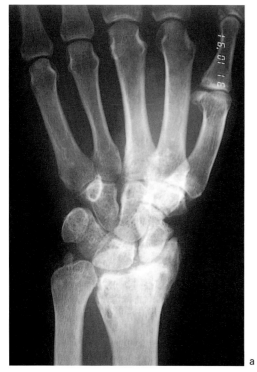
a

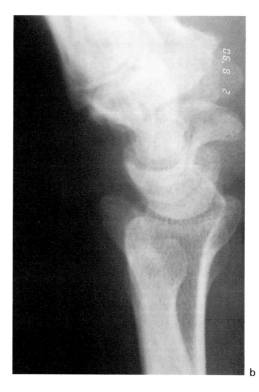
b

Figure 30.4

Indications for bone resection. a) Intra-articular malunion with a radial styloid fracture component. b) Dorsal fragment overlapping the carpus.

Intra-articular osteotomy

This was the most difficult procedure to perform. It requires careful preoperative planning for the approaches, the site of the lines of osteotomies, and for the type of grafts and the fixation (Figs 30.5, 30.6, 30.7). Ten patients were treated by this method: eight men and two women; six of the patients were manual workers. The mean age was 40.1 years (range 19–57 years). The average time elapsed since injury was eight months (range 1–12 months). Pain decreased from 2.33 to 0.55 (practically painless). ROM increased from 83–101° in flexion-extension and 42–45° in deviation. Strength increased from 9.3 kg to 16.8 kg (less than half the opposite side).

These results are comparable to those of the global series, even though the cases addressed were much more severe.

Radiolunate arthrodesis

This was performed using a dorsal approach on a total of 12 cases. After assessing the status of the cartilage and the carpal ligaments, a groove is cut from the posterior aspect of the distal radius, at the level of the lunate facet, and in the lunate. After distraction of the carpus, a graft is interposed between the radius and lunate to lengthen the distance between the two bones (Fig. 30.8). Note that the scaphoid will rotate back to a normal alignment if the carpal ligaments are intact. Another graft is inserted in the trough at the dorsal aspect of the radius and the lunate: the graft is fixed to the radius and lunate by two screws. This latter graft comes from the iliac bone or from the proximal radius (Fig. 30.9).

The procedure was performed on 12 men, nine of whom were manual workers. The mean age

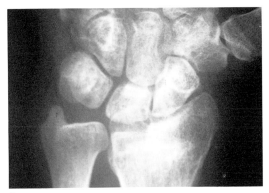
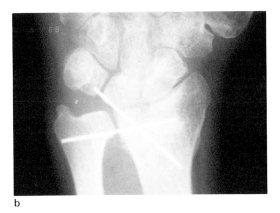
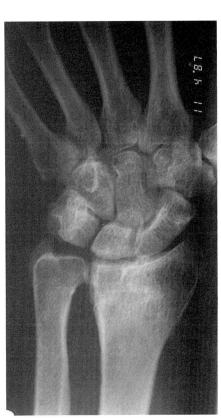

Figure 30.5

Displaced postero-medial fragment a) before operation; b) osteotomy and pinning; c) the result.

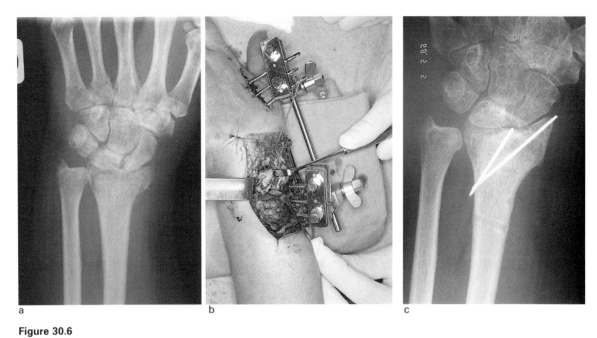

Figure 30.6
Complex intra-articular malunion treated by a) osteotomy, b) external fixation and c) pinning.

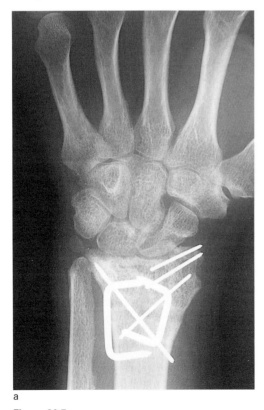

Figure 30.7
ab) Complex treatment of an intra-articular malunion and the result.

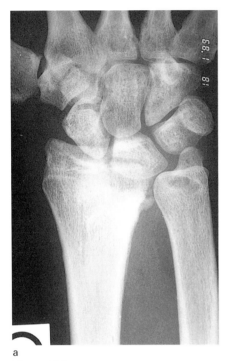 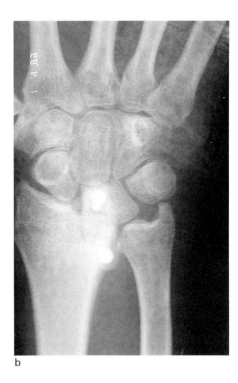

Figure 30.8

a) Intra-articular malunion with dorsal displacement. b) Radiolunate arthrodesis.

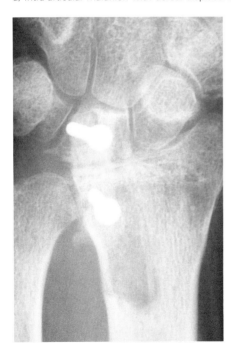

Figure 30.9

A sliding graft from the proximal radius fixed by two screws.

was 34.4 years (range 28–53 years). Five right hands and six dominant hands were involved (one patient was left-handed). The fractures were caused predominantly by high-velocity injuries. The time elapsed since injury was 23 months on average. The fractures were classified into two isolated die-punch fractures, one V-type fracture, and seven comminuted fractures. Two of the comminuted fractures had dorsal rim destruction resulting in dorsal carpal subluxation with a first carpal row in flexion and with a complete loss of extension (Fig. 30.10). The DRUJ was completely destroyed in three cases, in five it was incongruent and in one, irregular (Fig. 30.11). Preoperative ROM was on average 40° flexion, 24° extension, 10° radial deviation (RD) and 19° in ulnar deviation (UD). Pain was present for light strains (mean: 3) and grip strength was 50% of the opposite side.

Postoperatively, with a mean follow-up of 26.2 months, ROM was 34° in flexion, 40° in extension, 17° in RD and 22° in UD. Pain was absent or minimal (0.5) and grip strength was 70% of the opposite side. No progression of osteoarthritis was noted.

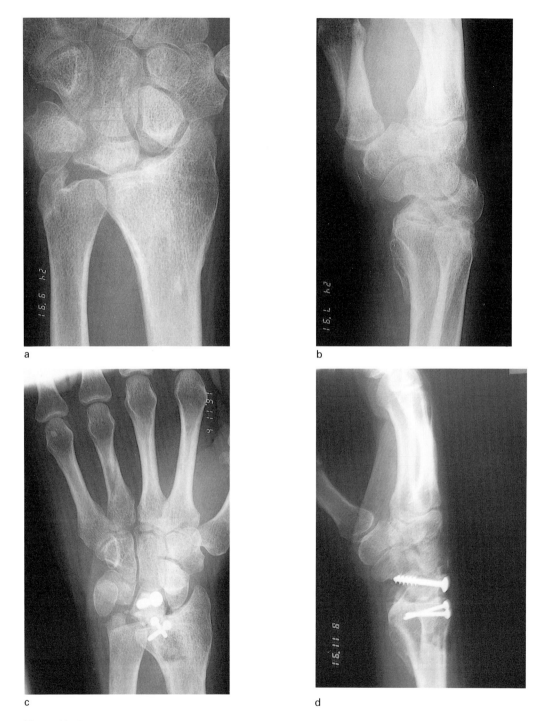

Figure 30.10

ab) AP and lateral views of a distal radial malunion with a carpal dorsal subluxation and dorsiflexion of the first row (stiff wrist). cd) Radiolunate limited arthrodesis.

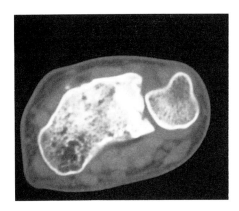 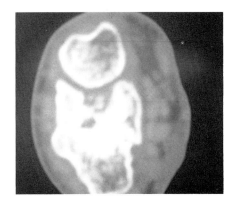

Figure 30.11

Transverse CT scan of the DRUJ. a) Irregularity of the sigmoid notch. b) Partial destruction of the sigmoid notch.

This procedure produces a slight increase in flexion-extension (10°) and radial deviation and ulnar deviation (10°) but more interestingly, there is a gain in extension relative to flexion, which is more functional, an increase of 20% in grip strength and a painless wrist. The patients returned to the same work in seven cases and to a lighter work in four cases (one case unknown.)

Indications

Total wrist arthrodeses were indicated when the articular surface was totally destroyed and at the beginning this series. In most of these cases, other procedures had been performed before total wrist arthrodeses. Extra-articular osteotomies were performed when the articular contour was relatively preserved, with a step-off less than 2 mm and with a significant dorsal angulation of the distal radius.

Bone resections were performed for localized impingements or early localized osteoarthritis in patients around 50 years of age, for whom an intra-articular step-off is more tolerable.

Intra-articular osteotomies were performed for complex and comminuted fractures in the absence of OA, when a short time had elapsed since injury (mean time: eight months) and in relatively young people (mean age: 40.1 years). Radiolunate limited arthrodesis was performed after die-punch fractures or comminuted fractures of the dorsal rim of the lunate facet with dorsal subluxation.

Discussion and indication by location of the step-off

Osteoarthritis of the radiocarpal joint is not always painful, in spite of the troubling radiological features. Even in manual workers, there is not always a progression of pain, as would be encountered in the SLAC (scapholunate advanced collapse) pattern of wrist osteoarthritis. The fact that there are different locations of the joint articular cartilage step-off can be easily tolerated in some cases. However, other patients complain of increasing pain related to daily activities and ask for relief. Some authors still recommend total wrist arthrodeses for painful osteoarthritis of the radiocarpal joint, but with a careful analysis of the localization of the deformities, a number of options for treatment can be performed to obtain a decrease in pain while keeping a good range of motion and increasing grip strength:

1. If the malunion predominates on the scaphoid facet, the choices include radial styloid excision (i.e. bone resection in cases of a very radial malunion), intra-articular osteotomy, or proximal row carpectomy.
2. If the lunate facet is completely involved in the malunion, the best choice is radiolunate arthrodesis. If only the postero-medial fragment is malunited, an intra-articular osteotomy is possible.
3. If the involvement is global an early intra-articular osteotomy is sometimes possible.

Wrist denervation is indicated in elderly people. Total wrist arthrodesis is indicated in young patients who perform manual labor. Total wrist prosthesis may be appropriate in older patients who do not require wrist motion.
4. For anterior or posterior rim malunion, a local bone resection may be the best treatment.

Longer follow-up will be necessary to judge whether these procedures are valuable in the long run, especially intra-articular osteotomies.

In conclusion, before planning wrist arthrodesis, which should be the last resort, a careful examination of the radiographs can suggest alternative procedures which will produce better results for the patient and the surgeon who wishes to preserve motion yet control pain and the progression of arthritis.

References

Altissimi M, Antenucci R, Fiacca C, Mancini GB. Long-term results of conservative treatment of fractures of the distal end of the distal radius. *Clin Orthop* 1986; **206**: 202–10.

Bradway JK, Amadio PC, Cooney WP. Open reduction and internal fixation of displaced comminuted intra-articular fractures of the distal end of the radius. *J Bone Joint Surg* 1989; **71A**: 839–47.

Cooney WP, Dobyns JH, Linscheid PL. Complications of Colles' fractures. *J Bone Joint Surg* 1980; **62A**: 613–19.

Fernandez DL. Correction of post-traumatic wrist deformity in adults by osteotomy, bone grafting and internal fixation. *J Bone Joint Surg* 1982; **64A**: 1164–78.

Knirk JL, Jupiter JB. Intra-articular fractures of the distal end of the radius in young adults. *J Bone Joint Surg* 1986; **68A**: 647–59.

Light TR. Salvage of intra-articular malunions of the hand and wrist: the role of realignment osteotomy. *Clin Orthop* 1987; **214**: 130–35.

31
Long-term follow-up of intra-articular fractures of the distal radius

Ph Kopylov

Fractures of the distal radius are among the most frequent fractures in adults. Distal radial fracture was described in 1814 by Colles as a fracture with good results, despite malunion and wrist deformity. More recently, however, different authors (Bengner and Johnell 1985, Cooney et al. 1980, McQueen and Caspers 1988, Pool 1973, Scheck 1962, Smaill 1965, Villar et al. 1987) have been less optimistic and have reported poor results associated with malunions; the intra-articular fractures are considered to be more severe.

In the light of these controversial results, this study attempts to trace the 'natural history' of this kind of injury and to analyse the long-term follow-up (30 years) of intra-articular fractures of the distal end of the radius.

Modern concepts put forth in studies of distal radial fractures lead us to distinguish two types:

1. fractures of osteoporotic bone;
2. fractures in young adults with good bone stock.

The second group was studied in this series (Kopylov et al. 1993). It is necessary to define these different types of fractures and to refer to a classification system, such as the Frykman classification (1967) which was chosen here (Table 31.1).

Patients and methods

The Department of Radiology at the Malmö General Hospital (Sweden) has kept radiographs since the beginning of the century. They are filed in relation to location and diagnosis. All wrist fractures from 1950 to 1959 were reviewed. Fractures of the distal radius were classified and the articular fractures distinguished. Patients between the ages of 18 and 50 years at the time of injury were invited to a clinical and radiographic examination. All these patients had been treated with cast for a period of five to six weeks after fracture reduction.

Clinical examination assessed subjective complaints, and wrist function was measured by grip strength and joint motion. Radiographs of both wrists (AP and lateral planes) were taken. Certain features were measured on these radiographs and on those taken in the 1950s:

- the axial compression, defined as the difference in length, between the radius and the ulna at the radio-ulnar joint level (ulnar variance);
- the radial compression, defined as the angle between the articular surface of the radius and the long axis of the radius on the AP view (radial slope);
- the dorsal compression, defined as the angle between the articular surface of the radius and the long axis of the radius on the lateral view (dorsal tilt).

Degenerative signs like subchondral cysts, sclerosis or narrowing of the joint space were noted. The clinical and radiographic results were compared to the non-fractured opposite side and to a group of extra-articular fractures.

Out of the 93 patients who fulfilled the necessary criteria, 47 agreed to come to the clinical and radiographic follow-up examination. This group showed no difference regarding age, sex, or type of fracture when compared with the patients who refused the follow-up examination. The control group of extra-articular fractures was composed of 29 patients with Frykman type I and II fractures.

Table 31.1 Frykman classification (1967)

Type	Distal fracture of the ulna	
	No	*Yes*
Extra-articular	I	II
Intra-articular		
Radiocarpal	III	IV
Radio-ulnar	V	VI
Radiocarpal and radio-ulnar	VII	VIII

Results

Clinical results

Thirty years after the fracture, 87% of patients noted no difference between the injured and the non-injured side. In 37% of cases, patients mentioned minor functional disability, such as cosmetic deformity or minor pain in relation to the weather. Clinical examination, in comparison with the non-injured side, showed a statistically significant decrease in grip strength (Table 31.2). Wrist motion was decreased in flexion (Table 31.3), while the other parameters of extension, pronation, supination, and radial or ulnar deviation showed no statistically significant difference.

No patient, regardless of the type of fracture, had changed occupational or recreational activities as a result of the wrist fracture.

Table 31.2 Grip strength measured in kg/cm^2

Non-fractured side	0.71 ± 0.23
Fractured side	0.65 ± 0.26
Difference	0.06 ± 0.13*

*$P < 0.01$

Table 31.3 Wrist mobility measured in degrees

	Flexion	*Extension*
Non-fractured side	72.0 ± 14.9	61.9 ± 16.1
Fractured side	$64.27 \pm 18.71 \pm$	59.5 ± 10.7
Difference	-7.73 ± 11.8*	-2.4 ± 10.7

*$P < 0.05$

Radiographic results

Thirty years after the trauma, the radiographs showed more degenerative changes in intra-articular fractures than in extra-articular fractures (Table 31.4). Radiographic signs of osteoarthrosis were in direct relation to axial compression, of which positive ulna variance is a sign (Table 31.5), and also in relation to the persistence of post-reduction incongruity in the radiocarpal or distal radio-ulnar joint (Table 31.6). Table 31.7 shows that, independent of axial compression, the persistence of joint incongruity is related to the presence of degenerative signs.

Discussion

Function

In this series, the long-term functional results, after a 30-year follow-up, seem to be excellent, with few complaints, in agreement with Frykman (1967). However, the delay between fracture and follow-up was too long as patients could never assess the duration of symptoms after trauma, and they seemed to have become accustomed to their eventual functional disability.

Motion

A decrease in wrist flexion has been reported by all previous authors, and appears to be related to the dorsal compression found in these fractures. This condition was evident in this series, but it was impossible to find a relation between the

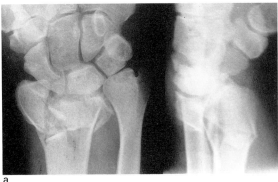 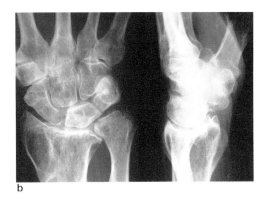

Figure 31.1

a) A 30-year-old manual worker, who sustained a Frykman type VII fracture of the non-dominant wrist in 1952. b) 34 years after the injury the patient has no complaints, despite a decreased flexion and supination. The radiographs show degenerative signs and significant axial compression.

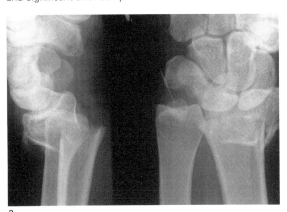 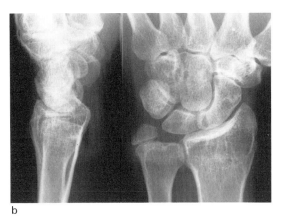

Figure 31.2

a) A 37-year-old truck driver, who sustained a fracture of the non-dominant wrist in 1956. b) 30 years later, the radiographic appearance of subchrondral sclerosis corresponds to a wrist with no functional disability. The patient had some discomfort but no axial compression was found.

diminution of joint range of motion and functional disability.

Grip strength

Reduced grip strength is most often recognized as a disability but the time elapsed since injury helped the patient to accept it.

Radioclinical correlations

Independent of the clinical results mentioned above, radiographic assessment showed a significant frequency of minor degenerative changes in intra-articular fractures after 30 years, with a higher rate in those fractures with a malunion. A relation was found between axial compression and eventual signs of osteoarthrosis on the radiographs, confirming the results of Lidström (1959) and Van der Linden and Ericsson (1981), who recognized radial shortening as a reason for poor results.

More interesting in this study is the relationship found between the persistence of incongruity of the radiocarpal joint and/or the distal radio-ulnar joint and the presence of degenerative signs on the radiographs taken 30 years after the injury. The poor prognosis associated with intra-articular fractures was confirmed,

Table 31.4 Frequency of degenerative signs in distal radio-ulnar joint (DRUJ) and radiocarpal joint (RCJ)

	Extra-articular fractures	Intra-articular fractures
DRUJ	25%	25%
RCJ	21%	40.5%*

*$P < 0.05$

Table 31.5 Relation between axial compression (in mm) and the presence of degenerative signs in the DRUJ and RCJ

	Extra-articular fractures	Articular fractures
No degenerative signs DRUJ	0.71 (SD 1.82)	1.35 (SD 1.92)
No degenerative signs RCJ	0.37 (SD 1.67)	1.5 (SD 1.99)
Degenerative signs DRUJ	1.5 (SD 2.35)	3.94 (SD 5.26)*
Degenerative signs RCJ	2.5 (SD 2.5)*	2.85 (SD 4.57)*

*$P < 0.05$

Table 31.6 Relation between degenerative signs and post-reduction persistence of DRUJ and RCJ incongruity

	Congruity	Incongruity
Degenerative signs in DRUJ	18%	46%
Degenerative signs in RCJ	29%	69%*

*$P < 0.05$

Table 31.7 Relation between axial compression (in mm) and degenerative signs DRUJ and RCJ in articular fracture

	Congruity	Incongruity
No degenerative signs DRUJ	1.06 (SD 1.58)	2.67 (SD 2.02)
No degenerative signs RCJ	1.18 (SD 1.56)	3.5 (SD 1.83)
Degenerative signs DRUJ	6.5 (SD 5.55)*	1.38 (SD 5.26)
Degenerative signs RCJ	4.42 (SD 5.45)*	1.25 (SD 3.19)*

*$P < 0.05$

emphasizing the importance of classification as described by Frykman (1967), Solgaard (1984), or Melone (1986). However, no correlation could be found between functional complaints and degenerative changes of the DRUJ and there was only a low correlation for the radiocarpal joint.

Aim of the treatment

The aim of treatment, if we refer to the results of this long-term follow-up, is two-fold:

1. to restore the radial length in relation to the ulna: the statistics show that 1 mm of shortening increases the risk of onset of degenerative changes to 20%, and 2 mm increases it to 50%;
2. to restore the congruity of both the radiocarpal and the distal radio-ulnar joints: an irregularity of more than 1 mm correlates with a higher frequency of degenerative changes.

For these reasons, a more aggressive treatment with open reduction, internal and/or external fixation and bone graft should be discussed.

However, it is necessary to assess the benefit of such treatment compared with the complications: fracture of the distal radius in young adults, with a good bone stock, is caused by a severe trauma which could, by itself, define the outcome. The influence of the direct trauma to the cartilage or to the other structures around the wrist is not discussed here.

Conclusion

The long-term results of intra-articular fractures of the distal radius, treated conservatively, show an increased risk of degenerative changes when compared with extra-articular fractures. There is a correlation between malunions and the presence of degenerative changes. The axial compression, which can be measured as positive ulnar variance, and the persistence, after reduction, of an incongruity of the articular surface, both correlate with the degenerative arthritis.

However, despite the increased frequency of osteoarthritic signs on the radiographs, the functional results are good and the complaints are few. There is no guarantee that the aggressive treatment that might have been proposed would improve on the results obtained by the conservative method of treatment.

References

Bengner U, Johnell O. Increasing incidence of forearm fractures, a comparison of epidemiologic patterns 25 years apart. *Acta Orthop Scand* 1985; **56**: 168–80.

Colles A. On the fracture of the carpal extremity of the radius. *Edin Med Surg J* 1814; **10**: 182–86.

Cooney WP, Dobyns JH, Linscheid RL. Complications of Colles' fractures. *J Bone Joint Surg* 1980; **62A**: 613–19.

Frykman G. Fracture of the distal radius including sequelae — shoulder-hand-finger syndrome, disturbance in the radio-ulnar joint and impairment of nerve function. *Acta Orthop Scand* 1967; **(Suppl)108**: 1–153.

Kopylov P, Johnell O, Redlund-Johnell I and Bengner U. Fractures of the distal end of the radius in young adults: a 30-year follow-up. *J Hand Surg* 1993; **18B**: 45–49.

Lidström A. Fracture of the distal end of the radius. A clinical and statistical study of end results. *Acta Orthop Scand* 1959; **41 (Suppl)**: 1–118.

McQueen M, Caspers J. Colles' fracture: does the anatomical result affect the final function? *J Bone Joint Surg* 1988; **70B**: 649–51.

Melone C. Open treatment for displaced articular fractures of the distal end of the radius. *Clin Orthop Rel Res* 1986; **202**: 103–11.

Pool C. Colles' fracture. A prospective study of treatment. *J Bone Joint Surg* 1973; **55B**: 540–44.

Scheck M. Long-term follow-up of comminuted fractures of the distal end of the radius by transfixation with Kirschner wire and cast. *J Bone Joint Surg* 1962; **44A**: 337–51.

Smaill GB. Long term follow-up of Colles' fracture. *J Bone Joint Surg* 1965; **47B**: 80–85.

Solgaard S. Classification of distal radius fractures. *Acta Orthop Scand* 1984; **56**: 249–52.

Van der Linden W, Ericsson R. Colles' fracture. How should its displacement be measured and how should it be immobilized? *J Bone Joint Surg* 1987; **63A**: 1285–88.

Villar RN, Marsh D, Rushton N, Greatorex RA. Three years after Colles' fracture. A prospective review. *J Bone Joint Surg* 1987; **69B**: 635–38.

32
Galeazzi and Essex-Lopresti fractures
G Herzberg

Previous studies have shown that fractures of the lower radius may be associated with distal radio-ulnar joint dislocation due to concomitant injury to the ligaments that stabilize this joint. Two other types of radial fracture, identified by eponyms, demonstrate this association: the Galeazzi fracture, where the radial diaphysis is fractured, and the Essex-Lopresti fracture, where the radial head is fractured. In both cases, the initial radiographs do not focus on the wrist and the distal radio-ulnar joint (DRUJ) dislocation may go unnoticed. These complex osteoligamentous lesions produce a double rupture of the antebrachial frame and can lead to severe limitation of prono-supination if anatomy is not restored. In this chapter, the pathology, initial diagnosis and the treatment of these two uncommon fracture–dislocations in adults will be reviewed.

Galeazzi fractures

First described at the beginning of this century, this fracture was named after Galeazzi in 1934. It combines a radial diaphysis fracture with a distal radio-ulnar joint dislocation. In most cases, the fracture occurs at the junction of the middle and distal third of the radius, but it can also be located slightly more distally or proximally. The fracture may be transverse, or sometimes oblique or comminuted, which influences the treatment. Variants of Galeazzi fractures present as fractures of both radius and ulnar in association with DRUJ dislocation and they are especially difficult to diagnose. The displacement of these highly unstable fracture-dislocations is always important and radiographs of the wrist must be taken whenever a distal radio-ulnar joint dislocation is suspected. The dislocation of the ulnar head is usually proximal and dorsal. In 1985, in a cadaveric study, Moore demonstrated that an isolated osteotomy of the radius with proximal traction on the distal fragment caused shortening of the radius compared to the ulna by an average of 3 mm. This can result in physiological laxity of the DRUJ. According to this study, only an apparent radial shortening of more than 5 mm is indicative of a true DRUJ dislocation with rupture of the triangular fibrocartilage complex (TFCC).

Galeazzi fractures represent approximately 7% of forearm fractures. On clinical examination, it is important to palpate the dorsal aspect of the DRUJ when faced with an apparently isolated radial fracture.

As early as 1957, Hughston mentioned the poor results observed after conservative treatment of Galeazzi fractures. Since that time, several studies have confirmed the need to fix the radius to achieve stabilization of these complex fracture-dislocations. The use of plates is generally preferred, as they provide anatomic reduction of the radius. It must be mentioned that although compression has proved useful in transverse fractures, it should be avoided in oblique and comminuted fractures. Thus, depending on the site of the radial fracture, non-compressive lateral or compressive anterior plating will be used. Cancellous bone grafting must be used if a bony defect is suspected.

Controversy surrounds the need for an additional approach to reduce the associated DRUJ dislocation. Alexander (1981) and Cetti (1977) recently reported three cases of Galeazzi fractures presenting with an irreducible DRUJ, despite fixation of the radial fracture. In each case, a surgical approach to the DRUJ revealed interposition of the extensor carpi ulnaris (ECU). The tendon was interposed between the radius and the ulna in two cases, and between the ulnar head and the fractured styloid process in the other. In all three cases, intra-operative radiographs taken after radial fixation suggested this interposition. Exact reconstruction of the anatomy of the radius must therefore be performed and intra-operative control radiographs, with the forearm in neutral prono-supination, must be checked carefully. When the DRUJ reduction is satisfactory, a long arm cast should be applied for six weeks. Otherwise, a direct dorso-medial approach to the joint is necessary to relieve a possible ECU interposition and/or to fix the ulnar styloid, or repair the TFCC itself.

Essex-Lopresti fractures

This fracture was named after Essex-Lopresti in 1951, in a classic article, although it was described first in 1946 by Curr and Coe. It is characterized by a displaced fracture of the radial head associated with a DRUJ dislocation. This injury is very rare and only about 10 cases have been published in the literature to date. The initial trauma must be strong enough to produce a compressive shearing force that can damage not only the radial head, but also the interosseous membrane and the DRUJ stabilizers.

The clinical signs appear primarily at elbow level, but it is just as important to X-ray and examine the injured wrist, which should be compared to the uninjured wrist.

This very unstable fracture-dislocation must be treated surgically; the aim is to restore the radial length and to allow soft tissue healing. The type of treatment chosen depends on the type of radial head fracture. Recently, Edwards and Jupiter suggested a classification which separates non-comminuted, large fragment fractures (type I), that are suitable for fixation, from comminuted fractures (type II) that can only be treated by excision.

In type I fractures, the fixation must restore the radial length. As in Galeazzi fractures, intra-operative radiographs in neutral prono-supination should be taken to check that the DRUJ has been properly reduced. A satisfactory reduction can be maintained with a long arm cast or by radio-ulnar pinning. An unsatisfactory reduction will require a direct approach to avoid a possible tendinous interposition, as well as to reduce and stabilize.

In a type II fracture, the only possible treatment is excision of the radial head, with or without replacement by a silastic implant. In this case, exact radio-ulnar relationships are difficult to restore and radio-ulnar pinning will be necessary. This should allow proper healing of the interosseous membrane and the DRUJ stabilizers. After healing, it is only these soft tissues that, in the absence of a radial head, can stop the progressive shortening of the radius and prevent ulnocarpal impingement. This complication affects mainly patients suffering from non-diagnosed Essex-Lopresti fractures, and is very difficult to treat. The best treatment is to shorten the ulna and replace the radial head with a silastic implant or a metal prosthesis. In cases of recurrent shortening of the radius, a radio-ulnar fusion in neutral prono-supination may be necessary. It is therefore essential to diagnose the Essex-Lopresti fractures at their early stage. It is preferable to avoid radial head resection when treating fractures of this type.

A possible connection between Galeazzi and Essex-Lopresti fractures should be mentioned. These extremely misleading variations are a reminder of how important it is to consider a possible lesion of each component of the antebrachial frame in every forearm injury, especially after high-energy trauma.

Conclusions

Galeazzi and Essex-Lopresti fractures are a combination of osseous and ligamentous lesions affecting the radius and the DRUJ. In each of these injuries, the fracture is obvious but it can hide the associated joint dislocation. The initial radiographs may provide a misleading impression because a partial spontaneous reduction is possible. Furthermore, the existence of possible variants of these rare lesions represents an additional risk of misdiagnosis. As surgical treatment will usually be planned, it is important, in both Galeazzi and Essex-Lopresti fracture-dislocations, to check the DRUJ on intra-operative radiographs after the treatment of the radial fracture. A radiographic suggestion of soft tissue interposition or poor reduction should be treated using a direct approach to the DRUJ.

References

Alexander AH, Lichtman DM. Irreducible distal radio-ulnar joint occurring in a Galeazzi fracture. Case Report. *J Hand Surg* 1981; **6A:** 258–61.

Cetti NE. An unusual cause of blocked reduction of the Galeazzi injury. *Injury* 1977; **9:** 59–61.

Curr JF, Coe WA. Dislocation of the inferior radioulnar joint. *Br J Surg* 1946; **34:** 74.

Essex-Lopresti P. Fractures of the radial head with distal radioulnar dislocation. *J Bone Joint Surg* 1951; **33B:** 244–47.

Galeazzi R. Di una particolare sindrome traumatica dello scheletro dell'avambracchio. *Atti Mem Soc Lombardi Chir* 1934; **2:** 12.

Galeazzi R. Uber ein besonderes Syndrom bei verltzunger im Berich der Unter armknochen. *Arch Orthop Unfallchir* 1934; **35:** 557–62.

Huten D. Fractures de l'extrémité supérieure du radius. In Cahiers d'enseignement de la SOFCOT, conférences d'enseignement 1991. Paris, Expansion Scientifique Française, 1991: 127–37.

Moore TM, Klein JP, Patzakis MJ, Harvey JP Jr. Results of compression-plating of closed Galeazzi fractures. *J Bone Joint Surg* 1985; **67A(7):** 1015–21.

Morrey BF, Chao EY, Hui FC. Biomechanical study of the elbow following excision of the radial head. *J Bone Joint Surg* 1979; **61A:** 63.

33
Radiocarpal dislocations and fracture-dislocations

C Dumontier, E Lenoble, Ph Saffar

Until the description of distal radius fractures by Pouteau (1783), radiocarpal dislocations were the only known wrist injuries, and it was Dupuytren who first recognized their rarity in 1834. Even the 70 cases of the preradiological era, quoted in Abadie's thesis (1901), are probably due to the usual confusion of radiocarpal dislocation with intracarpal dislocation, or even distal radial injuries. Moreover, the first radiographic interpretation of wrist injuries are unreliable. The case of a radiocarpal dislocation in a child reported by Peloquin in 1930, was in fact a very displaced epiphyseal injury.

In addition to radiological imprecision, there was some confusion in the classification of carpal dislocations. Dunn, who is frequently quoted, reported 6 cases in 1972. However, one case was a very comminuted distal radial fracture with severe displacement of the carpus but no dislocation, and the two other cases were subluxations, one secondary to a fracture of the anterior margin, and the other secondary to a fracture of the posterior margin (Barton's fracture). Most reports present the same problem with classification (Bianchi and Parenti 1956, Böhler 1930, Fantato 1966, Kireff 1933, Mouchet 1937, Russell 1949, Sgarbi and Sabetta 1968). Due to the rarity of radiocarpal dislocations and to the usual confusion in their classification, Dunn's estimated frequency of 0.2% is no more realistic than the 20% estimation of Moneim (1985).

One must consider three types of lesions: pure radiocarpal dislocations (Tables 33.1 and 33.2), radiocarpal dislocations with fracture of one or two styloids (Tables 33.3–33.8), and the different fractures of the distal radius, which may be associated with carpal subluxation or dislocation. Only the first two types will be discussed in this chapter. Incomplete reports in the literature, or reports without radiographs, will be excluded.

Historical review

Isolated radiocarpal dislocations are very rare. Without considering the cases reported before the radiographic era, Arcelin in 1921 seems to be the first to report a documented dorsal radiocarpal dislocation (Table 33.1). The first palmar radiocarpal dislocation was reported by Böhler in 1930 (Table 33.2). The first reported cases of proximal

Table 33.1 Isolated dorsal radiocarpal dislocations

	Author	Year	Side	Sex	Age	Comments
1	Arcelin	1921	R	M	?	
2	Destot	1923	?	M	50	open dislocation, death
3	Böhler	1930	R	M	54	fracture of the ulna
4	Wagner	1956	?	M	?	
5	Dumontier	1990	R	M	28	ulnar translation of the carpus, type I

Table 33.2 Isolated volar radiocarpal dislocations

	Author	Year	Side	Sex	Age	Comments
1	Böhler	1930	?	M	37	chronic subluxation
2	Trousseau	1953	R	M	34	fracture of the triquetrum
3	Rosado	1966	L	F	50	
4	Fehring	1984	L	M	50	
5	Moore	1988	L	M	23	
6	Dumontier	1985	R	F		immediate anterior and ulnar instability

Table 33.3 Dorsal fracture-dislocation type I, with fracture of the ulnar styloid but without fracture of the radial styloid

	Author	Year	Side	Sex	Age	Comments
1	Destot	1904	?	?	?	
2	Böhler	1930	R	M	64	
3	Weiss	1970	R	M	45	median nerve compression + distal radio-ulnar joint dislocation
4	Freund	1977	R	M	32	
5	Bilos	1977	L	M	25	scaphoid fracture
6/7	Bounds	1982	R+L	M	42	bilateral compression of the median nerves, avulsion of both rims of the radial epiphysis
8	Varodompun	1985	R	F	35	open dislocation + median nerve compression
9	Dumontier	1975	R	M		
10		1990	L	M	48	avulsion of the posterior rim of the radial epiphysis, secondary type II ulnar translation

radiocarpal instability, as a sequel of radiocarpal dislocation, were those of Dobyns (1975), Taleisnik (1985) and Rayhack (1987). Bellinghausen et al. (1983) reported the first cases of acute traumatic anterior subluxation of the radiocarpal joint. Radiocarpal dislocation with fracture of the ulnar or radial styloid are much more frequent, and yet less than 80 cases have been reported (Tables 33.3–33.8). Moneim (1985) described two types of dislocations: type I are radiocarpal dislocations with fracture of one or two styloids, in which the carpus remains intact (68 reported cases — Tables 33.1–33.6). In type II, there is an associated intracarpal dislocation (10 reported cases — Tables 33.7 and 33.8). The first case of type I radiocarpal dislocation seems to have been reported by Destot in 1904. Bounds (1982), Nyquist (1984) and Schoenecker (1985), each reported one case of bilateral fracture-dislocation. Type II radiocarpal fracture-dislocations were always anterior, except for one case reported by Klein (1986).

Table 33.4 Dorsal fracture-dislocation with fracture of the radial styloid

	Author	Year	Side	Sex	Age	Comments
1	Kireff	1930	L	M	23	
2		1930	L	M	28	
3	Rocher	1931	?	M	44	
4	(in Pouyanne)	1931	?	F	27	
5	Trousseau	1951	R	M	22	fracture of the ulnar styloid and
6		1951	L	M	?	posterior rim
7	Bianchi	1956	?	F	50	fracture of the ulnar styloid
8		1956	?	M	39	fracture of the ulnar styloid
9	Wagner	1959	?	?	?	
10	Fantato	1966	R	M	26	fracture of the ulnar styloid
11		1966	R	M	40	fracture of the ulnar styloid
12	Sgarbi	1968	?	M	29	fracture of the ulnar styloid
13		1968	?	M	54	lateral dislocation
14	Tanzer	1980	L	F	17	fracture of the anterior rim
15	Gerard	1981	6R	8M	26.5	8 fractures of the ulnar styloid
25			4L	2F		8 associated injuries
26	Fernandez	1981	L	M	20	open fracture, irreducible dislocation, fracture of the ulnar styloid, DRUJ dislocation, tendinous interposition, ulnar nerve and vascular injury
27	Moneim	1985	L	M	32	fracture of the ulnar styloid, median and ulnar nerve compressions.
28		1985	L	M	22	ulnar nerve compression
29		1985	?	M	30	fracture of the ulnar styloid
30	Schoenecker	1985	R+L	M	28	bilateral injuries
31						
32		1985	L	M	23	fracture of the ulnar styloid + radio-ulnar joint dislocation
33		1985	R	F	21	
34		1985	R	M	22	open dislocation, ischemia + nerve lesion, associated lesions
35		1985	L	M	51	fracture of the ulnar styloid + nerve lesions
36/40	Schweitzer	1987	?	?	?	5 fractures of the ulnar styloid
41	Rosson	1987	R	M	28	ipsilateral shoulder and elbow dislocation
42	Matthews	1987	L	M	24	fracture of the ulna. Ischaemia
43	Le Nen	1991	?	M	25	4 associated injuries, one ischaemia, fracture of the ulnar styloid or avulsion of the radial rim
44				M	30	
45				M	28	
46				M	22	
47				M	28	
48	Dumontier	1976	R	F	36	associated injuries, chronic dorsal subluxation
49		1977	L	M	38	fracture of the ulnar styloid + posterior rim
50		1986	R	M	29	fracture of the ulnar styloid + associated injuries
51		1988	L	F	45	complete brachial plexus palsy, associated injuries, fracture of the ulnar styloid
52		1990	R	M	?	open elbow dislocation
53		1991	?	M	25	
54		1992	L	M	32	

Table 33.5 Volar radiocarpal fracture-dislocations with fracture of the ulnar styloid but without fracture of the radial styloid

	Author	Year	Side	Sex	Age	Comments
1	Kaltsas	1982	L	M	21	associated injuries
2	Moneim	1985	L	F	37	
3	Thomsen	1989	?	M	62	distal radio-ulnar joint fracture
4	Penny	1989	R	F	68	fracture of the anterior rim with ulnar translation

Table 33.6 Volar radiocarpal fracture-dislocations with fracture of the radial styloid

	Author	Year	Side	Sex	Age	Comments
1	Böhler	1930	?	?	?	ulnar styloid
2	Fahey	1957	L	M	48	
3	Sgarbi	1968	?	M	45	fracture of the ulnar styloid
4	Dodd	1987	R	M	28	fracture of the ulnar styloid + shoulder and PIP joint dislocation
5	Le Nen	1991	?	M	21	
6	Dumontier	1984	R	F	30	fracture of the ulnar styloid
7		1992	L	M	26	fracture of the anterior rim

Table 33.7 Dorsal fracture-dislocations of Moneim type II (with intracarpal associated dislocation)

	Author	Year	Side	Sex	Age	Comments
1	Trousseau	1951	R	M	25	fracture of the radial and ulnar styloid
2	Bilos	1977	L	M	20	
3		1977	L	M	20	neurovascular and associated injuries
4		1977	L	M	21	neurovascular and associated injuries
5	Klein	1986	L	M	23	secondary necrosis of the lunate

Mechanism of injury

The lesions were always secondary to very severe trauma, and patients were unable to remember the precise wrist position during impact. Cadaver experiments have been inaccurate as well. If we discount the first experimental work of Abadie (1901), who obtained only dislocation with a 180° rotation of the wrist, the literature indicates that in posterior dislocations, there is associated hyperextension, pronation (Fernandez 1981, Gerard et al. 1987, Matthews 1987, Pouyanne 1933, Schoenecker 1985, Thomsen 1989, Weiss et al. 1970), and radial deviation (Gerard et al. 1981). This mechanism is consistent with the reported frequency of DRUJ injuries (Bilos et al. 1977, Fernandez 1981, Gerard et al. 1981, Le Nen et al. 1991, Schoenecker et al. 1985, Weis et al. 1970). Dodd (1987) is the only one who reported the possibility of a hyperflexion mechanism.

Table 33.8 Volar radiocarpal dislocations with fracture of the radial styloid and intracarpal dislocation (Moneim type II)

	Author	Year	Side	Sex	Age	Comments
1	Mullan	1980	R	M	35	associated carpometacarpal dislocation and radio and intracarpal dislocation
2	Lourie	1982	L	M	51	fracture of the ulnar styloid
3	Moneim	1985	?	M	29	
4			R	M	41	
5			R	M	51	fracture of the ulnar styloid

The anatomical lesions can be assessed only at surgery. The authors want to report, for clarity and elegance, the anatomical description of Voillemier (1839) of an almost pure radiocarpal dislocation: 'the lateral and posterior ligaments were ruptured; the anterior ligament, completely avulsed from the margin of the radius, only left some debris attached to the carpus; the medial ligament was the only one which resisted, and the ulnar styloid, attached to that ligament and to the sheath of the extensor carpi ulnaris, had been avulsed from the ulnar head. All the ligaments have been torn, and the forearm bones are solely attached to the carpus by few fibrous bundles, which form the posterior part of the radius, and from the discus articularis, go to the medial part of the carpus.'

The frequency of ulnar styloid fracture is evidence that those lesions seem to begin on the ulnar side of the wrist. The dislocation is made possible by a rotational movement, which lessens the bone surfaces in contact. In the few operated cases, the capsular tear is complete on the anterior margin of the radius, and may extend dorsally to the scapholunate interval (Fernandez 1981, Gerard et al. 1981, Moneim et al. 1985, Penny and Greene 1989, Pouyanne 1933, Rayhack et al. 1987, Thomsen and Falstie-Jensen 1989). This capsular tear is sometimes replaced by an avulsion fracture of the insertion of the ligaments (Le Nen et al. 1991, Schoenecker et al. 1985, Tanzer and Horne 1980). More often, there is impaction of the carpus, which may fracture the radial styloid (Fernandez 1981, Gerard et al. 1981, Le Nen et al. 1991). This fracture usually extends into the entire scaphoid fossa and may continue on the dorsal margin (Gerard et al. 1981, Le Nen et al. 1991). In Moneim type II fractures (1985), the radiocarpal lesions are dorsal, and the intracarpal lesions palmar. In one case, with a cadaver experiment, Matthews (1987) showed that tension forces could be lateral, and compression medial. Fehring (1984) thought that the patients who presented with a radiocarpal dislocation usually do so with a VISI (volar intercalary segment instability) position, but Varodompun (1985) reported a case with a bilateral DISI (dorsal intercalary segment instability) position. Due to the lack of precision in the reported cases, and the absence of strict radiographic criteria, it seems impossible to draw any conclusion.

In a case of palmar dislocation reported by Rosado (1966), the mechanism could have been hyperextension combined with a shearing force. According to Rosado, this type of lesion could produce a lunate dislocation, in which the lunate is found, at operation, entirely separated from the radius and the carpus. Penny (1989), describing an almost pure palmar dislocation, found an anteroposterior tear, extending from the scapholunate interval in a palmar to dorsal direction. Trousseau (1955) reported a case with a hyperflexion mechanism, but Le Nen (1991) considered that the anatomical lesions could be very similar to those encountered in dorsal dislocations.

Associated lesions reported in the literature

As for most violent trauma, these lesions have been reported mainly in males (62 males compared to 9 females), usually of young age (average 32 years old, age range 17–68 years). The only cases reported in children were before the discovery of radiography, and were probably epiphyseal injuries. Clinical description of these lesions is of little value. Due to the violence of the injury, associated lesions were frequently encountered in the same limb (35 cases). Dodd (1987) and Rosson (1987) reported three dislocations involving the same limb, and Mullan (1980) described three types of dislocation involving the same wrist (radiocarpal, intracarpal and carpometacarpal dislocation). Le Nen (1991) reported extensor carpi ulnaris and extensor digiti minimi injuries in the forearm; Fernandez (1981) and Nyquist (1984) reported a case of flexor tendon rupture, while Schoenecker (1985) reported avulsion of the pronator quadratus. Open dislocation (Bilos et al. 1977, Destot 1923, Fernandez 1981, Kireff 1933, Klein et al. 1986, Nyquist and Stern 1984, Schoenecker et al. 1985, Varodompun et al. 1985), ulnar nerve, or median plus ulnar nerve injuries (Bilos et al. 1977, Bounds 1982, Fernandez 1981, Gerard et al. 1981, Le Nen et al. 1991, Moneim et al. 1985, Nyquist and Stern 1984, Schoenecker et al. 1985, Varodompun et al. 1985, Weiss et al. 1970), or even acute hand ischaemia (Bilos et al. 1977, Le Nen et al. 1991, Matthews 1987, Nyquist and Stern 1984, Schoenecker et al. 1985) have also been reported.

Suggested treatment in the literature

Due to the rarity of these lesions, many treatment alternatives have been proposed. According to the literature, the reduction of the dislocation is easy. Only two cases of irreducible dislocation have been reported. They involved interposition of the flexor tendons in one case (Fernandez 1981), and of a bone fragment in the other (Weiss et al. 1970). After reduction, the joint is usually stable, and only one case of early anterior subluxation (Thomsen and Falstie-Jensen 1989) and one of ulnar translation (Penny and Greene 1989) have been reported after orthopaedic treatment. Both require surgical stabilization. In those two cases, there was no fracture of the radial styloid.

More often, non-operative treatment is considered the treatment of choice (Bianchi and Parenti 1956, Böhler 1930, Matthews 1987, Moneim et al. 1985), with forearm cast immobilization for four (Varodompun 1985) to six weeks (Fehring and Milek 1984, Moore and McMahon 1988). Schoenecker (1985) and Gerard (1981) both considered immediate surgery as a primary treatment to avoid displacement. They insisted, as did Le Nen (1991), Bilos (1977) and Weiss (1970), on fixation of the radial styloid to stabilize the lesions. This fixation can be difficult, owing to the comminution, and Schweitzer (1987) and Schoenecker (1985) suggested the use of a bone graft. According to Le Nen (1991), surgical exposure is also useful to remove chondral fragments. These cartilaginous lesions may heal under distraction by external fixator, as described by Schweitzer (1987). The surgical approaches employed have been very variable.

Results from the literature

Contrary to the severity of the injury, most of the results are apparently good, particularly after non-operative treatment, whatever the direction of the dislocation (Fehring and Milek 1984, Freud and Ovesen 1977, Matthews 1987, Moneim et al. 1985, Moore and McMahon 1988, Reynolds 1980, Rosado 1966, Varodompun et al. 1985). Functional recovery is usually complete in a few months (Varodompun et al. 1985), except for associated lesions (Bilos et al. 1977). However, Schoenecker (1985) reported four patients out of six with arthrosis at three year follow-up.

The results of surgical treatment were good, according to Gerard (1981), only if the radial styloid fragment was intact, which facilitated an anatomical reduction. Moneim (1985) reported one case with early stiffness and two fair results out of four operative cases. Although described as good, the results of Le Nen's patients (1991) showed limitation of motion (more than 90° of the flexion-extension arc), and one half suffered from pain during activity. One patient needed a distal radio-ulnar fusion (Sauvé–Kapandji procedure) for persistent pain. Five patients out of six had some narrowing of the radiocarpal interval with a follow-up ranging from 3 months to 11 years. The articular surface of the radius was irregular in three cases, and an ossification between the radiocarpal joint and the DRUJ was present in two cases. All the patients, however, returned to their previous jobs (Le Nen 1991). All

Table 33.9 Miscellaneous lesions

	Author	Year	Side	Sex	Age	Comments
1/6	Dunn	1972	?	?	?	3 dorsal, 2 volar and 1 unclassified dislocation
7	Reynolds	1980	L	M	31	dorsal dislocation with fracture of the posterior rim, fracture of the styloid
8	Bellinghausen	1983	R	M	73	anterior subluxation with fracture of the ulnar styloid
9			L	M	37	anterior subluxation with fracture of the ulnar styloid and of the anterior rim
10/20	Nyquist	1984	6L 4R	9M	42	10 associated lesions, 1 bilateral lesion

the patients reported by Nyquist (1984) had a poor functional result, with arthrosis and a flexion–extension arc limited to 57° on average. However, all had sustained very severe injuries, with open dislocation in each case (Table 33.9).

Radiocarpal instability, which theoretically should be very frequent, was seldom reported. Klein (1986) reported an ulnar translation of the carpus two months following injury, but this was secondary to a lunate necrosis in a Moneim type II injury. Taleisnik (1985) described two types of proximal instability: in type I, the entire carpus slides medially; in type II, the scaphoid remains under the scaphoid fossa, and ulnar translation reveals an increased scapholunate gap. Moore (1988) reported a secondary scapholunate dissociation, which may be a Taleisnik type II. Penny (1989) reported an early ulnar translation. Taleisnik type I, which required stabilization using K-wires. Even with persistent ulnar translation at 16 months follow-up, the functional result was excellent. Only Böhler (1930) and Schoenecker (1985) have reported a chronic ulnar translation. In both cases, the radial styloid was intact, but one patient was treated only up to the fifth week (Schoenecker 1985).

The authors' series

Although rare, radiocarpal dislocations are not exceptional, as we have observed 13 cases (Tables 33.1–33.5). The usual easy reduction of these lesions explains why some dislocations, which spontaneously reduce, are missed. Two patients presented with an isolated dislocation. The patient with a dorsal dislocation that spontaneously reduced, presented on the fourth day with a severe ulnar translation. The dislocation was reproduced at operation. Closed reduction with percutaneous wiring gave a good functional result at 6-month follow-up (Fig. 33.1). In the case of palmar dislocation, an anterior subluxation with ulnar translation persisted after reduction, and was stabilized with K-wires (Fig. 33.2). In one case of fracture-dislocation without fracture of the radial styloid, ulnar translation was obvious even when the patient was still in his cast. This patient refused further treatment, and at 2-year follow-up considered that he had a good functional result (Fig. 33.3). No ulnar translation was noted in the nine cases of dislocation with fracture of the radial styloid, and it has never been reported in the literature.

Two groups of dislocations should be distinguished. The first group includes pure dislocation, and the second dislocation with fracture of the ulnar styloid. In these cases, the radiocarpal ligaments are torn and, even if stable after reduction, the lesion will evolve to anterior and/or ulnar translation. If ulnar translation seems to be well tolerated initially, long-term evolution of problems is doubtful. The two cases of acute anterior subluxation reported by Bellinghausen (1983) had a fair functional result and early arthrosis. Rayhack reported two patients who had ulnar translation, which was probably the

274 FRACTURES OF THE DISTAL RADIUS

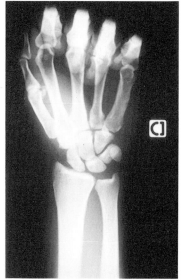

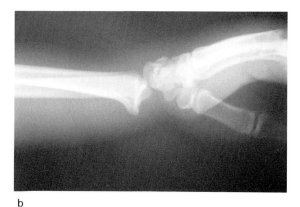

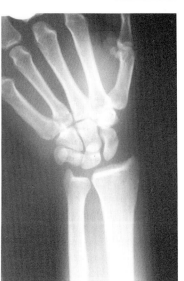

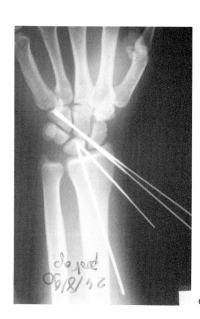

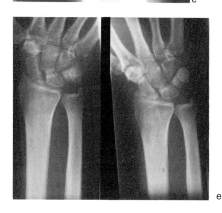

Figure 33.1

a) Acute ulnar translation (Case 5, Table 33.1), after spontaneous reduction of a pure dorsal radiocarpal dislocation. b) Perioperative reproduction of the dislocation. c) Radiograph taken in traction to show the ligamentous radiocarpal lesions. d) Radiocarpal fixation using K-wire to protect the radioscaphoid and radiolunate ligaments during 'healing'. e) Radiological results at 6 months. Good functional result.

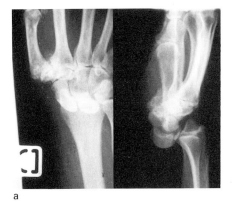

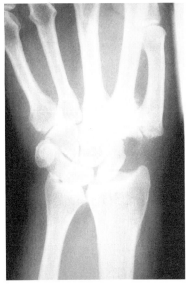

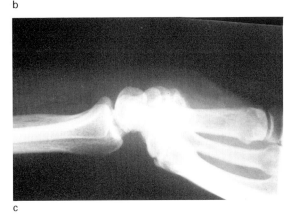

Figure 33.2

a) Pure palmar radiocarpal dislocation (Case 6, Table 33.2). b) Acute ulnar translation after reduction. c) Persistent anterior subluxation after reduction.

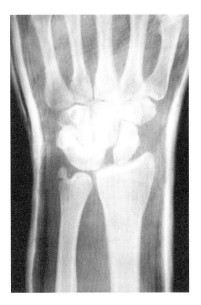

Figure 33.3

Early ulnar translation after closed treatment of a dorsal radiocarpal dislocation with fracture of the ulnar styloid (Case 10, Table 33.3). Good functional result at 2 years.

sequel of a radiocarpal dislocation, and who needed further treatment. The anterior subluxation is probably less well tolerated than the ulnar translation. We now believe that these patients should be operated on to reduce the dislocation and suture the ligaments. The addition of radiolunate K-wire fixation is needed to protect the repair. A surgical approach is mandatory, both to control the reduction of the lunate and to avoid persistent subluxation, as in one case in this series, in which there was a persistent subluxation following closed reduction, which needed surgery.

The second group of dislocations are the radiocarpal dislocations with fracture of the radial styloid. These are generally stable, as the ligaments are still attached to the styloid (Fig. 33.4). The long-term functional results in this group seem better, provided an anatomical reduction has been performed; this necessitates an anterior or lateral approach. Removal of osteochondral fragments, or bone grafting of a comminuted fracture can be performed using this approach. One month of immobilization seems to be adequate. Associated intracarpal dislocation should be surgically treated (Saffar 1989).

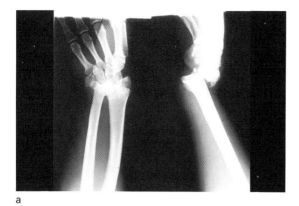 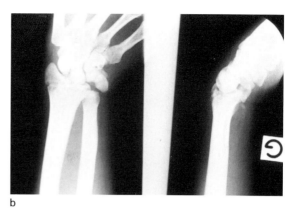

Figure 33.4

a) Dorsal dislocation with fracture of the radial styloid, still attached to the carpus (Case 36, Table 33.4). b) Radiographs taken after reduction. Note the avulsion of the posterior margin.

When the lesion presents as an ulnar translation, ligamentous reconstruction is inadequate (Rayhack et al. 1987, Thomsen and Falstie-Jensen 1989). A radiolunate arthrodesis, without shortening of the radiocarpal index (Youm et al. 1978), appears to be the best option.

References

Abadie J. Des luxations radio-carpiennes traumatiques. Thèse médecine. Montpellier, 1901.

Arcelin F. L'exploration radiologique du carpe. *J Rad Electrorad* 1921; **8**: 349–61.

Bellinghausen HW, Gilula LA, Young LV, Weeks PM. Post-traumatic palmar carpal subluxation. *J Bone Joint Surg [Am]* 1983; **65**: 998–1006.

Bianchi G, Parenti F. Le fratture-lussazioni della radio-carpica. *Bull Sci Med [Bologna]* 1956; **128**: 189–206.

Bilos ZJ, Pankovich AM, Yelda S. Fracture-dislocation of the radiocarpal joint. *J Bone Joint Surg [Am]* 1977; **59**: 198–203.

Böhler L. Verrenkungen des handgelenke. *Acta Chir Scand* 1930; **67**: 154–77.

Bounds TB. Bilateral radiocarpal dislocation. A case report. *Orthopaedics* 1982; **5**: 42–45.

Destot E. *Traumatismes du poignet et rayons X*. Paris: Masson Editions, 1923.

Dobyns JH, Linscheid RL, Chao EYS, Weber ER, Swanson GE. Traumatic instability of the wrist. In Instructional course lectures, the American Academy of Orthopaedic Surgeons. Vol 24. St Louis: CV Mosby, 1975: 182–99.

Dodd CAF. Triple dislocation in the upper limb. *J Trauma* 1987; **27**: 1307.

Dunn AW. Fractures and dislocations of the carpus. *Surg Clin North Am* 1972; **52**: 1513–38.

Dupuytren G. Des fractures de l'extrémité inférieure du radius simulant les luxations du poignet. In *Leçons orales du Baron Dupuytren*, Tome 4. Paris: Baillière, 1834: 161–231.

Fahey JH. Fractures and dislocations about the wrist. *Surg Clin North Am* 1957; **37**: 19–40.

Fantato S. Le fratture-lussazioni della radio-carpica. *Minerva Ortop* 1966; **17**: 92–95.

Fehring TK, Milek MA. Isolated volar dislocation of the radiocarpal joint. *J Bone Joint Surg [Am]* 1984; **66**: 464–66.

Fernandez DL. Irreducible radiocarpal fracture-dislocation and radioulnar dissociation with entrapment of the ulnar nerve, artery and flexor profundus II–IV: case report. *J Hand Surg [Am]* 1981; **6**: 456–61.

Freund LG, Ovesen J. Isolated dorsal dislocation of the radiocarpal joint. *J Bone Joint Surg [Am]* 1977; **59**: 277.

Gerard Y, Schernberg F, Elzein F. Les luxations-fractures postérieures de la radio-carpienne. *Rev Chir Orthop* 1981: **67 (suppl II)**: 92–96.

Kaltsas DS. Letter to the editor. *Injury* 1982; **13**: 351–52.

Kireff KM. Contribution à l'étude de la luxation traumatique de l'articulation radio-carpienne, Thèse médecine. Nancy, 1933.

Klein A, Bohrer SP, Wells M III. Dorsal dislocation of the radiocarpal joint with associated dorsal perilunar dislocation. *J Can Assoc Radiol* 1986; **37**: 201–2.

Le Nen D, Riot O, Caro P, Le Fevre C, Courtois B. Luxation-fractures de la radio-carpienne: Etude clinique de 6 cas et revue générale. *Ann Chir Main* 1991; **10**: 5–12.

Lourie JA. An unusual dislocation of the lunate of the wrist. *J Trauma* 1982; **22**: 966–67.

Matthews MG. Radiocarpal dislocation with associated avulsion of the radial styloid and fracture of the shaft of the ulna. *Injury* 1987; **18**: 70–71.

Moneim MS, Bolger JT, Omer GE. Radio-carpal dislocation — classification and rationale for management. *Clin Orthop* 1985; **192**: 199–209.

Moore DP, McMahon BA. Anterior radio-carpal dislocation: an isolated injury. *J Hand Surg [Br]* 1988; **13**: 215–17.

Mouchet A. Les luxations radiocarpiennes. In Ombredanne L, Mathieu P, eds. *Traité de chirurgie orthopédique*. Paris: Masson, 1937.

Mullan GB, Lloyds GJ. Complete carpal disruption of the hand. *Hand* 1980; **12**: 39–43.

Nyquist SR, Stern PJ. Open radiocarpal fracture-dislocations. *J Hand Surg [Am]* 1984; **9**: 707–10.

Peloquin, G. Luxation radio-carpienne traumatique en arrière. *Soc Med Milit Française* 1930.

Penny WH, Greene TL. Volar radiocarpal dislocation with ulnar translocation. *J Orthop Trauma* 1989; **2**: 322–26.

Pouteau C. *Oeuvres posthumes*. Paris, 1783.

Pouyanne PL. Contribution à l'étude des luxations traumatiques du carpe en arrière. Thèse médecine. Bordeaux, 1933.

Rayhack JM, Lindscheid RL, Dobyns JH, Smith JH. Posttraumatic ulnar translation of the carpus. *J Hand Surg [Am]* 1987; **12**: 180–89.

Reynolds ISR. Dorsal radiocarpal dislocation. *Injury* 1980; **12**: 48–49.

Rosado AP. A possible relationship of radio–carpal dislocation and dislocation of the lunate bone. *J Bone Joint Surg [Br]* 1966; **48**: 504–6.

Rosson JW. Triple dislocation of the upper limb. *J R Coll Surg Edinb* 1987; **32**: 122.

Russell TB. Inter-carpal dislocations and fracture dislocations. A review of 59 cases. *J Bone Joint Surg [Br]* 1949; **32**: 524–31.

Saffar P. *Les traumatismes du carpe*. Paris: Springer-Verlag, 1989.

Schoenecker PL, Gilula LA, Shively RA, Manske PR. Radiocarpal fracture-dislocation. *Clin Orthop* 1985; **197**: 237–44.

Schweitzer G. Letter to the editor. *Clin Orthop* 1987; **216**: 298.

Sgarbi G, Sabetta F. Considerazioni sul trattamento delle lussazioni complete della radiocarpica ed esiti a distanza. *Ospedali Ital Chir* 1968; **18**: 581–87.

Taleisnik J. *The wrist*. New York: Churchill Livingstone, 1985.

Tanzer TL, Horne JG. Dorsal radio-carpal fracture dislocation. *J Trauma* 1980; **20**: 999–1000.

Thomsen S, Falstie-Jensen S. Palmar dislocation of the radiocarpal joint. *J Hand Surg [Am]* 1989; **14**: 627–30.

Trousseau M. Etude clinique et radiologique des luxations du carpe: a propos de 59 cas originaux. Thèse médecine. Lyon, 1955.

Varodompun N, Limpivest P, Prinyaroj P. Isolated dorsal radiocarpal dislocation: case report and literature review. *J Hand Surg [Am]* 1985; **10**: 708–10.

Voillemier LC. Histoire d'une luxation complète et récente du poignet en arrière, suivie de réflexion sur le mécanisme de cette luxation et sur son diagnostic différentiel. *Arch Gen Med* 1839; 401–17.

Wagner CJ. Perilunar dislocations. *J Bone Joint Surg [Am]* 1956; **38**: 1198–207.

Wagner CJ. Fracture-dislocations of the wrist. *Clin Orthop* 1959; **15**: 181–96.

Weiss C, Laskin RS, Spinner M. Irreducible radiocarpal dislocation. *J Bone Joint Surg [Am]* 1970; **52**: 562–64.

Youm Y, McMurtry RY, Flatt AE, Gillespie TE. Kinematics of the wrist. *J Bone Joint Surg [Am]* 1978; **60**: 423–31.

34
Fractures and epiphyseal fracture-separation of the distal bones of the forearm in children

S Guero

The child is not an adult in miniature but the adult is a grown-up child. All the traumatology treatments for children are supported by two basic principles:

- the children's fractures are very specific compared to adult fractures, due in particular to the bone structure;
- depending on the injury type, growth can improve or conversely worsen the prognosis.

A classification of fracture types in children and treatments specific for these fractures are necessary. Distal forearm fractures are defined by their location at the distal quarter of the radius and ulna. They are situated at the metaphyseal or epiphyseal plate level (epiphyseal fracture-separation).

These very frequent injuries are supposed to be benign, but this is not always the case. Only a good knowledge of the child's bony physiology and the use of effective criteria of reduction and postoperative care will guarantee good results without sequelae.

Summary of distal forearm bones growth

The growth of the distal forearm bones equals 80% of the complete growth of the forearm bones which represent a length of 9 cm from birth to the growth end. This measurement is identical for both bones. At five years of age, the length of the two bones equals approximately half of the final length.

Growth rate is significant during the first year. It decreases afterwards to reach a plateau at around five years of age and stops at 11 to 14 years of age, depending on the sex (Bailey et al. 1989). In the distal ulna and radius epiphysis, there is no peak velocity of growth at puberty. It can then be assumed that a malunion can be extensively remodelled until five or six years of age, but less and less remodelling is possible afterwards. The bone maturation should be carefully assessed. The principal milestones of practical interest are as follows:

- at five years of age, the trapezium ossification center is present in the male child: the distal ulna epiphysis is appearing in the female child;
- at seven years of age, the latter is present in the male child;
- the thumb sesamoid is visible at 11 years of age in girls and 13 years of age in boys;
- the ulnar styloid is ossified at 12 years of age in girls and at 14 years of age in boys;
- the fusion of ulnar epiphyseal plates appears at 13 years of age in girls and at 15 years of age in boys.

These are average ages but are useful for surgical indications in the majority of cases.

Patients

A series of 105 cases was compared to the data in the literature. The patients were treated in 1989 and reviewed by radiographic assessment in 1991.

Distal forearm fractures are the most frequent type in children. Metaphyseal and epiphyseal fracture-separation represent 38% of upper limb fractures (Bedat and Kaelin 1989) and around one-quarter of all fractures in childhood (Bedat and Kaelin 1989, Landin 1983). Fractures occur at the metaphysis or metaphyseal-epiphyseal junction in 75% of cases and 25% involve epiphyseal fracture-separation. The ulna is fractured in 40% of cases (Collet 1982, Collet and Rigault 1985). Fractures occur more often in male children. In this series 73% of the patients were boys and 27% girls (compared to 58% versus 42% in the Bedat study, 1989). The mean age was 10 years (range 2 years 9 months to 15 years 10 months). In two-thirds of the cases, the injuries occurred between 9 and 14 years of age (Bedat and Kaelin 1989). The rate of fracture type relative to age and sex has been studied by some authors (Alffram and Bauer 1962, Bailey et al. 1989, Bedat and Kaelin 1989, Narod and Spasoff 1986). The maximum rate occurs between 9 and 10 years for girls and 13 to 14 years for boys. Fractures are caused by games in 24%, sport accidents in 21%, and traffic accidents (bicycle) in 12%. It is worth noting that 34% of the injuries happen in the absence of any definite physical activity (Landin 1983).

Pathophysiology

The increasing rate of fractures during puberty is usually explained by the physical activity at that age. The Bailey study (1989) has compared the mean age at which fractures occur with the maximum child growth peak. It is surprising to note a difference depending on the sex ($11\frac{1}{2}$ years of age for girls and 14 years of age for boys). A study in sport activities (Mirwald and Bailey 1983) shows no correlation between sport and the maximum rate of fractures. On the contrary, the mean fracture age does correspond to the decrease of physical and sports activity: there is conversely a strong correlation of the growth curves in both sexes with the maximum rate of fractures. The maximum increase of growth rate is at 11.9 years (range 11.5–12.5 years) in girls and 14.3 years (range 13.5–14.5 years) in boys. This suggests a correlation between the bone resistance during maximum growth and the onset of forearm fractures (Chan et al. 1984, Cook et al. 1987, Landin et al. 1983).

Mechanism

The history of accident and symptoms are always the same: a fall from a standing height onto a wrist in extension is the usual story.

The diagnosis is often evident with pain, disability of the distal upper limb and deformity. Associated vascular, nerve or skin injuries should be sought. AP and lateral comparative radiographs are taken, and at times oblique views are also obtained.

Fractures saving the epiphyseal plate

Impaction fractures or buckle fractures

The impaction fracture occurs through the metaphysis and is stable. The palmar and dorsal cortex are not interrupted but there is an impaction of the bony trabeculae on one side and distraction on the other (Fig. 34.1). Immobilization in a below elbow cast for three weeks provides an excellent result. In very young children an above-elbow cast is highly recommended.

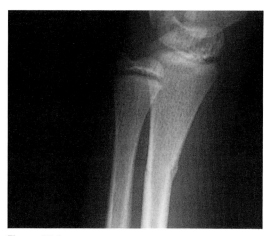

Figure 34.1

Impaction fracture of the distal radius.

Incomplete displaced fractures

One cortex is broken and commonly, a dorsal deformity is present on the opposite side (Fig. 34.2). Comminution can exist and secondary displacement is possible. Even if minimal, the deformity should be reduced. Reduction is easy but careful operative and postoperative care is mandatory: sometimes the operation is performed under general anaesthesia, mainly in cases of comminution, to obtain a stable reduction. A slight over-reduction may be necessary. An above-elbow cast with the wrist flexed at 45° (initial dorsal tilt) or extended at 15° (initial volar tilt) is applied. Radiographs are taken at the 8th and 15th days. In case of redisplacement, reduction is performed again at the second week. Cast immobilization is applied for four weeks; two more weeks with a below-the-elbow cast may sometimes be needed in older children.

Complete fractures

The fracture line goes through the metaphyseal-diaphyseal junction of the radius and more or less proximally through the ulna. Posterior tilt is most commonly observed (Bailey et al. 1989) with overlapping and rotation of the distal fragment (Fig. 34.3).

In contrast to the other fractures, reduction may be difficult and complete correction impossible. A correction of 1° each month and 10° each year may be obtained in malunions, but growth does not correct all the deformities. When judging the remodelling options, two factors should be considered: the child's age and the residual deformity after reduction. Several authors (Daruwala 1979, Fuller and MacCullough 1982, Gandhi et al. 1962, Nilsson and Obrant 1977) have studied the remodelling capabilities of the malunited forearm bones. All agree that the distal forearm capabilities of remodelling are better than those of the diaphyses. There is no concensus of opinion on the acceptable residual deformity in angulation.

A recent study (Roberts 1986) compared the loss of prono-supination motion with bone angulation in different planes, depending on the age of the child when the injury was sustained. The authors concluded that correction of radial angulation of the fracture is mandatory:

- In a child under five years, remodelling is total and there is no loss of prono-supination, even if residual radial deviation is significant.
- When growth is completed, any residual radial deviation will result in loss of prono-supination. Reduction should be perfect.
- Between 5 and 12 years, dorsal angulation does not alter prono-supination. Conversely, radial deviation can decrease prono-supination by as much as 30° in more than half the cases. Ulnar deviation, even if associated with dorsal deviation, does not result in any limitation.

Radial deviation should always be aligned after five years of age. After 12 years of age, the reduction should be perfect in all planes.

Treatment

The periosteum or the pronator quadratus may make the reduction difficult to perform. Pilcher's manoeuvre, combining traction with over-reduction, usually allows reduction. The reduction criteria should be precise and the anterior metaphyseal cortex should go beyond the anterior diaphyseal cortex (Fig. 34.4). Immobilization is achieved with an above-the-elbow cast, open at the anterior part of the elbow level, with the wrist in 45–60° flexion (Fig. 34.5).

If comminution of the radius lateral cortex is present, the wrist should be placed in ulnar deviation to prevent malunion in radial deviation. The cast is removed after five weeks for isolated fractures of the radius and after eight weeks if both forearm bones are fractured. Radiographs are taken at the 2nd, 8th and 15th days to assess and eventually treat any secondary displacement. Secondary displacement is frequent (30% to 40% according to this study). In this series, late secondary displacement occurred between the 15th and the 21st days. Half of these redisplaced fractures were correctly reduced at the first attempt. The cause of redisplacement was incorrect positioning in the cast.

An alternative method of reduction can be performed. Mobilization of the fragments is possible until the 21st day. Pinning should then

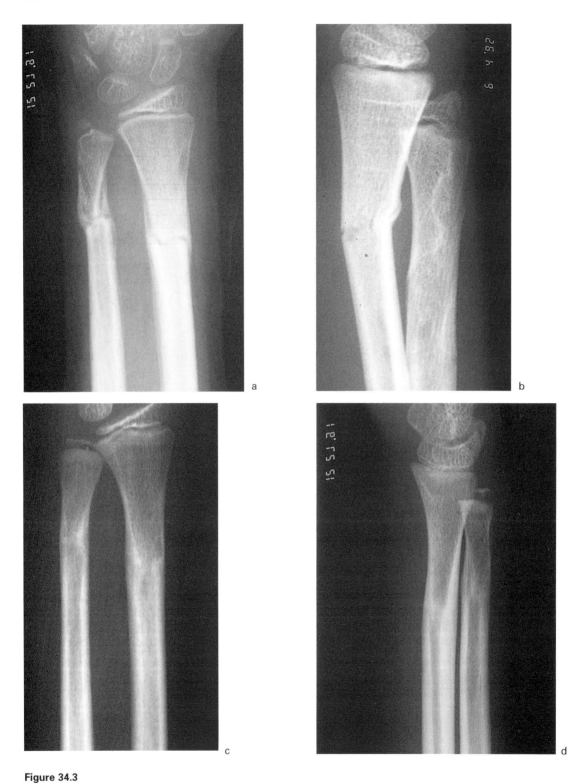

Figure 34.3

Metaphyseal radial and ulnar fracture with dorsal tilt, overlapping and lateral displacement of the distal fragment.

FRACTURES OF THE DISTAL BONES OF THE FOREARM IN CHILDREN 283

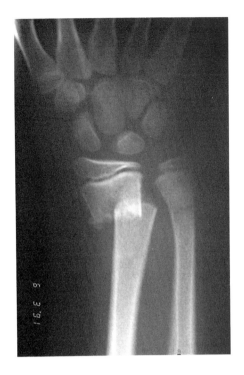
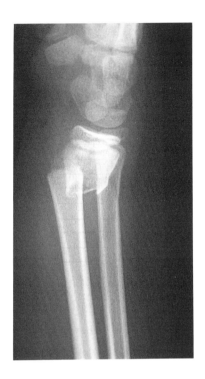
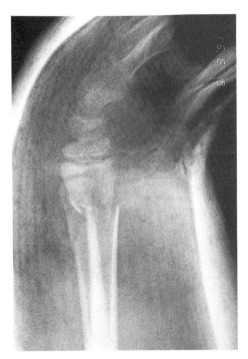
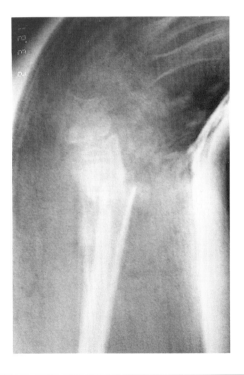

Figure 34.4

Metaphyseal fracture, showing secondary displacement after inadequate reduction.

284 FRACTURES OF THE DISTAL RADIUS

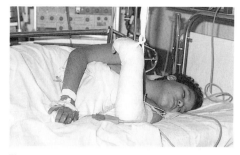

Figure 34.5
Above-the-elbow cast. Note the flexed position of the wrist.

be performed using the systematic Kapandji procedure (1976) (Fig. 34.6) or Metaizeau's procedure (1988) (Fig. 34.7). The important thing is to spare the epiphyseal plate. This possible risk of secondary displacement may indicate initial pinning in an unstable fracture with significant comminution, or if it impossible to regularly watch over the child (if the family circle is non-compliant).

Operative treatment is usually not necessary. Indications for operative intervention include

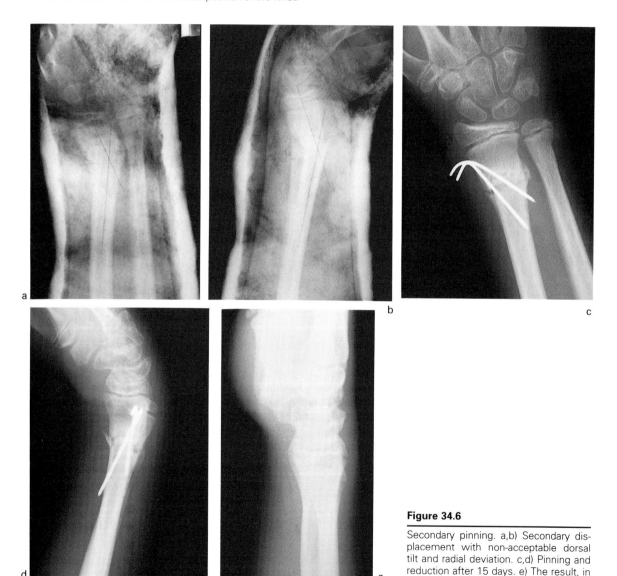

Figure 34.6

Secondary pinning. a,b) Secondary displacement with non-acceptable dorsal tilt and radial deviation. c,d) Pinning and reduction after 15 days. e) The result, in lateral view.

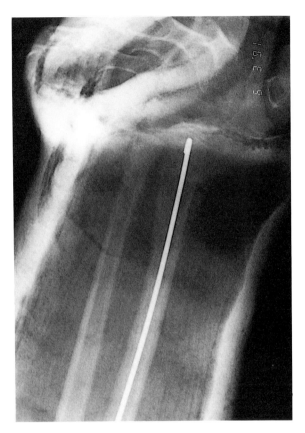 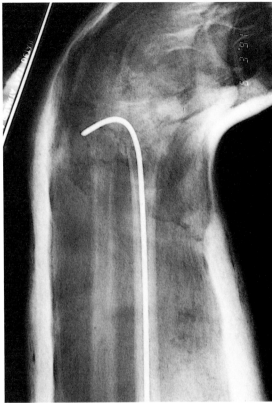

Figure 34.7

Internal fixation used after secondary displacement: intramedullary pinning after Métaizeau (1988).

irreducibility, inability to achieve closed reduction, and cases when closed reduction after redisplacement is unsuccessful. The approach is a small incision at the lateral aspect of the radius. The pronator quadratus is elevated, and osteotomy and reduction are then performed, with two pins inserted to preserve the epiphyseal plate. Above-the-elbow cast immobilization is necessary.

In the less frequent cases of volar displacement (10% in this series), a closed reduction and an above-the-elbow cast with the wrist in extension provide good stability. Other authors (Seriat-Gautier and Jouve 1988) favour Kerboul volar molded plate fixation with screws in the metaphysis and a buttress effect in front of the epiphysis. In this series, this treatment was performed in the only case of secondary displacement. Traditionally, this type of fracture was thought to be caused by a fall on the dorsal aspect of the hand. In fact, a fall on the palmar aspect of the hand or on a hand in forced flexion (bicycle handlebar) are more frequently encountered. Although neurovascular complications are possible, they are very rare in the literature and were absent in this series.

Open fractures are uncommon (Fig. 34.8) and command the same rules of wound care and prophylactic antibiotic therapy and prophylaxis as would be applied to the adult fracture. The usual closed reduction (Tachdjian 1972) might not be possible, indicating a larger approach (Manoli 1982).

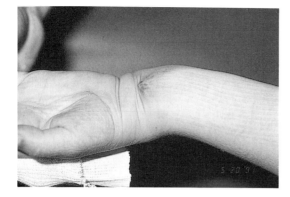
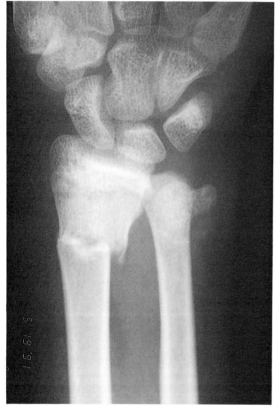
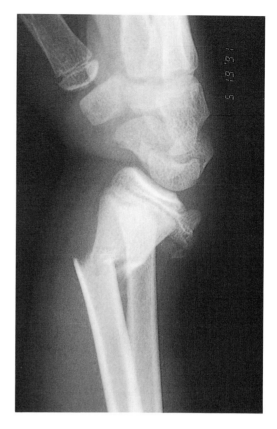

Figure 34.8

Open fracture stage 1: volar displacement of the proximal fragment causing bruising and skin necrosis.

Epiphyseal fracture-separations (EFS)

These are more common in boys and at the period of bone maturation, around puberty. An emergency closed reduction is mandatory. Types I and II of the Salter and Harris classification (1963) are the most frequent: the other types are rare.

Epiphyseal fracture-separation: Salter type I

The non-displaced type I fracture (Fig. 34.9) is relatively common but often overlooked in the small child, and has the potential to collapse. The usual mechanism is a fall on a hyperextended wrist. The child presents with functional inability of the limb. The radiographs are normal, but a

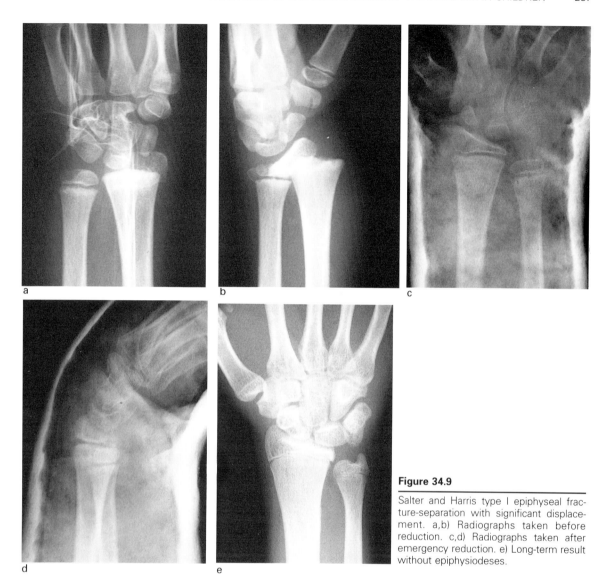

Figure 34.9

Salter and Harris type I epiphyseal fracture-separation with significant displacement. a,b) Radiographs taken before reduction. c,d) Radiographs taken after emergency reduction. e) Long-term result without epiphysiodeses.

careful analysis, with the aid of comparative views of the other wrist, reveals displacement of the fatty lines or of the pronator quadratus. A slight displacement of the ossification centre of the radius, which appears between 8 and 18 months, can also be detected on the comparative radiographs, but the great majority of Salter's type I fracture-separations are unrecognized in emergency.

The possibility of this fracture being present indicates systematic cast immobilization for all painful traumatic wrists in the child. At the tenth day, a radiograph taken after cast removal confirms the diagnosis showing a peripheral callus. Cast immobilization is maintained for a further two weeks.

Epiphyseal fracture-separation: Salter type II

This is the more common type of epiphyseal fracture-separation: 70% of the cases in this series were in this category (and more than 50% of all the epiphyseal fracture-separations according to Tachdjian, 1972). It occurs in children between the ages of 6 and 10. Clinically, there is a dorsal angulation resembling the 'dinner fork' deformity of displacement. An associated ulnar fracture is often present (Fig. 34.10), as well as DRUJ ligamentous lesions. The separation (triangular fibrocartilage tear) detaches a fairly large metaphyseal fragment.

Reduction of dorsal tilt is performed using slight traction combined with wrist flexion. Pressure at the dorsal aspect of the wrist realigns the epiphyseal fragment distal to the metaphysis. The initial reduction should be perfect. Cast immobilization with an above-the-elbow cast is mandatory. Healing in a stable position occurs in one month. Pinning is usually not necessary.

When the displacement is volar (20% of EFS cases), reduction is performed using a reverse process. Immobilization is achieved with an above-the-elbow cast, with the wrist in slight extension, for one month. Redisplacement should be carefully monitored because these fractures heal rapidly and a secondary reduction cannot be performed until the 15th day.

Epiphyseal fracture separation: Salter types III, IV and V

Salter type III and IV EFS provided only 10% of the cases each. Spontaneous epiphysiodesis is the main, though rare, complication which dampens the prognosis. Radiologic follow-up should be performed one year after healing.

Salter type V EFS is often not diagnosed in an emergency. A compression mechanism is present in all EFS types. At the distal radial level, this can result in a pseudo-Madelung deformity (Rang 1983, Saffar et al. 1991). An emergency reduction is the best way to prevent epiphysiodesis.

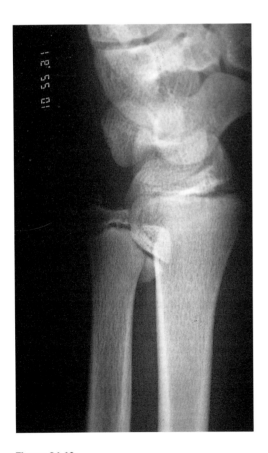

Figure 34.10

Salter and Harris type II epiphyseal fracture, showing separation of the radius and ulna.

Intermediate fractures

Some authors (Collet 1982 and 1985) have described 'intermediate fractures' between metaphyseal and EFS: they are composed of a horizontal metaphyseal line with a vertical line running in the direction of the epiphyseal plate, similar to the Salter type II line. One case was found in this series. Cast immobilization should be applied for 10 weeks if displacement looks like a metaphyseal fracture displacement.

Isolated ulnar fractures

Less than 1% of the total (Collet 1982 and 1985), these fractures occur away from the epiphyseal plate (Fig. 34.11). They are rarely displaced and the cause is a direct impact on the ulna. Reduction is usually not necessary. A three-week immobilization is sufficient.

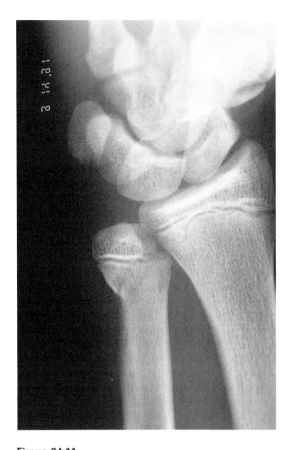

Figure 34.11

Isolated ulnar fracture (without radial head dislocation).

Epiphyseal ulna fractures

Fractures or injury involving the distal ulna epiphysis are not common, but subsequent observation should be prolonged during growth because a deformity can appear with time. Conversely, styloid process fractures are common and prono-supination movement should be prevented by cast immobilization because ulnar styloid pseudoarthrosis is frequent. DRUJ injuries can lead to some disabilities. In one case in this series, surgical treatment was necessary.

Conclusions

Fractures of the distal radius and ulna in children are considered benign, but some important points should be considered:

- Any epiphyseal separation should be reduced immediately as an emergency to save the epiphyseal plate.
- At any age, perfect reduction is mandatory and will provide a good result.
- Remodelling of malunion is not significant after 10 years of age.
- In displaced incomplete fractures, the possibility of secondary displacement demands a perfect reduction, good immobilization in a plaster cast, and radiographic follow-up.
- Complete fractures should be treated by closed reduction with strict criteria for reduction and immobilization.
- The family should be advised how to monitor the upper limb after cast immobilization to prevent cast complications as well as loosening of the cast and loss of reduction.

References

Alffram PA, Bauer GCH. Epidemiology of fractures of the forearm. *J Bone Joint Surg* 1962; **44A**: 105–14.

Aufaure P, Bendjeddou M, Gilbert A. Les fractures du poignet et de la main chez l'enfant. *Ann Chir* 1982; **36**: 499–506.

Bailey DA, Wedge JH, MacCulloch RG et al. Epidemiology of fractures of the distal end of the radius in children as associated with growth. *J Bone Joint Surg* 1989; **71B**: 1225–30.

Bedat Ph, Kaelin A. Fractures de l'extrémité distale du radius chez l'enfant *Med Hyg* 1989; **47**: 1679–82.

Chan GM, Hess M, Hollis J et al. Bone mineral status in childhood accidental fractures *Ann J Dis Child* 1984; **138**: 569–70.

Collet LM. Les fractures de l'extrémité inférieure des deux os de l'avant bras chez l'enfant, à propos de 500 cas. Thèse Médecine. Amiens, 1982.

Collet LM, Rigault P. Fractures de l'extrémité inférieure des deux os de l'avant bras chez l'enfant. In: *Encycl Med Chir (Paris). Appareil locomoteur*, 14045 C10,6. 1985.

Cook SD, Harding AF, Morgan E et al. Association of bone mineral density and pediatric fractures. *J Pédiat Orthop* 1987; **7**: 424–27.

Daruwala JS. A study of radioulnar movements following fractures of the forearm in children. *Clin Orthop* 1979; **139**: 114–20.

Friberg KSI. Remodelling after distal forearm fractures; Parts 1, 2 and 3. *Acta Orthop Scand* 1979; **5**: 537, 731, 741.

Fuller DJ, MacCullough CJ. Malunited fractures of the forearm in children. *J Bone Joint Surg* 1982; **64B**: 364–67.

Gandhi RK, Wilson P, Mason Brown JJ, MacLeod W. Spontaneous correction of deformity following fracture of the forearm in children. *Br J Surg* 1962; **50**: 5–10.

Kapandji A. L'ostéosynthèse par double embrochage intrafocal. *Ann Chir* 1976; **30, 11–12**: 903–8.

Landin LA. Fracture patterns in children. *Acta Orthop Scand* 1983; **202(Suppl)**: 1–109.

Landin L, Lennart C and Nilsson BE. Bone mineral content in children with fractures. *Clin Orthop* 1983; **178**: 292–96.

Manoli A II. Irreductible fracture-separation of the distal radial epiphysis. *J Bone Joint Surg* 1982; **64B**: 1095–96.

Métaizeau JP. *Ostéosynthèse chez l'enfant*. Montpellier: Sauramps Ed. 1988.

Mirwald RL, Bailey DA. *Maximal aerobic power. A congenital analysis*. London, Ontario: Sports Dynamics, 1983.

Narod S, Spasoff RA. Economic and social burden of osteoporosis. In Uhtoff HK, Stahl E eds. Current concepts of bone fragility. Berlin: Springer, 1986: 391–401.

Nilsson BE, Obrant K. The range of motion following fractures of the shaft of the forearm in children. *Acta Orthop Scand* 1977; **48**: 600–2.

Rang M. *Children's fractures*, 2nd ed. Philadelphia: JB Lippincott Company, 1983.

Roberts JA. Angulation of the radius in children's fractures. *J Bone Joint Surg* 1986; **68B**: 751–54.

Saffar P, Ducloyer P, Leclerc C, Lisfranc R. Spontaneous ruptures of the extensor tendons of the fingers in Madelung's deformity. *J Hand Surg* 1991; **16B**: 329–33.

Salter RB, Harris WR. Injury involving the epiphyseal plate. *J Bone Joint Surg* 1963; **45A**: 586–622.

Seriat-Gautier B, Jouve JL. Les décollements-fractures de l'extrémité inférieure du radius à déplacement antérieur chez l'enfant. *Chir Pediatr* 1988; **29**: 265–68.

Tachdjian MO. *Pediatric orthopaedics*. Philadelphia: WB Saunders, 1972.

35
Radial styloid fractures associated with scapholunate ligament sprains

Ph Saffar

A fall on an outstretched hand may cause a fracture of the distal end of the radius in an elderly woman, carpal ligament sprains in a young man and a combination of both injuries at intermediate ages in either sex.

The association of distal radial fractures with a scapholunate ligament tear has been described by many authors (Brown 1987, Hixson et al. 1989, Knirk and Jupiter 1986, Melone 1984, Rosenthal 1983, Saffar 1990, Taleisnik 1985). This tear occurs more frequently with intra-articular fractures, particularly with radial styloid fractures.

Isolated radial styloid fractures are rare: only 12 were found in a systematic review of 772 fractures of the distal radius. They should not be confused with other intra-articular fractures of the distal radius and antero-posterior, lateral and oblique radiographs should be carefully inspected. Comminution of the anterior or posterior rim of the radius is frequently present, indicating a mechanism of injury in flexion or extension: these are not pure radial styloid fractures. The fracture line may sometimes continue transversely up to the distal radio-ulnar joint; again, these are different fractures with different pathomechanisms. However, there are fractures with a radial styloid fragment which may be associated with carpal ligament sprains (Fig. 35.1).

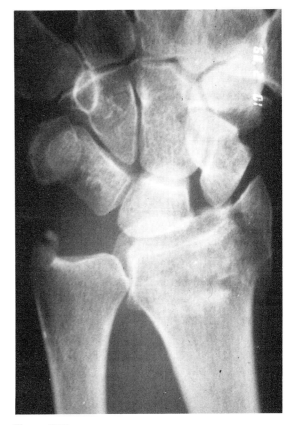

Figure 35.1

Scapholunate instability associated with a distal radial fracture.

Pathomechanism

This type of fracture occurs with the wrist in extension, slight radial deviation and neutral prono-supination. Radial styloid fractures are caused by a fall with the wrist in extension. It seems that slight radial deviation and neutral prono-supination are necessary to produce the associated scapholunate ligament tear. It is a shear fracture: the scaphoid detaches the radial styloid and displaces it proximally (Fig. 35.2). The fracture line is oblique, extending from the crest between the scaphoid and lunate fossae.

292 FRACTURES OF THE DISTAL RADIUS

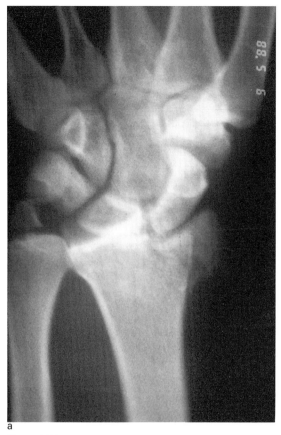
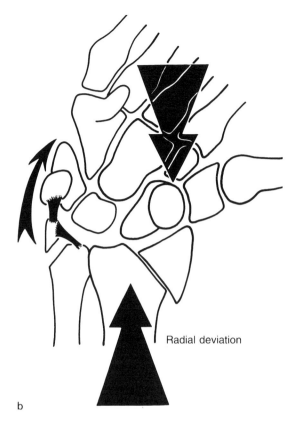

Figure 35.2

a, b) Mechanism of injury in a distal radial fracture with scapholunate ligament tear. The radiograph is of a recent injury.

Patients

This series consisted of 19 radial styloid fractures. There were 11 male and 8 female patients, which is not the usual ratio in distal radial fractures. The mean age was 49 years. An associated ulnar styloid fracture was present in seven cases. Nine cases of scapholunate instability (Fig. 35.3), five of a scapholunate gap of more than 2 mm, and two with a scapholunate angle of more than 70° were noted. Three cases showed no abnormalities in the scapholunate relationship.

Sixteen cases were reviewed in a retrospective study of radial styloid fractures to determine scapholunate instability, diagnosed on examination of the first post-injury radiographs. Three cases were diagnosed acutely: two on the radiographs and one by arthroscopy. Scapholunate dissociation may be visible on the first radiographs but more often, it becomes visible later, sometimes when still in the cast (Fig. 35.4). However in some cases, only the radial styloid fracture is obvious and the instability is missed, as in the case shown in Fig. 35.5.

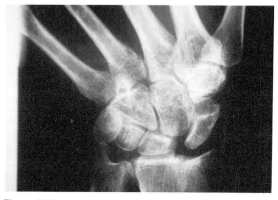

Figure 35.3

Scapholunate instability associated with malunion of a radial styloid fracture.

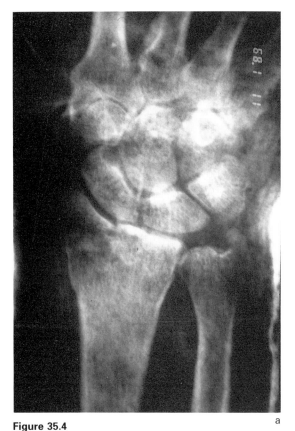 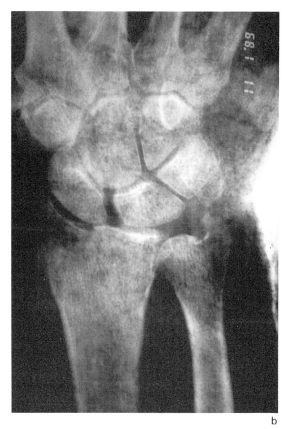

Figure 35.4
a) Radial styloid fracture. b) Displacement of the radial styloid fracture and appearance of a scapholunate gap whilst still in a cast.

Treatment

In the three cases seen in emergency or during the first month, two were treated by reduction, pinning and ligament suture, combined with pinning of the radial styloid fracture (Fig. 35.6). One case was treated on the 25th day, when displacement of the fracture and a scapholunate gap became evident when still in the cast. The other cases that presented were treated by limited arthrodesis (three cases), or ligamentoplasty (one case), or by no treatment when the symptoms were mild or absent.

Discussion

In one case, the injury that produced a radial styloid fracture was described by the patient as having been produced by wrist flexion; however, a single mechanism cannot account for all cases. Styloid fractures with little or no displacement are not usually associated with ligament tears. Certain information seems to point to a shear fracture as the cause of radial styloid fractures with associated scapholunate dissociation:

- scaphoid impaction fractures have been described, in which an impaction is seen on the scaphoid fossa reproducing the scaphoid contour (Fig. 35.7);
- these fractures have been reproduced experimentally. Using a pendulum released by an electromagnet at different heights, the force of impact needed to produce an injury can be calculated by dividing the height of the pendulum by the weight. This device can simulate weight-bearing and non-weight-bearing injuries on cadavers. In this study, 28

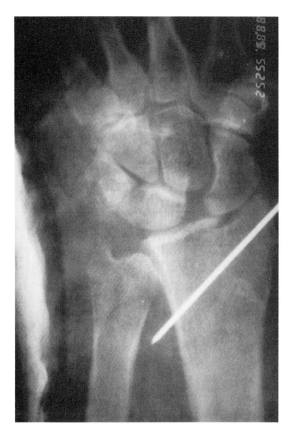

Figure 35.5

Missed scapholunate dissociation and incorrect reduction of a radial styloid fracture.

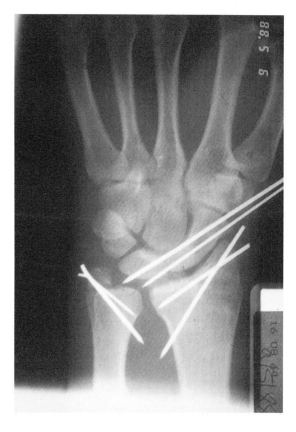

Figure 35.6

Emergency treatment of a radial styloid fracture associated with a scapholunate dissociation and an ulnar styloid fracture.

specimens were submitted to frontal impacts with the wrist in various positions. A radial styloid fracture was produced twice. A complete scapolunate interosseous ligament (SLIL) tear was associated in one case (Fig. 35.8) and a partial rupture in the other;

- immediate midcarpal arthography after reduction of distal radial fractures has been performed (Fontes et al. 1992). There was a very high incidence of associated carpal ligament injuries in this study: out of 12 intra-articular fractures with a radial styloid fragment, nine were associated with an SLIL tear (not included in this study). Control wrist arthrography performed after fracture healing showed there was no more abnormal passage of the dye in many cases. This could indicate that there is normal healing of the ligaments after immobilization. It could also explain the increase of the scapholunate gap or the scapholunate angle in the cases discovered by the author's retrospective study.

This information suggests that an impact of the scaphoid on the radius detaches the radial styloid, which is displaced radially and posteriorly, while the lunate stays in the lunate fossa. This movement produces the scapholunate interosseous ligament (SLIL) tear and can produce an avulsion fracture of the ulnar styloid.

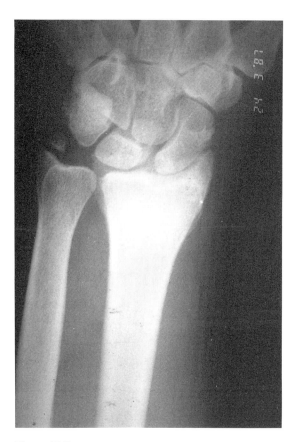

Figure 35.7

A scaphoid impression fracture.

Conclusions

The frequency of association of these two injuries demands a very careful examination of the carpus in all intra-articular fractures of the distal radius, especially the radial styloid fractures. A poor prognosis can be expected with insufficient treatment, because the combination of these two injuries causes wrist pain and later, osteoarthritis.

The recommended treatment is reduction and fixation of the radial styloid fracture if displacement is present. Dynamic radiography, arthroscopy, or midcarpal arthrography should then be performed, depending on the possibilities available to the surgeon.

Percutaneous pinning is advised if a ligament tear is found and there is no intracarpal displacement. If there is a scapholunate gap, an increased scapholunate angle, or a frank scapholunate

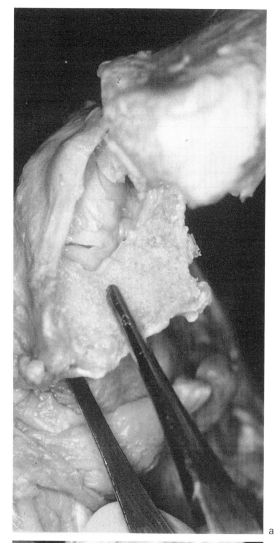

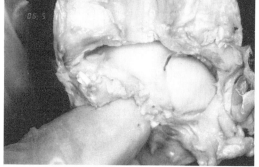

Figure 35.8

Cadaver studies. a) The radial styloid fragment is held by the forceps; b) the associated anterior scapholunate tear is demonstrated.

dissociation, a ligament repair is necessary. For a non-displaced fracture with normal carpal alignment, radiographs must be taken each week until the fifth week after presentation, checking all the time for a scapholunate or distal radial displacement.

Now that we are aware of the association between radial styloid fractures and scapholunate dissociation, careful consideration should be given when considering immediate mobilization of the wrist after intra-articular distal radial fractures, even after an osteosynthesis, as is recommended in some techniques.

References

Brown IW. Volar intercalary carpal instability following a seemingly innocent wrist fracture. *J Hand Surg* 1987; **12B**: 54–56.

Fontes D, Lenoble E, de Somer B, Benoit J. Lésions ligamentaires associées aux fractures distales du radius. *Ann Chir Main* 1992; **11,2**: 119–25.

Hixson ML, Fitzrandolph R, Andrew MM, Walker C. Acute ligament tears of the wrist associated with Colles' fracture. Presented at the Annual Meeting of the ASSH, No. 61. Seattle, 1989.

Knirk JL, Jupiter J. Intraarticular fractures of the distal end of the radius in young adults. *J Bone Joint Surg* 1986; **68A**: 647–59.

Melone CP. Articular fractures of the distal radius. *Orth Clin N Am* 1984; **15**: 217–36.

Rosenthal DI, Schwartz M, Phillips WC, Jupiter J. Fracture of the radius with instability of the wrist. *Am J Roentgenol* 1983; **141**: 113–16.

Saffar Ph. Radial styloid fractures associated with scapho-lunate sprains. Presented at the Annual Meeting of the ASSH. Toronto, 1990.

Taleisnik J. *The wrist*. New York: Churchill Livingstone, 1985: 243.

36
Fractures of the ulnar styloid
C Sokolow

Introduction

The anatomy of the distal part of the ulna has already been described, but it is important to emphasize several points. The ulnar styloid is a cone-shaped knob, situated medially and dorsally off the head of the ulna, from which it is separated by a groove which is the site of insertion of the triangular fibrocartilage complex (TFCC). The ECU tendon and tendon sheath support the ulna dorsally. The length of the ulnar styloid is variable; it continues on the medial side of the ulnar shaft and turns distally towards the triquetrum, offering a large insertional area to the triangular fibrocartilage complex (TFCC). The TFCC has been fully described by several authors (Palmer and Werner 1981, Kuhlmann 1984, Taleisnik 1986). It is composed of several fibrous elements, spreading from the radial and sigmoid notch towards the fifth metacarpal base and covers the ulna and the triquetrum. These elements are described below.

The triangular fibrocartilage is a large band of fibrocartilagenous tissue, which begins at the distal part of the sigmoid notch of the radius and ends at the base of the ulnar styloid. It has two thicker parts, situated anteriorly and posteriorly, composed of thick collagen fibres oriented to resist the compression and tension forces that occur during strong grip. These thicker parts adhere to the wrist joint capsule. There is also an intermediate thin portion, which frequently contains perforations (30–50% of the people 50 years old composed of cartilage (compression) forces). The TFC proper is reinforced anteriorly by ulnocarpal ligaments and dorsally by a looser dorsal radio-ulnar ligament which unites it to the carpus.

The ulnocarpal ligament is the main anterior reinforcement of the triangular fibrocartilage and is composed of two bundles, beginning at the base of the styloid with the TFCC attachment and spreading in a lateral and volar direction towards the lunate and the triquetrum; these two bundles are intimately blended with the anterior margin of the triangular fibrocartilage. This double ligament is necessary for the latero-palmar stability of the carpus and is also important to prevent dorsal displacement of the distal ulna.

The meniscal homologue is a structure beginning at the posterior part of the thickened triangular fibrocartilage (and therefore on the radius), which bridges the intra-articular facet of the triangular fibrocartilage and extends to the palmar aspect of the triquetrum. When it is identifiable, it presents a free articular border (compared to a meniscus) and forms an opening, leading to a space surrounding the styloid process (the prestyloid recess visible by arthrography).

Other stabilizing structures of the distal radio-ulnar joint include the dorsal carpal ligamentous complex, composed of the dorsal radiotriquetral ligament and the dorsal retinacular (extensor retinaculum structure), distal to the dorsal aspect of the ulnar head. Two structures protect this zone: one is a weak expansion of the radiotriquetral ligament (the radiolunotriquetral ligament), and the other is a stronger structure, and the only real posterior constraint, represented by the extensor carpi ulnaris sheath, which blends intimately with the posterior margin of the TFCC.

The other structures of the ulnar side of the wrist do not participate directly in the stability of the joint: these are the ulnar collateral ligament, the dorsal and the ulnar radio-ulnar ligaments.

The pronator quadratus acts as a dynamic stabilizer of the distal radio-ulnar joint.

The ulnar styloid is an intermediate link with these stabilizing structures of the wrist. It is the medial junctional point, often mentioned in the literature but functionally underestimated.

Ulnar styloid fractures are usually not considered, for example in the isolated cases or those associated with a distal radial fracture. This chapter will describe the so-called isolated fractures of the ulnar styloid, which are not always so benign as is generally thought.

History

Ulnar styloid fractures can occur in several circumstances, which are listed below.

- A fall on a fully pronated wrist with dorsiflexion results in a tear of the lunotriquetral ligament and extends to the triangular ligament and to the ulnar styloid, which can fracture at several levels.
- A forced radial deviation will lead to a partial or total avulsion of the ulnar styloid (usually at its distal portion) without any carpal injury. The triangular ligament can be torn in some circumstances.
- A direct impact on the ulnar styloid may produce a fracture. The level is variable, and in the case of a longitudinal force, significant impaction of the styloid can be produced.

The ulnar styloid fracture must be considered with care, and it must be stressed that it can be associated with carpal instability.

Conditions of occurrence

Ulnar styloid fractures can occur after wrist trauma which was described as a carpal sprain. We have analysed 13 charts from patients presenting with a so-called isolated ulnar styloid fracture. Patients with this injury were rapidly and incorrectly examined, and treated by cast immobilization for six to eight weeks. The patients complained of a painful wrist for a mean period of 1.5 years before being correctly treated.

Clinical examination

The typical patient complaint was of an ulnar pain, increasing in ulnar deviation, and a pain occurring when compression was applied to the ulnar styloid process. Other signs were noted less frequently:

- a decrease of grip strength without correlation between the anatomical aspect of the fracture and the degree of the decrease in strength;
- a decrease of supination (these patients presented no other distal radio-ulnar joint pathology);
- a click in ulnar deviation and pronation, without any correlation with any type of lesion. This was noted in over half of the patients in this series.

The clinical examination was usually deceiving. The patients were generally young (mean age 29 years), and had sustained violent trauma to the wrist in a position that usually was difficult to determine.

Radiological findings

Standard radiographs reveal the fracture type and stage. The following types must be distinguished:

- fractures of the base and of the proximal third of the styloid (located proximal to the insertion of the triangular ligament) are usually at the junction of the ulnar head and the styloid process; recent fractures have a clear-cut radiographic appearance, but if not treated, these fractures develop a hypertrophic and loose non-union;
- more distal fractures are similar to an ulnar styloid tip stripping, which is clean at first and later appears as a string of calcification at the tip of the styloid process; this has a lengthening effect.

Dynamic radiographs detect the possible mobility of the fracture or non-union of the fracture.

Arthrography of the wrist joint is mandatory to rule out an associated ligament tear, for example of the triangular ligament, or the lunotriquetral ligament. Injection of the radiocarpal and distal radio-ulnar joints is efficient, but cinearthrography is more precise, with injection of the mid-carpal and distal radio-ulnar joints followed, if necessary, by a radiocarpal injection.

A correlation was sought between the type of ulnar styloid fracture and the cinearthrography findings. In over one-third of the cases, there was an associated ligament injury without any positive correlation with fracture displacement. Thus, arthrographic exploration is mandatory for all types of fractures to decide whether the surgical approach should be intra- or extra-articular.

In this series of 13 patients the radiological findings were as follows:

- nine normal arthrographies: the ulnar styloid fracture was proximal in five cases and distal in four cases;
- four pathological arthrograms with ligament tears (in all four cases, a tear was detected in either the triangular or the lunotriquetral ligament): the ulnar fracture was proximal in two cases and distal in the other two cases.

Treatment

Treatment should be instigated as soon as possible, and so the clinical and paraclinical investigations must be performed immediately.

Proximal ulnar styloid fractures

A surgical approach is mandatory to fix the fracture. An intra-articular approach should be used to check the triangular and the lunotriquetral ligaments.

If the fracture is seen after a delay, a complete clinical and paraclinical investigation must be performed. In the case of an isolated fracture of the ulnar styloid, an internal fixation should be performed, providing the fragment is sufficiently large. In other cases, the fragment is excised, taking care to reattach the peripheral structures to the medial border of the TFCC.

Distal ulnar styloid fractures

In these cases, the fragments are usually too small to be fixed. They are usually seen after a delay and should be treated in exactly the same manner as proximal fractures seen after a delay. During the operative approach, a zone of chondromalacia was frequently seen on the triquetrum facing the abnormally long fractured ulnar styloid: this zone may heal after the removal of the small styloid fragments.

Conclusions

Ulnar styloid injury must be considered carefully in cases of wrist trauma because it can jeopardize the ulnar stability of the wrist. A simple methodology leads to complete evaluation of these lesions and allows formulation of a complete therapeutic plan.

References

Kuhlmann JN, Fahrer I, Kapandji IA, Tubiana R. La stabilité du poignet normal. In *Traité de la chirurgie de la main*, Tome II. Paris: Masson Ed, 1984: 808–21.

Palmer AK, Werner FW. The triangular fibrocartilage complex of the wrist. *J Hand Surg* 1981; **6A**: 153–61.

Taleisnik J. *The Wrist*. New York: Churchill Livingstone. 1986.

37
Acute and chronic neurovascular complications of distal radial fractures

Arnold-Peter C Weiss, James B Steichen

Introduction

Fractures of the distal radius represent one of the most common injuries treated by orthopaedic surgeons. In general, they can be treated with closed reduction and casting without long-term disability. Patients who have undergone appropriate treatment usually require only a short period of immobilization to allow consolidation of the fracture fragments prior to a return to normal wrist function. The recognition of specific sub-groups of distal radial fractures has led to the use of newer techniques of treatment in more complicated fracture patterns (Melone 1984). Moreover, these techniques can be modified to suit a particular fracture pattern in an individual patient, but with these specific fracture patterns and modified techniques, unique complications have arisen.

Complications described after the treatment of distal radial fractures have included peripheral compression neuropathy, Volkmann's ischemic contracture, pin-tract infections, tendon ruptures, malunion of fracture fragments, secondary degenerative joint disease, secondary adjacent joint dystrophy, and other associated injuries (Abbot and Saunders 1933, Bacorn and Kurtzke 1953, Bauman et al. 1981, Cooney et al. 1990, Gartland and Werley 1951, Smaill 1965, Stark 1987, Steichen and Eckenrode 1988, Sumner and Khuri 1984, Zoega 1966). A review of the neurovascular complications secondary to fractures of the distal radius and their treatment will be described in this chapter. Three main factors tend to influence the incidence of complications and their severity after distal radial fractures: fracture pattern and displacement, the type of treatment undertaken for maintenance of fracture reduction, and the position of immobilization. By far the majority of complications described deal with compressive neuropathies or direct contusion to the median, radial, or ulnar nerves (Kozin and Wood 1993). Relatively few complications related to disturbance of the vascular supply of the upper limb, such as ischemia, have been described (Fernandez 1981).

Fracture pattern and displacement

The fracture pattern and its relative displacement, either during the injury or at presentation, is probably the most common cause of neurovascular complications following fractures of the distal radius. Non-comminuted extra-articular fractures can result in neurologic injury, nearly always involving the median nerve, if the displacement is of a significant magnitude to cause a transient compression, or if the distal fragment heals in a shortened and angled position with prominent volar callus or excessive dorsal tilt, causing a stretch phenomenon with subsequent neuropathy (Abbot and Saunders 1993, Bauman et al. 1987, Bourrel and Ferro 1982, Cooney et al. 1980, Dickson 1926, Fernandez 1981, Kumar 1990, Lynch and Lipscomb 1963, McClain and Wissinger 1976, Paley and McMurtry 1987, Rychak et al. 1991).

The median nerve lies in the fixed carpal tunnel, approximately 3 mm away from the distal radius. After simulated distal radial fractures, this distance decreases to 2 mm and includes an angulation of the nerve over the bone, if angulation of the bone persists (Vance and Gelberman 1978). Injury to the median nerve is far more common than ulnar neuropathy; the central location of the median nerve contrasted to the relatively greater excursion available to the ulnar nerve, proximal to Guyon's canal, is thought to account for this difference (Cooney et al. 1980, Kozin and Wood 1993, Vance and Gelberman 1978). Nerve compression is most frequently seen in the elderly, since aggressive surgical treatment of distal radial fractures is often not employed in these patients. This is due to many factors, including significant osteoporosis (eliminating certain forms of treatment that would otherwise be appropriate to the fracture pattern) and possible limited functional demands in this age group. Traditionally, these considerations may have led the orthopaedic surgeon to accept a borderline result regarding fragment reduction. Frequently, shortening and dorsal angulation of the distal radius are noted, with resultant stretch of all the volar structures, including the median and ulnar nerves (Fig. 37.1).

Secondary injury due to chronic compression of the median nerve can often occur months after the fracture itself. The carpal tunnel is relatively inflexible in its potential volume. A decrease in absolute volume caused by fracture fragment displacement, hematoma, chronic edema, or exuberant callus may cause carpal tunnel syndrome (Cooney et al. 1980, Frykman 1967, Paley and McMurtry 1987). In general, carpal tunnel decompression or removal of osseous impingement reduces the symptoms substantially.

Comminuted, high-energy, intra-articular distal radial fractures involving several bony fragments with sharp spikes often directed volarly can impart a mechanical injury to the median or ulnar nerves, either during acute impaction of the fracture or by prolonged bony impingement on the nerve by an unreduced fracture fragment (Abbot and Saunders 1933, Paley and McMurtry 1987). Fractures with the greatest comminution or displacement have a higher likelihood of direct injury (Kozin and Wood 1993). In a similar fashion, although far less commonly encountered, injury to the intrinsic blood vessels supplying the hand can occur with a sharp, bony spike fragment causing intracompartmental bleeding with a secondary ischemic phenomenon, or median nerve compression from a hematoma (Paley and McMurtry 1993). This mechanism of injury is often seen in the younger patient, who has excellent bone quality, but falls from a significant height and sustains a high-displacement fracture with very sharp, strong bony fragments, which dis-

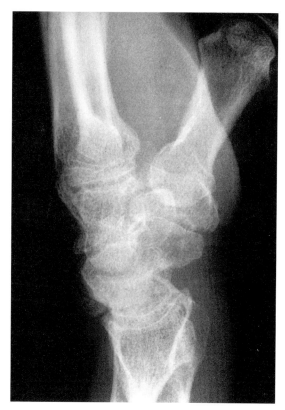

Figure 37.1

A 76-year-old female who was treated with short arm cast application. The fracture healed in dorsal angulation with shortening of the distal radius. The patient began to experience numbness and paresthesias in the median nerve distribution 14 months later. A carpal tunnel release was performed, with good symptomatic relief. Reproduced courtesy of Manus (1993).

place volarly due to forced wrist hyperextension (Fig. 37.2).

Aggressive management of these fractures is required not only to provide anatomical alignment, in the hope of preventing secondary traumatic arthritis, but also to reduce to an absolute minimum the amount of damage sustained by the median or ulnar nerve due to direct pressure or prolonged impalement by the bony fragments (Melone 1984). Frequently, this requires operative intervention utilizing some form of external fixation device with a limited arthrotomy for fracture fragment alignment and joint congruity (Melone 1984, Sanders et al. 1991, Schuind et al. 1984). Occasionally, in addition to an external fixator, internal fixation with Kirschner

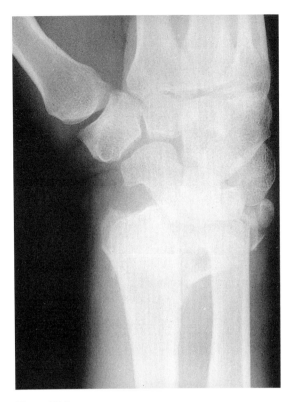

Figure 37.2

A 33-year-old male construction worker fell 10 m onto his right upper extremity, sustaining a high-energy distal radial fracture. The patient noted median nerve paresthesias prior to external fixation and open reduction. A carpal tunnel release was performed at the same time as the reduction and fixation, with excellent symptomatic relief. Reproduced courtesy of Manus (1993).

wires or rigid plating is necessary. If there is bone loss after reduction, bone grafting may also be necessary.

Preoperative neurologic examination is mandatory in high-energy injuries, and if the patient presents with evidence of either a median or ulnar neurapraxia, immediate decompression of either nerve is quite appropriate to ensure that no frank laceration has occurred and that no bony fragments remain impinging upon the nerves after reduction. If a patient is unresponsive during examination and operative treatment of the fracture is required, then a carpal tunnel release is mandatory. Similarly, should an acute bleeding disorder in any compartment of the forearm or hand be suspected, based on the patient's symptoms, or the presence of unexplained acute swelling or deep ischemic pain, then exploration and hemostatic control is essential to prevent any increased pressure on the adjacent nerves or secondary ischemic problems due to lack of appropriate blood flow to the intracompartmental tissues (Kozin and Wood 1993). Intraosseous entrapment of the ulnar artery has been reported and can represent an impediment to complete fracture reduction (Fernandez 1981).

Rarely, patients with a distal radial fracture form significant amounts of callus about the healing fracture, which may result in local compression of the median nerve with secondary neuropathy (Cooney et al. 1980, Frykman 1967). Very rarely, a flexor tendosynovitis can develop due to irritation after a distal radial fracture. This can elicit median nerve paresthesias based on local pressure increases in the carpal tunnel. With highly displaced fractures, or in patients who are not compliant with post-reduction extremity care, edema of the hand and wrist can often increase carpal tunnel pressure, producing secondary paresthesias (Kozin and Wood 1993).

In any of these situations involving extra- or intra-articular displaced distal radial fractures, the treatment protocol should involve reduction of the fracture fragments to their anatomic location by whatever means are required and appropriate to that particular patient. If symptoms of nerve compression are noted at initial presentation or persist post-treatment, an exploration and decompression of the median and/or ulnar nerves is appropriate to ensure that no further compression and subsequent damage are sustained.

If the radial fracture is allowed to heal with excessive shortening, angulation and dorsal tilt, the ulna may become displaced anteriorly. As time progresses, this malunion may cause chronic problems of ulnar nerve compression and flexor tendon rupture (Fig. 37.3).

Position of immobilization

The demonstration that intracarpal pressure increases with significant wrist flexion during reduction of distal radial fractures has alerted the orthopaedic surgeon to avoid this particular position (known as the Cotton–Loder position) when undertaking closed manipulation and casting (Abbot and Sanders 1933, Bauman et al. 1981,

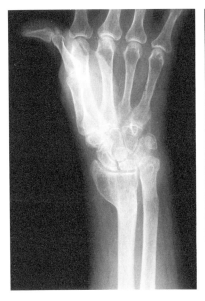 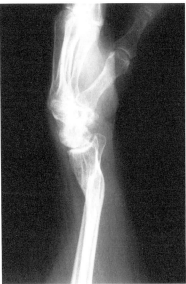 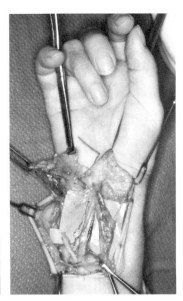

Figure 37.3

a,b) This 65-year-old woman had sustained an open fracture of the distal wrist with laceration over the anterior surface of distal ulna 5 years before these radiographs were taken. The fracture initially healed with asymptomatic malunion. The patient presented with 6-month history of a 2.5 × 3.5 cm anterior ulnar wrist mass, associated with progressive numbness. There was loss of two-point sensory discrimination of the long, ring and small fingers and of the dorsal surface of the hand, associated with decreased grip and weakness of flexion. c) Surgical exploration of the anterior ulnar wrist revealed marked circumferential scarring about the ulnar nerve and artery with additional compression from a large synovial-fluid-filled sac deep to the neurovascular bundle and encasing the flexor tendons of the ring and small fingers. There was an attritional rupture of the flexor digitorum profundus tendons to the ring and small fingers secondary to motion over an anteriorly displaced irregular distal ulna. The distal flexor digitorum profundus to the ring and small fingers had attached to the intact flexor digitorum profundus of the middle finger. Surgical excision of the sac, Darrach resection of the distal ulna, neurolysis of the ulnar nerve and tendolysis eventually produced return of sensation to the involved digits with improved flexion and relief of all symptoms. Reproduced courtesy of Manus (1993).

Cassebaum 1950, Lynch and Lipscomb 1963, Zemel 1987). Patients undergoing reduction who have been placed in excessive wrist flexion will often present with median nerve sensory changes, as well as pain, and should be repositioned immediately in a more favorable position that produces less compression of the carpal canal. In fact, the use of the Cotton-Loder position for fracture reduction should be avoided, since the theoretical advantage of maximal wrist flexion in obtaining or maintaining volar tilt is not supported anatomically. The magnitude of wrist flexion required to produce any meaningful ligamentotaxis via the dorsal ligament complex to the distal fracture fragment is extreme, and would never be accomplished clinically without significant morbidity (Bartosh and Saldana 1990).

Appropriate alignment of the volar cortical fragments in the reduction is essential to eliminate the need for the Cotton-Loder position. If a manipulation is undertaken so that the volar cortical fragments are aligned in a longitudinal fashion, then an adequate reduction can be obtained using this fulcrum as an appropriate lever arm without positioning the wrist in excessive flexion. If appropriate volar cortical abutment is not obtained, the dorsal tilt can only be corrected with excessive wrist flexion, due to the relative shortening of the volar radius as the reduction dorsiflexion maneuver is undertaken and, as noted, this should be avoided. During the reduction maneuver, one should avoid attempts at multiple, forced manipulations, thereby reducing the amount of soft tissue trauma and edema (Cassebaum 1950, Cooney et al. 1980, Frykman 1967).

Significant swelling is frequently seen during the early post-fracture period. If there is any indication that the patient is experiencing significant continued swelling, then a circumferential cast should be avoided, since these can produce an external compressive effect on any of the peripheral nerves and, in the extreme case, loss of blood flow to the distal extremity with a secondary Volkmann's ischemia. If a circumferential cast is required to maintain reduction, yet the risk of significant swelling exists, the surgeon should bivalve the cast, including the underlying padding. This provides an axis along the cast, which can then be displaced by any subsequent swelling, thereby avoiding internal constriction. Alternatively, a well-molded splint can be applied in a bivalved fashion to the upper extremity. Usually, this provides almost the same degree of immobilization as a circumferential cast. This type of splint application in the acute period can often reduce the risk of secondary complications due to compression of the soft tissues by plaster or fiberglass.

Type of fracture treatment

Modifications to the standard cast treatment of distal radial fractures, as well as technical advances in the treatment of these fractures with external fixation devices, have led to unique complications related to the neurovascular structures. The most obvious form of injury to any of the neurovascular structures involves the use of percutaneous pinning devices, either in a pins-in-plaster technique (Melone 1984) or through an external fixation device which can directly impale these structures, causing acute and often irreversible damage (Cooney et al. 1980, Sanders et al. 1991, Schuind 1984). Injury during pin placement (Fig. 37.4) is most often seen in the sensory branch of the radial nerve, which is located in the region where external fixation pins are frequently placed (Cooney et al. 1980, Linscheid 1965, Steichen and Eckenrode 1988). This complication can be extremely annoying to both the patient and

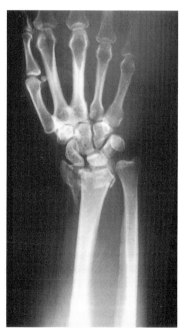
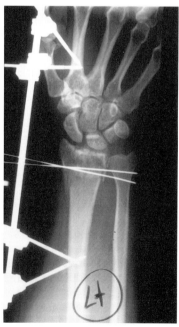
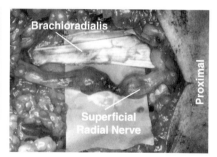

Figure 37.4

a) A 46-year-old woman with a closed comminuted intra-articular fracture of the left distal radius. b) Closed reduction and percutaneous pinning was performed through puncture wounds without open exposure of the radius or metacarpal. Percutaneous Kirschner wires were also inserted. c) The patient presented $4\frac{1}{2}$ months after the fracture with pain, hypersensitivity and loss of sensation in the distribution of the superficial radial nerve with a painfully positive Tinel's percussion test at the site of the radial external fixator puncture wound. The symptoms were present immediately following the insertion of the external fixator. She also developed a painful malunion of the distal radiocarpal and radio-ulnar joints. At the time of wrist fusion, exploration of the site of insertion of the proximal radial external fixator pin revealed that the superficial radial nerve had been impaled by the pin. The neuroma-in-continuity was treated with excision and the proximal superficial radial nerve was buried deep to the brachioradialis muscle, with eventual resolution of the pain and hypersensitivity.

surgeon and can cause significant pain and sensory changes resulting in permanent disability. The placement of external fixation pins should always be performed in a limited open fashion, allowing appropriate identification and visualization of the neurovascular structures and thus avoiding any direct injury to the nerves or vessels. This form of placement is easily accomplished through a limited incision, with careful retraction of the soft tissues to allow direct visualization of the bone to which the pins will be fixed. Using this technique, damage to nerves or vessels can be eliminated or greatly reduced.

In rare instances, some form of sensory radial nerve damage, on a transient basis, can still be seen. This is most frequently secondary to a 'tenting phenomenon' of the sensory branch of the radial nerve over the placed pin after the retraction devices are removed. This local irritability of the nerve frequently resolves after the fracture has healed and the pins are removed. The placement of external fixation or other percutaneous pins distally must also be undertaken with care. This is also frequently performed using a limited open approach to avoid any damage to the surrounding intrinsic musculature of the hand, or to volar blood vessels, which might cause an acute intracompartmental bleed.

Radial sensory dysesthesia may also be noted if cast application is too tight (Stewart et al. 1985). This nerve is quite prominent in the subcutaneous fat above the hard, immobile radial styloid. Excessive swelling in a non-compliant case or application of a tight cast will cause an increase in local pressure to the nerve, with resulting transient or permanent neuritis.

Discussion

Acute injury of the median nerve, which represents the most frequent distal radial fracture complication, has been reported in anywhere from 0.2% to 3.2% of cases undergoing fracture management (Bacorn and Kurtzke 1953, Lynch and Lipscomb 1963). In any patient presenting with a distal radial fracture, a careful neurologic examination is essential, not only to document the prereduction and pretreatment status of the neurovascular supply to the hand, but also to provide a baseline by which to judge any subsequent changes in these structures. A careful examination involving two-point discrimination measurements along both borders of all digits of the median and ulnar nerve distribution is mandatory. Less important, although occasionally helpful, is the Semmes–Weinstein evaluation, which can also provide significant data regarding the function of either the median or the ulnar nerve. A sensory examination along the dorsal aspect of the proximal thumb should also be documented, as this area is nearly always accessible, even with cast treatment, and can be used to follow post-treatment changes in the sensory branch of the radial nerve.

In patients who present with extremely high-energy fractures, or fractures involving significant volar comminution and 'spike' formation, a heightened awareness of the possibility of a median nerve, ulnar nerve, or vascular injury is essential for proper assessment (Paley and McMurtry 1987). Should symptoms be present on initial evaluation of a neuropathy, an acute vascular bleed, or a progressive ischemic event, immediate open surgical intervention involving decompression and stabilization of the injured structure is essential to avoid any secondary and progressive damage to the nerves or vessels. Iatrogenic compression of the median or ulnar nerve should be avoided by the surgeon during reduction of the fracture fragments, by carefully positioning the hand and wrist in the immobilization device, so that volar flexion is less than 45° (Abbott and Saunders 1933, Cassebaum 1950, Lynch and Lipscomb 1963). Appropriate attention to the fracture anatomy, with reconstitution of the volar cortical alignment, can provide an appropriate lever arm for reduction, and eliminate the need for significant palmar flexion to be used in the reduction technique and maintenance of that reduction. If a patient undergoes a fracture reduction and cast immobilization, but is found to have an acute change in the status of the median or ulnar nerve sensation after post-reduction examination, then another form of fixation and maintenance of fracture reduction is required, for example external fixation (Sanders et al. 1991, Schuind et al. 1984).

Not all injuries to the median or ulnar nerve occur immediately after the fracture. Several can be rather progressive in nature, usually due to the stretch phenomenon of the nerves themselves following inadequate or, on occasion, over-reduction. This type of complication is frequently seen in the elderly, where a distal radial fracture reduction that might not be appropriate in the younger age group, is accepted due to tradition, or possibly due to the patient's decreased daily functional requirements, significant osteopenia, or poor medical status. Occasionally, an electromyographic, or nerve conduction velocity study is appropriate in these patients to assess the condition of the median or ulnar nerve. This is not always required, as the symptoms tend to be classically distributed, leaving little doubt as to the exact site of chronic compression. As with acute cases, surgical decompression of the carpal tunnel in the case of the median nerve, or of Guyon's canal in the case of the ulnar nerve, is warranted in an attempt to relieve as much pressure upon the nerve as possible, despite the fact that the fracture malunion is not addressed. Even if a surgical decompression is undertaken, the symptoms in these patients are generally prolonged and very slow to resolve, with this observation most frequently being attributed to a stretch injury and secondary intraneural fibrosis, which appears less likely to recover than compression alone. On rare occasions, osteotomy of the malunited distal radius may be required to adequately relax the volar structures, including the median and ulnar nerves (Bourrel and Ferro 1982).

References

Abbott LC, Saunders JBCM. Injuries of the median nerve in fractures of the lower end of the radius. *Surg Gynec Obstet* 1933; **57**: 507–16.

Bacorn RW, Kurtzke JF. Colles' fracture. A study of two thousand cases from the New York State Workmen's Compensation Board. *J Bone Joint Surg* 1953; **35A**: 643–658.

Bartosh RA, Saldana MJ. Intraarticular fractures of the distal radius: a cadaveric study to determine if ligamentotaxis restores radiopalmar tilt. *J Hand Surg* 1990; **15A**: 18–21.

Bauman TD, Gelberman RH, Mubarak SJ, Garfin SR. The acute carpal tunnel syndrome. *Clin Orthop* 1981; **156**: 151–56.

Bourrel P, Ferro RM. Nerve complications in closed fractures of the lower end of the radius. *Ann Chir Main* 1982; **1**: 119–26.

Cassebaum WH. Colles' fracture. A study of end results. *J Am Med Assn* 1950; **143**: 963–65.

Cooney WP III, Dobyns JH, Linscheid RL. Complications of Colles' fractures. *J Bone Joint Surg* 1980; **62A**: 613–19.

Dickson ED. Peripheral nerve injuries associated with fractures of the long bones. *Southern Med J* 1926; **19**: 37–42.

Fernandez DL. Irreducible radiocarpal fracture-dislocation and radioulnar dissociation with entrapment of the ulnar nerve, artery, and flexor profundus II–V — a case report. *J Hand Surg* 1981; **6A**: 456–61.

Frykman G. Fracture of the distal radius including sequelae — shoulder-hand-finger syndrome, disturbance in the distal radio-ulnar joint and impairment of nerve function. A clinical and experimental study. *Acta Orthop Scand* 1967; **18 (Suppl)**:1–153.

Gartland JJ, Werley CW. Evaluation of healed Colles' fractures. *J Bone Joint Surg* 1951; **33A**: 895–907.

Kozin SH, Wood MB. Early soft-tissue complications after fractures of the distal part of the radius. Instructional Course Lectures, AAOS. *J Bone Joint Surg* 1993; **75A**: 144–53.

Kumar A. Median and ulnar nerve injury secondary to a comminuted Colles fracture. *J Trauma* 1990; **30**: 118–19.

Linscheid RL. Injuries to radial nerve at wrist. *Arch Surg* 1965; **91**: 942–46.

Lynch AC, Lipscomb PR. The carpal tunnel syndrome and Colles' fractures. *J Am Med Assn* 1963; **185**: 363–66.

McClain EJ, Wissinger HA. The acute carpal tunnel syndrome: nine case reports. *J Trauma* 1976; **16**: 75–78.

Melone CP Jr. Articular fractures of the distal radius. *Orthop Clin N Am* 1984; **15**: 217–36.

Paley D, McMurtry RY. Median nerve compression by volarly displaced fragments of the distal radius. *Clin Orthop* 1987; **215**: 139–47.

Rychak JS, Kalenak A. Injury to the median and ulnar nerves secondary to fracture of the radius. A case report. *J Bone Joint Surg* 1977; **59A**: 414–15.

Sanders RA, Keppel FL, Waldrop JI. External fixation of distal radial fractures: results and complications. *J Hand Surg* 1991; **16A**: 385–91.

Schuind F, Donkerwolcke M, Burny F. External fixation of wrist fractures. *Orthopedics* 1984; **7**: 841–44.

Smaill GB. Long-term follow-up of Colles' fracture. *J Bone Joint Surg* 1965; **47B(1)**: 80–85.

Stark WA. Neural involvement in fractures of the distal radius. *Orthopedics* 1987; **10**: 333–35.

Steichen JB, Eckenrode JF. Management of the neuroma-in-continuity. In: Brunelli G, ed. *Textbook of microsurgery*. Milan: Masson, 1988: 665–70.

Stewart HD, Innes AR, Burke FD. The hand complications of Colles' fractures. *J Hand Surg* 1985; **10B**: 103–6.

Sumner JM, Khuri SM. Entrapment of the median nerve and flexor pollicis longus tendon in an epiphyseal fracture-dislocation of the distal radioulnar joint: a case report. *J Hand Surg* 1984; **9A**: 711–14.

Vance RM, Gelberman RH. Acute ulnar neuropathy with fractures at the wrist. *J Bone Joint Surg* 1978; **60A**: 962–65.

Zemel NP. The prevention and treatment of complications from fractures of the distal radius and ulna. *Hand Clin* 1987; **3**: 1–11.

Zoega H. Fracture of the lower end of the radius with ulnar nerve palsy. *J Bone Joint Surg* 1966; **48B(3)**: 514–16.

38
Extensor pollicis longus tendon rupture after distal radial fractures

J Sallerin, P Bonnevialle, M Mansat

Extensor pollicis longus (EPL) tendon rupture during the course of distal radial fractures is an infrequent but well-known complication. This spontaneous rupture was first described by Duplay in 1876. In 1946, Smith estimated its frequency at 0.2–0.3%.

Patients and methods

Twenty patients were reviewed for this study: 16 females and 4 males. The mean age was 63 years (range 24–74 years). Fourteen fractures were treated conservatively with a short or long arm cast for four to six weeks. Six patients were treated by intrafocal pinning with two to three pins.

In each case, the time lapse until rupture, the previous symptoms and the mechanism were recorded. Ulnar variance, radial inclination, and the situation of the fracture line relative to the distalmost point of the radial styloid process were noted on the radiographs. When pinning was performed, the pin length was also measured. Fifteen patients were operated on by extensor indicis proprius (EIP) transfer to the distal part of the ruptured EPL tendon.

Results

The time lapse between distal radial fracture and EPL rupture was short. After conservative treatment (14 cases), 10 tendons were ruptured between the first and second months, one at the fifth and one at the eighth month. Two patients suffered rupture after two years. Among the fractures treated surgically by pinning (six cases), all the ruptures were present before the second month.

In most cases, there were no symptoms before rupture. Three patients presented with dorsal swelling over Lister's tubercle and three others had moderate pain before rupture. Tendon rupture was spontaneous, sometimes still under cast, a minimal strain was noted in four cases. The fractures treated conservatively were minimally or non-displaced (Table 38.1). After surgical treatment, reduction was good in all cases. In one case, a long pin migrated proximally, causing tendon rupture.

Mechanism

Conservative treatment

Two theories are proposed. Both recognize the fact that the dorsal retinaculum is left intact in non-displaced or slightly displaced distal radial fractures (Helal et al. 1982).

Vascular theory

Engkuist in 1979 and, more recently, Hirasawa in 1990 have studied the EPL tendon vascular supply. A progressive decrease in the vascular supply to the tendon and synovium is noted after the musculotendinous junction. A very poor supply of around 5 mm in length is noted, beginning at 11 mm and ending at 16 mm distal to this junction. This section is situated near Lister's tubercle, at the distal part of the dorsal retinaculum (Fig. 38.1).

Table 38.1 Radiologic study of 20 patients

Sagittal plane	ulnar variance	−1 − +2 mm
		0° (+20 − −15°)
Fracture line	radial inclination	18° (−30 − +10°)
	situation	17 mm (10–25 mm)

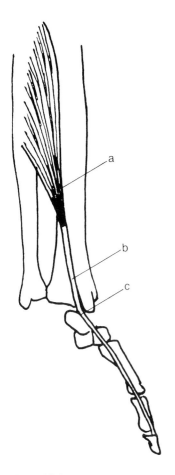

Figure 38.1

EPL vascular supply (after Hirasawa et al 1990). a) Musculotendinous junction; b) 11 mm distal to the junction; c) 16 mm distal to the junction. The hypovascularized area is between b) and c), near Lister's tubercle.

At the time of rupture, the hematoma penetrating the third dorsal compartment and local oedema causes an increase in pressure, and impedes the vascular supply to the tendon and synovium. This produces tendon ischaemia and necrosis. Heavy constraints applied at Lister's tubercle will cause tendon rupture.

Mechanical theory

Helal (1982) has pointed out that the third compartment volume is decreased by the presence of callus on the radial fracture or by a moderate malunion. Periosteal hypertrophy accentuates this phenomenon. The intact dorsal retinaculum compresses the tendon on the callus or the malunion. Mechanical wear of the tendon during repetitive movements eventually causes rupture (Fig. 38.2).

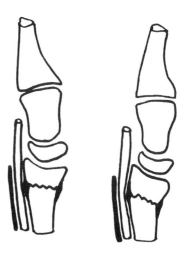

Figure 38.2

Mechanical theory of EPL rupture. The dorsal retinaculum compresses the EPL tendon against a callus or a slight malunion. Repetitive movements of the tendon over either of these results in tendon rupture.

Other theories

Rupture can occur by tendon injury against bony spurs. Denman (1979) explained the tendon rupture as a result of compression between the distal radius and the third metacarpal tubercle during the hyperextension movement causing the fracture. Stahl (1988) described delayed ruptures following tendon wear on a non-united Lister's tubercle.

Surgical treatment by pinning

The pin causing rupture is always in a postero-lateral position. Direct injury is possible when drilling or removing the pin. Rupture occurs more often due to repetitive rubbing of the tendon on a pin that is cut too short (Fig. 38.3).

After either conservative or surgical treatment, rupture is always situated near Lister's tubercle.

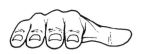
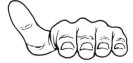

Figure 38.4

With the hand at rest on a flat plate, adduction of the thumb is impossible owing to EPL tendon rupture.

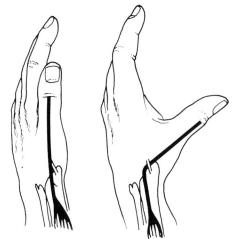

Figure 38.3

During thumb motion, the tendon rubs the dorsal aspect of the wrist.

Clinical examination

The dorsal prominence limiting the anatomical snuffbox dorsally has disappeared. It is impossible to extend the distal phalanx of the thumb when the metaphalangeal (MP) joint is in extension. A certain amount of extension is possible when the MP joint is in flexion. This is due to the action of the thenar muscles and may delay the diagnosis. Loss of thumb adduction is observed. This is obvious when the hand is resting on a flat plane (Fig. 38.4). On radiographic examination, displacement is minimal or has been correctly reduced.

Technique

Several techniques have been proposed to treat EPL rupture:

1. End-to-end sutures (McMaster 1932) are difficult to perform due to tendon retraction and attrition.

2. Tendon grafts may be performed, using a toe extensor or palmaris longus, both tunnelled subcutaneously (Hamlin and Littler 1977, Magnell et al. 1988).

3. Tendon transfer is the most common technique. The EIP is passed either through the fourth or third dorsal compartment (Magnussen et al. 1990, Schneider and Rosenstein 1983), or subcutaneously, and a pulley can be reconstructed (Saffar and Fakhoury 1987). The tendon can also be left in place in the fourth compartment (Tubiana 1986) and sutured to the distal stump of the EPL. This latter technique was used in this study, with good results for thumb motion and strength (Table 38.2). A cast was applied for an average of 24 days (15–35 days). Retropulsion was decreased by 30% compared with the opposite side. At the level of the index, the extensor lag was only 5° when isolated index extension was performed. Extension and flexion associated with other fingers was normal.

Conclusions

This infrequent complication should be considered following a non-displaced distal radial fracture with a dorsal swelling at Lister's tubercle. Some authors recommend a preventive release of the third dorsal compartment in this case.

Pin placement and removal should be performed, if possible under tourniquet, and stab incisions are used to ensure that no conflict exists

Table 38.2 Restoration of thumb motion after EIP transfer to EPL: review of 15 patients

	MP	IP
Extension	normal: 12 cases −20°: 1 case −25°: 2 cases	normal: 12 cases −10°: 1 case −15°: 1 case −25°: 1 case
Flexion	normal: 13 cases −5°: 1 case −30°: 1 case	normal: 15 cases

between the tendons and the pins, which should be cut not too short.

References

Denman E. Rupture of the extensor pollicis longus — a crush injury. Hand 1979; II: 295–98.

Duplay M. Ruptures sous cutanées du tendon du long extenseur du pouce au niveau de la tabatière anatomique. Bull Mem Soc Chir [Paris] 1876; 2: 788.

Engkvist O, Lundborg G. Ruptures of the extensor pollicis longus tendon after fracture of the lower end of the radius. A clinical and microangiographic study. The Hand 1979; II, I: 76–86.

Hamlin C, Littler JW. Restoration of the extensor pollicis longus tendon by an intercalated graft. J Bone Joint Surg 1977; 59A,3: 412–14.

Helal B, Chen SC, Iwegbu CG. Ruptures of the extensor pollicis longus tendon in undisplaced Colles'-fracture. The Hand 1982; 14,2: 41–47.

Hirasawa Y, Katsumi Y, Akiyoshi T, Tamai K, Tokioka T. Clinical and microangiographic studies on rupture of the EPL tendon after distal radial fractures. J Hand Surg 1990; 15B,1: 51–57.

McMaster PE. Late rupture of the extensor and flexor pollicis longus tendon following Colles' fracture. J Bone Joint Surg 1932; 14: 93.

Magnell TD, Pochron MD, Condit DP. The intercalated tendon graft for treatment of extensor pollicis longus tendon rupture. J Hand Surg 1988; 13A: 105–9.

Magnussen PA, Harvey FJ, Tonkin A. Extensor indicis proprius transfer for rupture of the extensor pollicis longus tendon. J Bone Joint Surg 1990; 72B,5: 881–83.

Saffar Ph, Fakhoury B. La réparation secondaire du long extenseur du pouce. Ann Chir Main 1987; 3: 225–29.

Schneider LH, Rosenstein RG. Restoration of extensor pollicis longus function by tendon transfer. Plast Reconst Surg 1983; 71: 533–37.

Smith FM. Late rupture of the extensor pollicis longus tendon following Colles' fracture. J Bone Joint Surg 1946; 28: 49.

Stahl S, Wolff TW. Delayed rupture of the extensor pollicis longus tendon after nonunion of a fracture of the dorsal radial tubercle. J Hand Surg 1988; 13A: 338–42.

Tubiana R. Lésions des tendons extenseurs du pouce. Traité de la chirurgie de la main, 111. Paris: Masson Ed, 168–73. 1986.

INDEX

Note: References in *italics* refer to illustrations, those in **bold** to tables. In most cases there will be textual references on these pages too.

Abductor pollicis brevis, anatomy, 4
Abductor pollicis longus, anatomy, 2, *3*, 5
Adductor pollicis, anatomy, 4
Anterior interosseous artery, anatomy, 4, 6, *7*, *8*, *9*
Anterior tilt, fractures with intrafocal pinning with arum pins, 75, 77, *78*, 80, 160, *161*, *162*
  see also Smith's fracture
Anterior (volar) plates
  Mathoulin type 1 fractures, 240
  Mathoulin type IV fractures, *242*, 243
Anteriorly displaced fractures, 149–50
  children, 285–6, 289
  classification of, *148*
  intrafocal pinning with arum pins, 161, *163*, *164*
  mechanisms, 21, *22*, 23, 24, *25*, 148, 151
  treatment by plates, 151–2
  volar rim fractures and trabeculae alignment, 2
Antero-lateral/medial pins, intrafocal pinning, Smith's fracture, 77, *78*
Antero-medial fragments, flexible double pinning, 67, *68*, *69*, *70*
AO classification, 14, **15**, *169*
  Barton's fracture in, 141, 194
  open reduction of intra-articular fractures and, 193, *194*, 195

shortcomings, 42, 131
Arteries, distal radius anatomy, *3*, 5–10
Arthritis, post-traumatic see Post-traumatic osteoarthritis
Arthrodesis
  DRUJ, 111, 113
  radiolunate, 253, *255–7*, 276
  wrist, 99, 250–1, 257, 258
Arthroscopy, 14
  computerized tomography compared, 144
  percutaneous pinning, 197
Arum pins, *73*, *74*
  arum nut, *71*
  intrafocal pinning with extra-articular fractures, 71–82
  intra-articular fractures, 160–5
Avulsion fractures, classification and treatment, **16**, 211, **212**, **220**, 225
Avulsion theory, intra-articular fractures, 19, 20
Axial forces, intra-articular fractures, *24*, 26, 43, *45*
Axial scaphoid shift sign, scapholunate disruption, 219, *222*

Barton's fracture
  classifications, 131–2, 141

AO classification and, 141, 194, 195
dorsal, 131, **134**, *135*
  combined chauffeur's fracture, *132*, 133, *134*, *135*, **136**, *139* *140*, 141
  dorsal plate fixation, 195
  incidence of, **136**
  treatment, 136, *137*, *139*, *140*
palmar, 131–2, **134**, *135*
  combined chauffeur's fractures, *133*, *134*, *135*, **136**, 139, *140*, 141
  incidence of, **136**
  treatment, 136, 139, *140*
  see also Volar Barton's fracture
Bending fractures, classification and treatment, **16**, 43, *44*, 211, **212**
Biomechanical studies
  external fixation, 30–4, 53–4, 203
  extra-articular fracture malunions, 89–90, *98–9*, 100, 105–6, *107*, 108
Blood vessels
  distal radius anatomy, 5–10
  extensor policis longus rupture and, 308, *309*
  neurovascular problems, 301, 302, 305
Bone cementing, elderly patients, 13, 84–8
  bone window, 84, *85*
  results, 85, *86–7*

Bone grafting, 13
 comminuted fractures, 13, 184–92, 197–8, *199*, 213, *214*
 Galeazzi fractures, 264
 historical review, 104–5
 long-term follow-up recommendations, 262
 open fractures, 204–5
 placement in comminuted Colles' fracture, *138*
 with radial wedge osteotomies, *93*, 96, 101, 109, 110–11
 radiocarpal fracture-dislocations, 272
Bone morphology, intra-articular fractures, 24
Bone resection
 Essex-Lopresti fractures, 265
 intra-articular malunions, 252, 257
 see also Darrach's procedure; Osteotomy
Bone strength, Sennwald and Segmüller classification, 42
Bones, distal radius anatomy, 2–3
 in children, 279
 vascularization of, 7–10
Brachioradialis tendon, anatomy, 3

Campbell, WC, radial osteotomy, 104
Carpal ligament tears, 219–20
 frequency rates, 14
 see also Scapholunate instability
Carpal tunnel syndrome, 301, *302*, 303, 306
 corrective osteotomies and, 96
 with external fixation, 207–8
 or median nerve compression with extra-articular malunions, 91
Carpus
 consequences of malunions, 90
 mechanism of injury, 41, 43, 44
 malangulation and, 47
 position of in deciding treatment, 14
 subluxation
  Barton's fracture, 131
  combined dorsal Barton's and chauffeur's fracture, 133
  extra-articular deformity, 105–6
  types of instability in, 105–6, *107*
 vascularization of, *7*, *8*, *9*
 see also Lunate; Scaphoid
Cast immobilization
 children, 280–1, *282*, *284*, 288, 289
 comminuted fractures, 171
 excessive swelling and, 304
 intrafocal pinning and, 75
 ligament tears, 14
 Mathoulin type II fractures, 241

 neurovascular complications with, 302–3, 304, 305
 radiocarpal fracture-dislocations, 272
 redisplacement and, 12
Castaing classification, 14, **16**, 126
 'potential fracture', 153–4
 T-fractures, 128, 129
Cauchoix, J, anterior rim fracture classification, 148
Chauffeur's fracture
 combined dorsal Barton's, *132*, 133, *134*, *135*, **136**, *139*, *140*, 141
 combined palmar Barton's, 133, *134*, *135*, **136**, 139, *140*, 141
 definition, 132
 incidence of, **136**
 mechanics of, 44
 Saito classification, **134**, *135*
 treatment, 136, *139*
 see also Radial styloid
Children, 279–89
 complete fractures, 281, *283*
 distal forearm bone growth, 279
 epiphyseal fracture-separations, 287–9
 fracture classifications, **212**
 frequency of fractures, 280
 impaction fractures, 280, *281*
 incomplete displaced fractures, 280–1, *282*
 injury mechanisms, 280
 pathophysiology of fractures, 280
 Salter II fractures, **212**, *288*, 289
  arum pins, 81
 treatment, 281, *283*–7
 two-bone fractures, arum pins, 81, *82*
C-Hoffman external fixator, 184, 198, 203–4
Clancey, G, radial pinning, 29, *52*, 53
 comminuted fractures, 175, *177*
Classification systems, 14–17, 126–30
 comminuted fracture management, 169–70
 epiphyseal fracture-separations in children, 287–9
 eponymous, 131–41
 for external fixation and pinning, 210–11, **212**
 open reduction and, 119–22, 193–5
 for percutaneous pinning, 50, *51*
Closed reduction
 intra-articular fractures, 193
 Mathoulin type I fractures, 240
 Mathoulin type II fractures, 241
 radiocarpal fracture-dislocations, 273, 275

Closing wedge osteotomies *see* Radial wedge osteotomies
Codivilla, A, percutaneous pinning, 28, 29
Colles' fracture
 chauffeur's fracture compared, 132
 classification of, **17**, 126, 131
  Saito, 133, **134**
 dorsal plate fixation, 195
 incidence of, **136**
 intra-medullary pinning, 238
 intrafocal pinning with arum pins, 77, 80
 malunions, *107*, 111, *113*, *114*
 outcome evaluation system, **123**
 ulnar styloid process fracture with, *165*
 unstable intra-articular fractures differentiated, 155
 see also Comminuted Colles' fracture; PouteauColles' fracture
Combined dorsal Barton's and chauffeur's fracture, *132*, 133, *134*, *135*, **136**, *139*, *140*, 141
Combined palmar Barton's and chauffeur's fracture, 133, *134*, *135*, **136**, 139, *140*, 141
Comminuted Colles' fracture
 definition, 132
 Gartland and Werley classification, **17**
 incidence of, **136**
 Saito classification, 133, 134–5
 subtypes, 134, *135*
 treatment, 136, *137–8*, 141
Comminuted fractures
 bone grafting, 13, 184–92
 classification by degree of comminution, 15, **17**, 193, *194*, 195
 classification by mechanism of comminution, 43, 44, 45, 46
 external fixation, 13, *172–3*, 178, *179*, 203–8, 210–24
 intra-articular, 13, 14
  computerized tomography evaluation of, 143–7
  internal distraction plates, 246–8
  Saito classification, **134**
 management of, 167–82
 McMurtry classification, 169, *170–6*
 open reduction and internal fixation, 178–82, 193–201
 see also Comminuted Colles' fracture; Comminuted Smith's fracture; Malunions
Comminuted Smith's fracture, 132, 133, *135*, **136**, 139

Compression fractures, classification and treatment, 211, **212**, **220**, 225
Compression impaction (crush) theory, intra-articular fractures, 19, *20*
Computerized tomography, 143–7
 after closed reduction, *145*, *146*
 evaluation of comminuted fractures, 167
 scan through cast, *143*
 scout film, *144*
Cooney (Universal) classification system, 15, **17**, **42**, *43–5*, 118, *119*, **120**, 121–3
Cotton-Loder position, neurovascular complications with, 302–3
Crenshaw, AH, radial pinning, *52*, 53
Crush (compression impaction) theory, intra-articular fractures, 19, *20*
CT (computerized tomography), 143–7, 167

Darrach's procedure
 background to, 92, 104, 105
 indications for, 96, 100, *101*, 111, 113
 radial neck pseudoarthrosis, *92*
De Oliveira, JC, Barton fracture classification, 141
DePalma, A, percutaneous pinning, 29, 50, *52*
Diaphysis, anatomy, 2
Die-punch fractures
 bone grafting, 13, *188*
 indications for open reduction, 118, 121–2
 Mathoulin classification, 128
 radial pinning, 29
 Saito's comminuted Colles' fracture and, 135
 treatment, *137*
 see also Lunate and lunate fossa, fractures
DISI (dorsal intercalated segment instability) deformity, 105–6, 161, *164*
Distal articular facet, anatomy, 2
Distal carpal facet, anatomy, 2
Distal fragments, proximal displacement, 46–7
Distal radio-ulnar difference (DRUD), extra-articular malunions, 99
Distal radio-ulnar fusion *see* Sauvé–Kapandji procedure
Distal radio-ulnar joint *see* DRUJ
Distraction
 internal distraction plates, *246–8*
 Mathoulin type IV fractures, 243–4
 see also Ligamentotaxis

Dorsal Barton's fracture, 131, *132*
 and combined chauffeur's fracture, *132*, 133, *134*, *135*, **136**, *139*, *140*, 141
 dorsal plate fixation, 195
 incidence of, **136**
 Saito classification, *134*, *135*, 141
 treatment, 136, *137*, *139*, *140*
Dorsal carpal arch, distal radius anatomy, 8, *9*
Dorsal cortex injuries, classification by, 43, *44*
Dorsal displacement fractures
 incurvation theory, 21
 plate fixation, 13–14
Dorsal intercalated segment instability (DISI) deformity, 105–6, 161, *164*
Dorsal (posterior) intra-articular fragment, Mathoulin type IV fracture, 129
Dorsal (posterior) marginal fractures, Mathoulin type I, 127, 240
Dorsal (posterior) rim fragments, anteriorly displaced fractures, *148*, *149–50*, 151, 152
Dorso-medial fragments, flexible double pinning, 69, 243
Dorsoradial displacement, dorsal ligamentotaxis and, 46–7
Double pinning
 crossed type, Mathoulin type II fractures, *241*
 double elastic spring (flexible double) type, 29, 62–70
 standard, 56, *57*
Dowling, JJ, percutaneous pinning, *52*
Drahextension (wire extension), 29
DRUD (distal radio-ulnar difference), extra-articular malunions, 99
DRUJ (distal radio-ulnar joint)
 anatomy, 3
 bone grafting in comminuted fractures, 186, *187*
 classification and treatment indications, *121*, 122, 217, **218**, 219
 Essex-Lopresti fractures and, 265
 extra-articular malunions, 89–90, 99, 106
 corrective osteotomy, 92, *93*, *95*, 96, *100–1*, 108–9, 111, 113
 radiography, 91
 Frykman classification, 140–1
 with Galeazzi fracture, 47, 264–5
 intrafocal pinning and, 80
 long-term follow-up, 260, 261, **262**
 pinning postero-medial fragment and, 160
 Py isoelastic pinning and, 57, *58*

radiolunate arthrodesis and, 255, *257*
 stabilizing structures of, 297–8
 TFCC dislocation and, 161–2, *165*
Durman, CD, radial osteotomy, 104

Elastic pinning
 double elastic spring (flexible double) type, 29, 62–70
 Py procedure, 56–61
 treatment trends, 13
 see also Intrafocal pinning
Elderly patients
 bone cementing, 13, 84–8
 contraindications to open reduction, 213
 neurovascular complications, *301*, 306
 treatment trends, 12, 13, 14
Epiphyseal arteries, distal radius vascularization, 8–9
Epiphyseal displacement, pathomechanism of extra-articular malunions, 89, *90*
Epiphyseal fracture-separations, children, 287–9
Epiphyseal ulna fractures, 289
Epiphysiodesis, spontaneous, 289
Epiphysis, anatomy, 2
Eponymous classification systems, 131–41
Essex-Lopresti fractures, 264, 265
Extensor carpi radialis brevis (ECRB), anatomy, *3*
Extensor carpi radialis longus (ECRL), anatomy, *3*
Extensor carpi ulnaris (ECU)
 anatomy, *3*, 297
 Galeazzi fractures and, 264–5
Extensor digiti minimi (EDM), anatomy, *3*
Extensor digitorum communis (EDC), anatomy, *3*
Extensor indicis proprius (EIP)
 anatomy, *3*
 extensor pollicis longus rupture and, 308, 310, **311**
Extensor pollicis brevis (EPB), anatomy, 2, *3*, 5
Extensor pollicis longus (EPL)
 anatomy, 1–2, *3*
 frequency of injury to, 2–3, 10, 308
 rupture, 308–11
  mechanical theory of, *309*
  pinning treatment, *310*
  tendon transfer, *3*, 310, **311**
  thumb adduction, 310
  vascular theory of, 308, *309*
External fixation, 13, *172–3*
 biomechanics of, 30–4, 203
 complications, 207–8

External fixation (*continued*)
  indications for, 178, 184, 205–6
  long-term follow-up
    recommendations, 262
  Mathoulin type IV fractures, 243–4
  postoperative treatment, 205
  radial wedge osteotomy, 93, 96
  results, **206, 207**
  techniques, 178, *179*, 203, *204–5*, 213–24
    4-part fracture, 213, *214*
    bone grafting and, 184–92, 197–8, *199*, 204–5
    pitfalls, 220, 222–4
    radiocarpal fracture-dislocation, 215, *216*
    wrist fixator, 215, *217*
  versus intramedullary pinning, 229–39
    results, 230–1, *232–8*
    techniques, 229, *230*, *231*
  see also Ligamentotaxis; Percutaneous pinning
Extra-articular fractures
  biomechanical studies of percutaneous pinning in, 30, *31*, *32*, *33*, 34
  Cooney type I and II, injury mechanisms, 43, *44*
  elastic intrafocal/extrafocal pinning, 13
  flexible double pinning, *64*, 65–6, 69
  intrafocal pinning with arum pins, 71–82
  intramedullary pinning or external fixation, 231–2, *233*, 235, 237, *238*, 239
  Mathoulin type IV classification and, 129, 242
  neurovascular complications, 300–1, 302
  palmar displacement, 44–5, *46*, 47
  Py isoelastic pinning, 56–61
  treatment indications, **120**, 121
  see also Colles' fracture; Smith's fracture
Extra-articular malunions
  historical review, 104–5
  indications for surgical correction, 90–1, 100–1, 108
  pathomechanisms, 89–90, *98*, *99*, 100, 105–6, *107*, 108
  treatment options, 92–6, 100–3, 108–13
Extra-articular osteotomy, intra-articular malunions, 251, 257
Extrafocal pinning, treatment trends, 13

FDP (flexible double pinning), 29, 62–70
Fernandez classification system, 14, **16**, 211, **212**
Fernandez and Geissler, percutaneous pinning, *52*, 53
Flexible double pinning (FDP), 29, 62–70
Flexor tendons
  anatomy, 1, *3*, 4–5
  neurovascular complications, 303
  redisplacement and, 12
  tendosynovitis, 302, *303*
Fracture lines
  factors affecting, *21*, 22–3, 24, *25*
  Mathoulin classification by, 127–30
Frykman classification, 14, **15**, 42, 126
  ligamentotaxis of type VII fracture, 37, *38–9*, 40
  Pouteau–Colles' fracture, 42
  shortcomings, 42, 121, 140–1, 169

Galeazzi fractures, 41, 47, 264–5
Gartland-Werley classification, 15, **17**, 42
  Colles-type fractures, 139–40
  fracture outcome evaluation, **123**, 200
  modified *see* Cooney (universal) classification system
Goyrand fracture, 131
  see also Smith's fracture
Grafts *see* Bone grafting
Graham, TJ, percutaneous pinning, 53–5
Green and O'Brien, fracture outcome evaluation, 123, **124**, 200
Greenstick fractures, children, 280, *282*
Grip strength, long-term follow-up, **260**, 261
Guyon's canal
  anatomy, 5
  ulnar nerve compression and, 91, 301, 306

Harris epiphyseal fracture-separations, children, *287–8*
High-velocity fractures
  classification and treatment, **16**, 211, **212**, 213, **220**, *221*, 225
  forces acting in, 23, 26
  injury mechanisms, 47
  neurovascular complications, 301, *302*, 305
Hobart and Kraft, radial osteotomy, 104
Hoffman external fixator, 184, 198, 203–4

Hutchinson's fracture *see* Chauffeur's fracture

Iliac bone grafts *see* Bone grafting
Impaction fractures, children, 280, *280*
Implants, Essex-Lopresti fractures, 265
Incurvation theory, pathomechanism of fractures, 19, 20, *21*
Injury mechanisms, classification by, 14, **16**, 41–7, 126, 211, **212**
'Intermediate fractures', children, 289
Internal fixation
  comminuted fractures, 178–82, 197–8, *199*, 210–24
  internal distraction plates, *246–8*
  long-term follow-up recommendations, 262
  see also Plate fixation
Intra-articular fractures
  external fixation, 13, *172–3*, 178, *179*, 203–8, 210–24
  incidence of, **136**
  injury mechanisms, 19–26, 43–4, *45*, *46*
  intrafocal pinning with arum pins, 160–5
  intramedullary pinning or external fixation, 232–4, *235*, 238, 239
  ligamentotaxis and radiopalmar tilt, 37, *38–9*, 40
  long-term (30 years) follow-up, 259–63
  Mayo classification, **16**
  Melone classification, **16**
  neurovascular complications, 301–2
  open reduction of, 118–24, 193–201
  percutaneous direct pinning and, 13
  Saito classification, 133, **134**
  see also Anteriorly displaced fractures; Barton's fracture; Comminuted fractures; Postero-medial fragment
Intra-articular malunions, 249–58
  bone resection, 252, 257
    posterior rim fragment, *252*
    radial styloid, *252*
  extra-articular osteotomy, 251
  intra-articular osteotomy, 253, *254*, 257
    displaced postero-medial fragment, *253*
  with intra-articular step-off, *249*
  proximal row carpectomy, 251–2
  radiolunate arthrodesis, 253, *255–7*

Intra-articular malunions (*continued*)
  wrist arthrodesis, 250–1, 257, 258
Intrafocal pinning
  with arum pins, *73*, *74*
    arum nut, *71*
    extra-articular fractures, 71–82
    intra-articular fractures, 160–5
    percutaneous pinning evolution, 29
    principles of, 71, *72*, *73*
    treatment trends, 13
    triple, for Mathoulin type III fractures, 241, *242*
Intramedullary pinning
  fractures and epiphyseal fracture-separation in children, *285*
  versus external fixation, 229–39
  results, 230–1, *232–8*
  techniques, 229, *230*, *231*
Ischemic pain, neurovascular complications, 302, 305
Isoelastic pinning, Py procedure, 56–61

Jenkins classification, 15, **17**

Kerboul plates
  anteriorly displaced fractures, 151
  Mathoulin type 1 fractures, 240
King's method closed reduction, dorsal Barton's fracture, 136, *137*, 141
Kirschner, M, drahextension, 29
K-wires
  anteriorly displaced fractures, 151
  arthroscopically controlled fracture reduction, 197
  bone cementing, 84–5
  classic intrafocal pinning, 71, *73*
  elastic pinning, 13
  flexible double pinning, 62–4, *63*, *64*, *67*, *68*, 70
  Mathoulin type IV fractures, 243
  postero-medial fragment fixation, 156, *157*
  radial pinning, 53, *54*, 175
  radial wedge osteotomies, 93, 109, 110–11, *112*, 113
  severely comminuted fractures, *176*, 180, 195, 197–8, *199*
  wrist arthroscopy, 14

Lambotte, A, percutaneous pinning, 29
Laugier's sign, 3
Lidström classification, 14, **15**
Ligamentotaxis, 13
  anatomic status post-fracture, 46–7
  and bone grafting in comminuted intra-articular fractures, 184–92
  indications for open reduction, 118
  postero-medial fragment and, 156
  to restore radiopalmar tilt, 37–40, *38–9*
Linscheid classification, 14
Lister's tubercle
  anatomy, 1, 2–3, *7*
  extensor pollicis longus rupture and, 308, *309*, 310
Lucas and Sachtjen, radial pinning, *52*, 53
Lunate and lunate fossa
  anatomy, 2, 41
  fractures
    definition, 132
    indications for open reduction, 118, 241
    Mathoulin type II, 127, 128, 241
    Saito classification, **134**, *135*
    treatment, 136, 141
  incurvation theory, 21
  mechanism of injury, 43, 44, *45*, 46, 47
  radiocarpal fracture-dislocations, 271
  ulnar impingement, postero-medial fragment, 154, *155*
  see also Die-punch fractures

Malunions
  carpal kinematics and, 47
  extra-articular fractures
    historical review, 104–5
    indications for surgical correction, 90–1, 100–1, 108
    pathomechanisms, 89–90, *98*, *99*, 100, 105–6, *107*, 108
    treatment options, 92–6, 100–3, 108–13
  intra-articular, 249–58
  intrafocal pinning with arum pins, 80
  neurovascular complications, 300–6
  postero-medial fragments (PMF), 154, *155*
Mathoulin, Letrosne and Saffar classification, 15, **16**, *127–8*, *129*, *130*
  indications for open reduction, 240–5
Mayo classification, 15, **16**
  modified, fracture outcome evaluation, 123, **124**
  universal classification and, 120, *121*, 122
McMurtry and Jupiter classification, 15, **16**, 169, *170–6*
  universal classification and, 120, 121, *122*
Medial cuneiform (lunate fossa) fracture *see* Lunate and lunate fossa, fractures
Medial cutaneous nerve, anatomy, 3
Medial lunate fossa, anatomy, 2
Median nerve
  anatomy, *3*, 4, *5*
  compression with extra-articular malunions, 91
  neurovascular complications, 300–2, 305–6
Median nerve artery, anatomy, 7
Melone classification, 15, **16**, 42, 126, 169
  comminuted Colles' fracture and, 134, 135
  shortcomings, 141
  universal classification and, 120, *121*, 122
Meniscal homologue, anatomy of, 297
Merle D'Aubigné and Joussemet, multi-facet curved osteotomy, 105
Metaphalangeal (MP) joint, extensor pollicis longus rupture and, 310, **311**
Metaphyseal arteries, distal radius vascularization, 8–9
Monoblock fractures, 42
  see also Extra-articular fractures
Multi-facet curved osteotomy, 105
Multiplanar spherical osteotomy, 101–3
Munson and Gainor, percutaneous pinning, *52*, 53
Muscular contractions, pathomechanism of intra-articular fractures, 25
Musculocutaneous nerve (MC), anatomy, 3, 5, *6*

Nagelextension (nail extension), 29
Nerves, distal radius anatomy, 3–5
Neurapraxia, decompression for, 302
Neurosympathetic dystrophy (NSD)
  corrective osteotomies and, 96
  external fixation and, 13
  extra-articular malunions, 90, 91
  intrafocal pinning with arum pins and, 80
Neurovascular complications, 300–6
  extra-articular malunions, 91
  fracture pattern and displacement, 300–2
  fracture treatments and, 304–5
  immobilization position, 302–4
Non-articular fractures *see* Extra-articular fractures

OA *see* Post-traumatic osteoarthritis
Older classification, 15, **17**
Open fractures
  bone grafting, 204–5
  children, *286*
  indications for surgery, 219
Open reduction, 118–24
  anteriorly displaced fractures, 151
  classification of intra-articular fractures, *119*, **120**, *121–2*, 193, *194*, 195
  comminuted fractures, 178–82, 193–201
    internal distraction plates and, 246–8
  Essex-Lopresti fractures, 265
  functional assessment, 123
  indications for, 118–19, 178–9, 193–5, 211, **212**, 213
    using computerized tomography, 143–7
    using Mathoulin classification, 240–5
  long-term follow-up recommendations, 262
  postoperative management, 224
  radiocarpal fracture-dislocations, 272
  techniques, 195–8, 213–24
    anterior approach, 179, *180–2*
    arthroscopically controlled, 197
    bone grafting, 197–8, *199*
    dorsal approach, 180, 195
    pitfalls, 220, 222–4
    volar plate fixation, 195, *196*
Opening wedge osteotomies *see* Radial wedge osteotomies
Opponens pollicis (OP), anatomy, 4
Osteoarthritis, post-traumatic *see* Post-traumatic osteoarthritis
Osteoporosis
  bone cementing and, 84–8
  bone grafting, 13
  contraindication to open reduction, 213
  contraindication to percutaneous pinning, 54
  corrective osteotomies and, 96
Osteosynthesis
  by flexible double pinning, 29, 62–70
  by intrafocal pinning, 71–82, 160–5
  see also Percutaneous pinning; Plate fixation
Osteotomy
  extra-articular malunions, 92–6, 100–3, 104–15
  intra-articular malunions, 251, 253, *254*, 257
    displaced postero-medial fragment, *253*
  see also Bone resection

Palmar Barton's fracture, 131–2
  combined chauffeur's fractures, *133*, *134*, *135*, **136**, 139, *140*, 141
  incidence of, **136**
  Saito classification, **134**, *135*
  treatment, 136, 139, *140*
Palmar capsule, anatomy, 41
Palmar carpal arch, anatomy, *7, 8*
Palmar cutaneous nerve, anatomy, 4
Palmar displaced fractures, 44–5, *46*, 47
Palmar radiocarpal dislocation, 271, 273, *275*
Paresthesias, causes of, 301–2, *303*
Percutaneous pinning
  anteriorly displaced fractures, 151
  arthroscopically directed, 197
  biomechanical studies, 30–4, 53–4
  comminuted fractures, 171, *172*, *174*, 175, *177*, 178, *179*
  contraindications, 54
  evolution of, 28–9
  extensor pollicis longus injury, 3, 10
  flexible double pinning, 62–70
  fracture classification, 50, *51*
  indications for, 54
  literature review, 50, 52–3
  neurovascular complications with, *304*, 305
  postero-medial fragment fixation, *156*, 157, *158*
  Py procedure, 56–61
  radial nerve and, 5, 10
  treatment rationale, 50
  treatment trends, 12–13
Periosteal plexus, anatomy, 8
Peristyloid vascular loop, 9, *10*
Pin loosening, 224
Pin-tract infection, 224
Plate fixation, 13–14
  anteriorly displaced fractures, 151–2
  dorsal approach, 195
  Galeazzi fractures, 264
  internal distraction type, 246–8
  Mathoulin type 1 fractures, 240
  radial wedge osteotomy, 93, *94*
  volar approach, 195, *196*
PMF *see* Postero-medial fragment
Posterior (dorsal) intra-articular fragment, Mathoulin type IV fracture, 129
Posterior (dorsal) marginal fractures, Mathoulin type I, 127, 240
Posterior (dorsal) rim fragments, anteriorly displaced fractures, *148*, *149–50*, 151, 152
Posterior interosseous artery, anatomy, *7, 9*

Posterior tilt, fractures with, intrafocal pinning, 74–5
Posteriorly displaced fractures, bone morphology, 24
Postero-medial fragment (PMF), 153–8
  bone morphology and, 24
  diagnosis, 154–5
  flexible double pinning, K-wires, 62, *63*
  intra-articular osteotomy, 253, 257
  intrafocal pinning with arum pins, *160*, *161*
  intramedullary pinning or external fixation, 232, 233, 235, *238*
  malunions, 154, *155*
  modification to Py pinning, *59*, *60*
  pathomechanics of, 153–4, *155*
  treatment, 155–8
Post-traumatic osteoarthritis
  DRUJ disorders and, 122
  following open reduction, *200*
  frequency of, 118, 143, 210, 225
  intra-articular malunions and, 249, 250, 527
  long-term follow-up, 260, *261*, 263
  treatment trends, 14
'Potential fracture'
  Castaing classification, 153–4
  see also Postero-medial fragment (PMF)
Pouteau, Claude, 126
Pouteau–Colles' fracture
  classifications, 41–2, 131
  malunions, 98, 105–6, 110–11
  see also Colles' fracture
Pronator quadratus, anatomy, 2, *3*, 4, 41
Prostheses, Essex-Lopresti fractures, 265
Proximal row carpectomy, intra-articular malunions, 251–2
Py isoelastic pinning, 56–61

Radial artery, anatomy, 1, 2, *3*, 5, *6, 7, 8, 9*, 10
Radial diaphysis, Galeazzi fracture, 264–5
Radial head, Essex-Lopresti fractures, 264, 265
Radial nerve
  anatomy of, 3, 4, 5, *6*, 10
  extra-articular malunions, 91
  neuroma in, *304*
  percutaneous pinning and, 223–4, 304–5
Radial pinning
  comminuted fractures, 175, *177*
  percutaneous pinning evolution, 29, *52*, 53
Radial styloid
  anatomy, 1, 2, *3*, 9, *10*

bone morphology and, 24
injury mechanisms, 43, 44, *45*, 154, 291, *292*
intrafocal pinning with arum pins, 161, *163–4*
intramedullary pinning or external fixation, 235, *238*
plate fixation, 148, 151–2
postero-medial fragment and, 154, *156*
radiocarpal fracture-dislocations, 268, **269–71**, 272, 275, *276*
resection, *252*, 257
scapholunate instability, 44, *45*, 291–6
see also Chauffeur's fracture
Radial superficial vein, anatomy, 1
Radial wedge osteotomies, extra-articular malunions, *93*, *94*, 101, 108
historical review, 104–5
Pouteau–Colles' fracture, 110–11
results, 113, **114**, 115
Smith's fracture, *109*, 111, *112*
Radiocarpal joint
anatomy, 4
dislocations and fracture-dislocations, 267–76
associated lesions, 271–2
historical review, 267–70
injury mechanisms, 270–1
treatments, 272–3
incurvation theory, 21
long-term follow-up, 260, 261, **262**
Radiocarpal subluxation, extra-articular deformity, 105–6
Radiodorsal type Barton fractures, 133, *134*, 139, *140*
Radiography
AO classification, 14, **15**
computerized tomography compared, 144, *145–6*
criteria for reductions, 78, *79*
evaluating comminuted fractures, 167
extra-articular malunions, 91
Lidström classification, 14, **15**
long-term follow-up, 260, *261*, **262**
measurements in long-term follow-up, 259
Sarmiento classification, 14, **15**
Radiolunate arthrodesis, 253, *255–7*, *276*
Radiometacarpal external fixation versus intramedullary pinning, 229–39
results, 230–1, *232–8*
techniques, 229, *230*, *231*
Radiopalmar tilt, ligamentotaxis to restore, 37–40, *38–9*
Radiopalmar type Barton fractures, 133, *134*, 139, *140*

Radio-ulnar fractures, Mathoulin type II, 127, 128, 241
Radio-ulnar fusion
Essex-Lopresti fractures, 265
see also Sauvé–Kapandji procedure
Radio-ulnar inclination, 2, 10
Radio-ulnar joint, distal *see* DRUJ (distal radio-ulnar joint)
Radio-ulnar pins, modification to Py pinning, 59–60, *60*
Radio-ulno-carpal space, location of, 1
Ramus carpeus volaris, anatomy, 5, 6
Ramus volaris superficialis, anatomy, 5
Rayhack, JM, percutaneous pinning, *52*, 53
Redisplacement, treatment trends, 12–13, 14
Reductions, radiographic characteristics, 78, *79*
Remodelling, fractures and epiphyseal fracture-separation in children, 279, 281
Reverse Barton's fracture, 132
Rixford operation, 105
Rush, LV and HC, percutaneous pinning, 29, *52*

Sagittal plane fractures
Mathoulin type II, 127–8, *241*
with postero-medial fragment, 160, *161*
Saito classification system, 133, **134**, *135*, 136–41
Salter fractures, children, 81, **212**, 287–8, 289
Sarmiento, A
classification system, 14, **15**
fracture outcome evaluation, 123
Sauvé–Kapandji procedure, DRUJ disorders, *95*, 96, 100, *101*, *102*
Scaphoid impression fractures, with radial styloid fractures, 293, *295*
Scaphoid and scaphoid fossa
anatomy, 2, 41
fractures, 220
correspondence with comminuted Colles' fracture, 135
injury mechanisms, classification by, 42, 44, *45*
Mathoulin type II, 127, 128
incurvation theory, 21
indications for open reduction, 118, 241
Scapholunate instability, *127*, 128, 129, *130*, 136, 219–20
axial scaphoid shift sign, 219, *222*
double crossed pinning, *241*

intrafocal pinning with arum pins and, 161, *164*
radial styloid fractures and, 44, *45*, 291–6
emergency treatment, 293, *294*
late visibility, *293*
malunion, *292*
missed case of, 292, *294*
Scapholunate interosseous ligament (SLIL) tears, 294, *295*
Seitz, WH, percutaneous pinning, 53, *54*
Sennwald and Segmüller classification system, 42
Shearing fractures
classification and treatment, **16**, 211, **212**, **220**, 225
forces in, *23*
radial styloid fractures with scapholunate sprains, 291, 293–4
Sigmoid notch
anatomy, 2, 3
DRUJ disorders and, 89–90
see also DRUJ (distal radio-ulnar joint)
Skin, distal radius anatomy, 1–2
Smith's fracture
classifications, 42, 126, 131, 194
comminuted, 132, 133, *135*, **136**, 139
flexible double pinning, 69, *70*
incidence of, **136**
intrafocal pinning with arum pins, 75, 77, *78*, 80, 81, 160, *161*, *162*
malunions, 106, 108
radial wedge osteotomy, *109*, 111, *112*
plate fixation, 13–14, 195, *196*
Thomas type 2, 131, 194, 195, *196*
'Snuff-box', 2
Spherical multiplanar osteotomy, 101–3
Split block fractures, 42
Stein and Katz, radial pinning, 29, *52*, 53
Steinman, F, nagelextension, 28–9

Tendon transfers, extensor pollicis longus repair, *3*, **308**, 310, 311
Tendosynovitis, flexor, 302, *303*
TFCC *see* Triangular fibrocartilage complex (TFCC)
T-fractures
intramedullary pinning in, 233–4, *235*
Mathoulin classification and, 128, 129, 241, *242*
with postero-medial fragment, 160, *161*

Thomas classification, Smith's
  fracture and, 131, 194, 195, *196*
Tomography, computerized *see*
  Computerized tomography
Tomography, trispiral, evaluating
  comminuted fractures, 167, *168*
Trans-ulnar pinning
  biomechanical study of, 30–4
  flexible double pinning, 29, 62–70
  percutaneous pinning evolution,
    29, *52*
  see also Intrafocal pinning
Transverse carpal ligament,
  anatomy, 1
Triangular fibrocartilage complex
  (TFCC)
  anatomy of, 2, 3, 297
  in Barton fractures, 133, 139
  deformity in extra-articular
    fracture malunions, 99, 106
  injury mechanisms, 45, 47
  intrafocal pinning of ulnar styloid
    process and, 161–2, *165*
  postero-medial fragment and, 154
Triple elastic procedure, Py pinning,
  57, *58*, *60*, 60
Triple intrafocal pinning, for
  Mathoulin type III fractures, 241,
  242
Trispiral tomography, evaluating
  comminuted fractures, 167, *168*
Two-bone fractures, children, arum
  pins, 81, *82*

Ulnar artery
  anatomy, 5–6, 7
  entrapment of, 302
  ulnar nerve course and, 5
Ulnar fractures, isolated, children,
  288, *289*
Ulnar head
  anatomy, 1
  dislocation in Galeazzi fractures,
    47, 264

  lunate impingement, postero-
    medial fragment, 154, *155*
  partial resection, 111, 113, 114–15
  resection *see* Darrach's procedure
Ulnar head fractures, 129
  bone grafting, 189, *191*
  Frykman classification, 42
  intramedullary pinning, 232, *233*
Ulnar neck fractures, 47, 129
  intramedullary pinning, 232, *233*
Ulnar nerve
  anatomy, 3, 4–5
  compression with extra-articular
    malunions, 91
  neurovascular complications,
    300–2, 305–6
Ulnar osteotomy, extra-articular
  malunions, 92–3, *100*, 101–2,
  103, 111, 113, 115
  historical review, 104, 105
Ulnar styloid
  anatomy of, 297–8
  bone grafting, 189, *191*
  extra-articular malunions, 106
  intrafocal pinning with arum pins,
    161–2, *165*
  Laugier's sign, 3
  pain with flexible double pinning,
    69
Ulnar styloid fractures, 129, 297–9
  children, 289
  clinical signs, 298
  Frykman classification, 42
  incurvation theory, 21
  injury mechanisms, 47, 154, 298
  radiocarpal fracture-dislocations
    with, **268**, **270**, 271, 273, *275*
  radiological findings, 298–9
  scapholunate interosseous
    ligament (SLIL) tears and, 294
  treatment, 299
Ulnar superficial vein, anatomy, 1
Ulnar translations, with radiocarpal
  fracture-dislocations, 273, *274–
  5*, 276

Ulnar variance, 2, 10
  axial compression and
    osteoarthritis, 260, **262**
  radiographic criteria, 78, *79*
Ulnocarpal ligament, anatomy of,
  297
Ulnodorsal type Barton fractures,
  133, *134*, *139*, 141
Ulnolunate impingement, postero-
  medial fragment, 154, *155*
Ulnopalmar type Barton fractures,
  133, *134*, *139*, 141
Universal classification system *see*
  Cooney (universal) classification
  system

V plates, Mathoulin type 1 fractures,
  240
Vascular system
  anatomy, 5–10
  extensor policis longus rupture
    and, 308, *309*
  neurovascular complications, 301,
    302, 305
Veins, anatomy, 7
Volar Barton's fracture, 42, 44, 194
  plate fixation, 13–14, 195, *196*
  see also Anteriorly displaced
    fractures; Barton's fracture
Volar plates *see* Anterior (volar)
  plates

Willeneger and Guggenbuhl, radial
  pinning, 29
Wrist arthrodesis, intra-articular
  malunions, 99, 250–1, 257, 258
Wrist arthroscopy, 14, 144, 197
Wrist flexion, neurovascular
  complications with, 302–3
Wrist motion, long-term follow-up,
  260, 261